S0-CQT-433

Biomedical polymers

Edited by
Mike Jenkins

Published by Woodhead Publishing and Maney Publishing
on behalf of
The Institute of Materials, Minerals & Mining

CRC Press
Boca Raton Boston New York Washington, DC

WOODHEAD PUBLISHING LIMITED
Cambridge England

Woodhead Publishing Limited and Maney Publishing Limited on behalf of
The Institute of Materials, Minerals & Mining

Woodhead Publishing Limited, Abington Hall, Abington
Cambridge CB21 6AH, England
www.woodheadpublishing.com

Published in North America by CRC Press LLC, 6000 Broken Sound Parkway, NW,
Suite 300, Boca Raton, FL 33487, USA

First published 2007, Woodhead Publishing Limited and CRC Press LLC

British Library Cataloguing in Publication Data
A catalogue record for this book is available from the British Library.

Library of Congress Cataloging in Publication Data
A catalog record for this book is available from the Library of Congress.

Woodhead Publishing ISBN: 978-1-84569-070-0 (book)
Woodhead Publishing ISBN: 978-1-84569-364-0 (e-book)
CRC Press ISBN: 978-1-4200-4451-5
CRC Press order number: WP4451

The publishers' policy is to use permanent paper from mills that operate a sustainable forestry policy, and which has been manufactured from pulp which is processed using acid-free and elementary chlorine-free practices. Furthermore, the publishers ensure that the text paper and cover board used have met acceptable environmental accreditation standards.

Typeset by SNP Best-set Typesetter Ltd., Hong Kong
Printed by TJ International Limited, Padstow, Cornwall, England

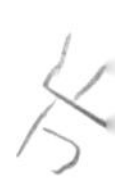

Contents

Contributor contact details

Editor

Dr M J Jenkins
Metallurgy and Materials
School of Engineering
The University of Birmingham
Edgbaston
Birmingham
B15 2TT
UK
email: m.j.jenkins@bham.ac.uk

Chapters 1 and 2

K Harrison
Physical Properties and Developability
HW8924A
GlaxoSmithKline R&D Ltd
New Frontiers Science Park
Third Avenue
Harlow
Essex
CM19 5AW
UK
email: Katherine.l.harrison@gsk.com

Chapter 3

A Hillel
Department of Biomedical Engineering
Johns Hopkins University
3400 N. Charles Street
Clark Hall, Room 102
Baltimore
MD 21218
USA
email: ahillel@jhmi.edu

Chapter 4

G S Kwon* and D Y Furgeson
School of Pharmacy
University of Wisconsin-Madison
777 Highland Avenue
Madison
WI 53705-2222
USA
emails: gskwon@pharmacy.Wisc.edu
dfurgeson@pharmacy.wisc.edu

Chapter 5

D Espino
Department of Mechanical and Manufacturing Engineering
School of Engineering
University of Birmingham
B15 2TT
UK
email: daniel.m.espino@gmail.com

Chapter 6

F-W Shen
The J Vernon Luck Research Center
Orthopaedic Hospital/UCLA
2400 S. Flower Street
Los Angeles
CA 90007
USA
email: fshen@laoh.ucla.edu

Chapter 7

F Davis and S P J Higson*
Cranfield Health
Cranfield University
Barton Road
Silsoe
MK45 4DT
UK
email: f.davis@cranfield.ac.uk
s.p.j.higson@cranfield.ac.uk

Chapter 8

Vitor M Correlo
3B's Research Group
Department of Polymer Engineering
University of Minho
Campus de Gualtar
4710-057 Braga
Portugal
email: vitorcorrelo@dep.uminho.pt

Preface

This book is concerned with biomedical applications of polymeric materials. Its purpose is to explore several key applications of polymers in bioengineering, including drug delivery, tissue scaffolding, joint components and cardiovascular devices. The intention is to highlight the relationship between polymers, the way they are processed and their resulting properties. The content should therefore appeal to a broad range of reader from industrial to academic.

The rationale for the work stems from the premise that the use of polymers in the human body is important. Polymers have transformed the quality of life for many patients, as demonstrated in the following examples. In a total hip replacement, the use of PMMA as a bone cement and PE as a replacement cup has offered patients with osteoarthritis near complete mobility and relief from the pain associated with this degenerative disease. The impact of the use of PET in cardiovascular prosthetics is even more profound as these biomedical devices offer the possibility of saving life.

The structure of the book is as follows. Chapters 1 and 2 provide an introduction to tissue engineering and drug delivery systems. The intention in these introductory chapters is to provide a background to these key themes from an interdisciplinary perspective. Chapters 3 and 8 develop the tissue engineering theme by considering the application of hydrogels and natural polymers as tissue scaffolds. The theme of controlled release is developed in Chapter 4 by considering the use of synthetic biodegradable block copolymers in drug delivery. While each chapter concludes with a section that considers the future in each area, Chapter 7 offers a view of the future based on the concept that polymers can be used as sensors in the body.

The application of polymeric materials in the human body is clearly an exciting area, one which offers the potential of profound benefits for society. I hope this book provides a way of facilitating the reader's entry into this rapidly expanding, interdisciplinary area. Finally, I would like to thank the contributors for all their time and effort during the preparation of the chapters.

M. J. Jenkins

1
Introduction to polymeric scaffolds for tissue engineering

K HARRISON, GlaxoSmithKline R&D Ltd, UK

1.1 Introduction

Tissue engineering is a strategy for the repair or replacement of damaged tissues or organs, involving the culture of living cells *in vitro* on a synthetic structure and the subsequent implantation of the construct into patients.[1] This is termed morphogenesis.[2] The aim is to harvest a relatively small piece of tissue, to remove the cells and then to expand the cell population. The cells can subsequently be reimplanted using a carrier material to assist in the generation of a substantial amount of tissue. As such, tissue engineering is a multidisciplinary area, which requires considerable biological input to gain insight into the behaviour of cells during *in vitro* culture and *in vivo* implantation. It also requires extensive engineering knowledge to fabricate and process materials that are suitable for guiding tissue development.

Tissue-engineered constructs (TECs) are typically composed of two components: a group of cells and a material scaffold on which they can grow.[3] The cellular component is responsible for the generation of new tissue through the production of an extracellular matrix (ECM), which is imperative for the synthesis of healthy functional tissue. The scaffold material initially provides mechanical stability and also provides a template to guide three-dimensional cellular growth. The interaction of these two components, such as the coordination of polymer degradation rate with cellular synthesis rate, is critical for the success of tissue engineering.[3]

1.2 Cells used in tissue engineering

Cells used in tissue engineering may be drawn from a variety of sources including primary tissues or cell lines.[4] Primary tissues may be xenogeneic (from different species), allogeneic (from different members of the same species), syngeneic (from genetically identical individuals) or autologous (from the same individual). The majority of TECs have employed primary autologous cells to prevent eliciting a foreign body response.[5]

One of the most critical elements of tissue engineering is the ability to mimic the body's natural scaffold that normally serves to organise cells into tissues.[6] The natural scaffolding biomaterial is the ECM.[6] The ECM is a composite tissue composed of a variety of macromolecules, which can be grouped into four major classes, each of which is responsible for specific ECM characteristics.[7] The four classes of macromolecules are collagens, proteoglycans, cell interactive glycoproteins and elastic fibres. Furthermore, although all ECMs share these components, the organisation, form and mechanical properties of ECMs can vary widely in different tissues depending on the chemical composition and three dimensional organisation of the specific ECM components that are present.

Collagens are the most abundant proteins in the body and are primarily responsible for the structural role of the cell. Proteoglycans, however, are complex macromolecules that each contain a core protein with one or more covalently bound linear polysaccharide chains known as glycosaminoglycans (GAGs).[7] Proteoglycans such as hyaluronic acid are found within the cell or on the cell surface. These macromolecules are able to self-associate to produce entangled networks that trap large amounts of water, are highly elastic and yet easily deformed. Owing to the elastic properties, proteoglycans define a space in which cells can move and differentiate and also form new matrices.

Within the ECM, there are domains containing specific amino acid sequences called cell-interactive glycoproteins that are recognized by cell–surface receptors. These polypeptide sequences often serve as adhesion recognition signals and may provide cell-type specificity.[7] Cell adhesion is critical for the assembly of cells into tissues and the maintenance of tissue integrity. In order to form a three-dimensional structure, cells must adhere not only to one another but also to the underlying support structure. Cell adhesion is usually accomplished by receptors such as integrin, which responds to the adhesion recognition signals.[7] The final component of ECM is elastic fibre, which provides tissue flexibility.

The primary function of the ECM in tissue development is its role as a physiological substratum for cell attachment.[6] Furthermore, most cells only grow when attached and spread on a solid substrate. As such, cells attach and spread *in vitro* by either depositing new ECM components or by binding to exogenous ECM. Likewise, if cells are detached from the ECM, they rapidly lose viability and can undergo programmed cell death such as apoptosis.[7]

Cell adhesion is a very important factor, which plays a role in tissue and organ formation and in the generation of traction for the migration of cells; it is also important in determining the biocompatibility of synthetic implant materials.[7] In animal cell adhesion, cells first attach to a surface by pseudopodial extensions. Subsequently, the cells spread to form focal contacts.

Both stages involve the cell *probing* the surface for protein ligands.[7] Transmembrane glycoproteins such as integrins may link extracellular proteins to the cytoskeleton inside the cell.

As such, specific cell–surface and cell–cell interactions are mediated by receptor molecules, which have an extracellular domain at the surface of the cell and adsorbed or soluble proteins or peptide sequence ligands, which bind to these receptors.[7] It is thought that the subsequent adsorbed protein layer influences events at the solid–liquid interface, as cells must interact with this protein layer. Adhesive proteins may act as bridging molecules between the cell and artificial surface.

The ECM also serves to organise cells spatially. The basement membrane forms anchorage points, which provide an initial point of orientation and stability. Moreover, it has been shown that orderly tissue renewal following injury or ageing is successfully achieved by the presence of insoluble ECM scaffolds. The ECM acts as a template that maintains the original architectural form and ensures accurate regeneration of pre-existing structures. Therefore, in order to engineer any organ or tissue successfully, a suitable substratum must be used to replicate the ECM and to provide initial support and guidance for tissue regeneration.

A number of different therapies have been developed to aid the regeneration of damaged tissue. One area that has received much interest is cartilage tissue engineering. Once damaged, adult cartilage has a limited intrinsic capacity for repair, particularly if the defect is confined to cartilage.[8,9] This arises because chondrocytes, the sole cellular component of cartilage, are unable to migrate to the site of injury, because of the absence of repair elements such as the ingrowth of mesenchymal cells and a fibrin clot scaffold into which the cells can migrate and because of the avascular and alymphatic nature of cartilage.[1] As such, external therapies have been developed to regenerate cartilage with appropriate functionality.

Cartilage has the lowest cellular density of any tissue in the body with less than 5% cells by volume.[1] It is an avascular mesenchymal connective tissue, which exists in three histological types.[4] Hyaline cartilage is present in walls of respiratory passages, ventral ends of ribs and articular surfaces of joints. Elastic cartilage is present in the walls of the external auditory canal, as well as in the epiglottis and the cuneiform cartilage of the larynx. The final type of cartilage is fibrocartilage, which is located in vertebral discs and is involved in attachment of certain ligaments to bone.

Articular cartilage, a type of hyaline cartilage, has a complex three-dimensional structure, which gives it the ability to bear and distribute loads.[1] The ability to withstand loads and to act in a poroelastic manner is an integral part of the functionality of articular cartilage and is partly determined by the presence of type II collagen.[9] Type II collagen makes up 15–22% of cartilage and is present when cartilage is in the differentiated state.

The differentiated state is when cells have a particular gene expression, which determines the specific function that the cell is able to perform such as load bearing for differentiated chondrocytes.

However, chondrocytes readily dedifferentiate and transform into fibroblast-like cells. Consequently, collagen type II switches to collagen type I. Dedifferentiation to the fibroblastic state causes cartilage to not possess the correct physical attributes such as a weight-bearing capacity.[5] The cartilage will instead be histologically similar to fibrocartilage, which is a non-weight-bearing tissue.

The propensity of articular cartilage to dedifferentiate into fibrocartilage can be limited by the culturing conditions. Chondrocytes grown on monolayers dedifferentiate with passaging and lose both the chondrogenic phenotype and their redifferentiation potential.[10] However, chondrocytes grown in conditions that support their round morphology and prevent spreading, such as three-dimensional constructs, can maintain the differentiated phenotype.[5]

The use of specific growth factors such as basic fibroblast growth factor (FGF-2) and transforming growth factor β1 (TGF-β1) has also been found to increase the rate of cell proliferation and to maintain the cellular ability to redifferentiate upon transfer to a three-dimensional environment.[11] As such, the incorporation of growth factors into the scaffold environment can successfully assist in the maintenance of the chondrocytic phenotype of engineered cartilage.

In addition to collagen, cartilage is composed of proteoglycans (4–7 wt%) and water. The proteoglycans are composed of sulphated glycosaminoglycans (sGAGs) attached to a protein core. These monomers bind to long chains of hyaluronate and form aggregates. Furthermore, proteoglycan aggregates or aggrecans are typically indicative of differentiated cartilage and the ability to weight bear.[12] The collagen and proteoglycans interact non-covalently to form a fibre-reinforced composite matrix, which has mechanical strength and stiffness.

Inherent to the success of cartilage is the interaction between chondrocytes and the ECM.[13] The ECM provides structural support and also consists of specific protein sequences that chondrocytes attach to via heterodimeric transmembrane receptors, namely integrins.[5,13] These mediate reciprocal interactions between the ECM and the intracellular cytoskeleton, resulting in functional organisation of the ECM and cytoskeleton. The binding of specific integrin complexes to ECM components also initiates signal transduction cascades that regulate chondrocyte survival, proliferation and gene expression.[5,13]

Under compression, articular cartilage behaves like a poroelastic material, whereby its response to compressive loads is frequency and strain dependent.[9] This is governed by the interrelationship between solid ECM constituents, namely collagen type II and interstitial fluid flow (e.g. water). As such, tissue-engineered cartilage needs to have a distinct molecular composition and architecture that is optimised for the unique mechanical functions the tissue is required to carry out. Various considerations therefore need to be made to minimise the proclivity of chondrocytes to dedifferentiate into fibroblast-like cells, which do not possess the correct physical attributes.

In contrast with cartilage, bone is continuously remodelled during the lifespan of most vertebrates.[10] Bone remodelling is a result of the balance between the activities of two different cell populations: osteoblasts and osteoclasts. Osteoblasts are responsible for bone deposition and are derived from mesenchymal lineage cells.[7] However, osteoclasts are multinucleated giant cells and are involved in bone resorption. When osteoblasts disperse as local lining cells on a bone surface, an exposed runway is provided for osteoclasts to attach to and, following expression of a soluble factor or second messenger from the osteoblasts, osteoclasts are prompted to resorb bone.[7] The dynamic reciprocal relationship between osteoblasts and osteoclasts, therefore, carefully controls resorptive–appositional activities.

Bone injuries are common and, although, unlike cartilage, bone can readily repair itself, certain injuries and defects do still require external therapies to regenerate bone effectively.[10] Common therapies have included permanent replacement of the bone tissue with a foreign material such as a metal plates or pins. However, restoration of bone tissue at the site using transplanted biological material such as autograft and allograft bone is becoming more widespread.[4]

Constructs implanted with bone cells can be osteoinductive (inducing new bone formation) in addition to being osteoconductive (permitting bony ingrowth) whilst also providing a source of osteogenic cells.[4] Bone formation consists of a complex series of events that begins with the recruitment and proliferation of osteoprogenitors from mesenchymal stem cells followed by cell differentiaton, osteoid formation and ultimately mineralisation.[14] Human bone remodels at a rate of approximately 2–10%/year and packets of cells, i.e. osteoblasts, osteoclasts and osteocytes, known as the basic multicellular unit (BMU) function as instruments for remodelling.[7] The BMU is responsible for the sum activities of cell activation, resorption and formation.

Bone is unique as it has a vast potential for regeneration from stem cells.[14] Autogenous osteoblasts or progenitor cells can therefore be derived from stem cells in the bone marrow.[4] Mesenchymal stem cells are subsequently capable of differentiating along multiple lineages and assist in bone remodelling and fracture repair.[15] This is extremely promising as it provides an additional source of donor cells that can successfully assist in producing functional bone.

Bone is a highly complex organ consisting of two distinctive integrated tissue types interspersed with multiple cell phenotypes. Bone is also dynamic; it is highly vascularised; it fulfils rigorous biomechanical roles and responds to physiological demands. As such, the aim to successfully engineer bone poses many difficult problems, which need to be considered to produce viable bone substitutes.

The liver is the largest organ in the body. The mass of the average adult liver is 1.5 kg or roughly 2.5% of the body mass.[7] The liver holds approximately 30% of the resting cardiac output at any one time and uses about 20% of the oxygen in the body. The liver performs a variety of functions including synthesis and regulation of a variety of molecules, the inactivation of hormones and the storage of glucose as glycogen; it is also involved in lipid metabolism.

Hepatocytes, the parenchymal cells of the liver, perform most of the metabolic functions of the liver. They account for 90% of cell mass and 60% of cell number in the liver.[7] Although generally considered to be epithelial cells, hepatocytes are not supported by a traditional basement membrane; however, they do contact ECM proteins such as collagen, laminin and proteoglycans at their basal surface. Hepatocytes also have an immense capacity for regeneration. In response to partial hepatectomy or toxic injury, liver cells are quickly stimulated to divide to replace lost cell mass.[7] This restoration can take up to 6 months but, provided with the correct structural support, a liver could recover from acute liver failure within a much shorter period of time.

Given the accelerated recovery rate of damaged liver with external support structures and the shortage of organ donors, a number of therapeutic methods are being explored to assist in liver regeneration.[4] One such method involves seeding isolated hepatocytes on to polymeric meshes. However, hepatocytes have high oxygen and nutrient requirements that cannot always be met by a TEC. Therefore, prevascularisation of the polymer scaffold is required to augment the supply of essential oxygen and nutrients. Furthermore, primary hepatocytes have been found to lose their differentiated function in 3–4 days and viability within 1 week when cultured as monolayers.

To overcome the problems associated with culturing hepatocytes, novel bioreactors have been designed. These include features such as the introduction of patient blood or plasma into the bioreactor, the use of a polymeric three-dimensional membrane or gel matrix to act as a cell microcarrier and also the supplementation of media with growth factors, hormones and ECM components.[16] These adaptations offer promising methods for successful liver regeneration.

Skin represents the body's first tissue-engineered organ to receive Food and Drug Administration (FDA) approval for clinical application.[4] The skin is a highly organised, complex structure that provides the boundary between vertebrates and their environment. As a barrier, the skin must be physically tough and yet must also be flexible and elastic to permit free movement.[7] The barrier must also be impermeable to toxic substances and must prevent the loss of excessive water to the environment. Moreover, the skin regulates body temperature by secretion from sweat glands and by regulating blood flow through superficial capillaries.

Skin consists of two layers. Firstly, the epidermis consists primarily of keratinocytes, which are constantly proliferating and replacing themselves.[7] Also present in the epidermis are melanocytes, which distribute melanin to protect the epidermis against ultraviolet radiation. Secondly, the dermis, a deeper layer that is rich in connective tissue, provides a high tensile strength and flexibility. It also supports the extensive vasculature, lymphatic system, nerve bundles and other structures in skin.[7] It is relatively acellular, consisting primarily of an ECM of interwoven collagen fibrils interspersed with elastic fibres, proteoglycans and glycoproteins. Fibroblasts are the major cell type in the dermis and are responsible for producing and maintaining most of the ECM.

When skin is damaged, if the wound extends only partially through the dermis, the dermis is able to provide cells for its own reconstitution.[4] Furthermore, deep skin appendages such as hair follicles and sweat glands can provide sources of epidermal cells to recreate the dermis. However, if the wound extends throughout the dermis, such as full-thickness burns or skin ulcers, there are no sources of cells for regeneration. This has led to the development of tissue-engineered skin equivalents.

Tissue-engineered strategies have involved autogenous epidermal keratinocytes seeded on a wound bed, bovine collagen-based skin replacement materials and bioengineered dermis using cell–polymer constructs.[17] While matrix scaffolds have shown some improvement in scar morphology, no acellular matrix has yet been shown to lead to true dermal regeneration. In order to replicate skin successfully, a bilayered composite skin structure may be required to reproduce the synergistic behaviour of the epidermis and dermis.

1.3 The scaffold structure

Polymer matrices need to provide a number of key functions in order for them to be successful in tissue-engineering applications. To enable scaffold conduits to be successful in recruiting reparative cells in an organised manner, a number of key characteristics need to be achieved. Scaffolds ideally need to provide the following.

1 A biocompatible and biodegradable matrix with controllable degradation kinetics.

2 Suitable surface chemistry for cell attachment, proliferation and differentiation.
3 An interconnected and permeable pore network to promote nutrient and waste exchange.
4 A three-dimensional and highly porous structure to support cell attachment, proliferation and ECM production.
5 Appropriate mechanical properties to match those at the site of implantation.
6 An architecture which promotes formation of native anisotropic tissue.
7 A reproducible architecture of clinically relevant size and shape.[9,18]

Polymers can replace diseased organ function by acting as a cellular nucleus for tissue regeneration or as a source of molecular signals to control host cell growth and tissue regeneration.[19] The formation of tissue produced by implanted cells is influenced greatly by the scaffold on to which they are seeded.[3] The choice of polymer is therefore vitally important in determining the success of the TEC.

1.3.1 Polymeric scaffold materials

Natural polymers such as collagen and hyaluronic acid are widely used for organ regeneration since they facilitate cell attachment and growth.[10,20] Collagen is the most abundant protein in the body and can be prepared in solution or shaped into threads, sponges or hydrogels. Furthermore, although it is derived from xenogeneic sources, purification techniques enable it to be used without eliciting a foreign body response. Bovine chondrocytes, which had been cultured in gels derived from collagen type I isolated from rats, increased in density initially but, from day 6 onwards, they dedifferentiated into fibroblast-like cells.[6]

Alginate, a naturally derived polysaccharide typically purified from seaweed, is a biocompatible polymer widely used in the food and chemical industry. In addition, it has more recently been developed as a cell transplantation material for a variety of cell types, including chondrocytes.[21] Studies have shown that chondrocytes seeded on alginate gels decrease in initial cell density.[22] However, chondrocytes typically retain their rounded morphology, an indication of the maintenance of chondrocyte phenotype.

Fibrin is also a commonly used natural polymer.[10] It originates during blood coagulation and plays an important role in wound healing. Fibrin is typically used as a glue or a hydrogel, which can controllably deliver growth factors with heparin binding affinity. Hyaluronic acid is also able to deliver biological agents.[23,24] It binds specifically to proteins in the ECM and on the cell surface. Partial esterification of hyaluronic acid stabilises the molecule and makes it suitable for controlled peptide release or protein delivery.[6]

Chitosan is a biosynthetic polysaccharide that is the deacylated derivative of chitin.[6] Chitin is a naturally occurring polysaccharide that can be generated via fungal fermentation processes. Chitin and chitosan can be degraded by lysozyme, which acts slowly to depolymerise the polysaccharide.[25] The biodegradation rate of the polymer is determined by the amount of residual acetyl content, a parameter than can be varied easily. Chitosan can be formed into membranes and matrices that are well tolerated by the body and are useful in a number of tissue-engineering applications.

Although naturally occurring biomaterials closely simulate the native cellular milieu, there is often a large variation between batches upon isolation from biological tissues as well as a restricted versatility in designing devices with specific biomechanical properties.[4] Therefore, synthetic polymers are more commonly used as they afford greater control over physicochemical properties and delivery kinetics of the scaffold.[10]

Early synthetic polymers were derived from adaptations of commodity plastics such as polyethylene, polyurethane and silicone rubbers.[7] Such synthetic polymers have been successfully used in tissue engineering; however, they are not biodegradable and the non-resorbed polymer remains an integral part of the tissue. This is not inappropriate for the successful implantation of a tissue-engineered product and yet the benefit of polymeric biomaterials that degrade to leave behind the biological component has been realised in the synthesis of bioerodible polymers.

Previously, synthetic bioerodible polymer scaffolds for cell seeding and tissue regeneration have focused on the poly(α-hydroxy acid) family of polymers such as poly(lactic acid) (PLA), poly(glycolic acid) (PGA), and the copolymer poly(lactic-co-glycolic acid) (PLGA).[14,22,26–28] These materials have the advantage of FDA approval and are currently used as biodegradable suture materials and drug delivery vehicles.[26]

PLA and PGA can be polymerised directly from lactic acid and glycolic acid, respectively, and the chemical structures are shown in Fig. 1.1.[7] A ring-opening polymerisation, typically catalysed by organometallic catalysts such as stannous octoate leads to polymerisation.[29] PGA is a linear aliphatic polyester which is highly crystalline and has a high melting temperature and low solubility in organic solvents.[6] Because of its relatively hydrophilic nature, surgical sutures made of PGA tend to lose their mechanical strength rapidly, typically over a period of 2–4 weeks post-implantation.[30]

The presence of an additional methyl group in lactic acid causes PLA to be more hydrophobic than PGA.[31] The rate of backbone hydrolysis is therefore much lower and is also more soluble in organic solvents. Furthermore, lactic acid is a chiral molecule and therefore exists in two stereoisomeric forms, D-PLA and L-PLA as well as the racemic polymer, D,L-PLA.[6] This enables products derived from lactic acid to exhibit a wide range of properties. D,L-PLA is an amorphous polymer and as such is

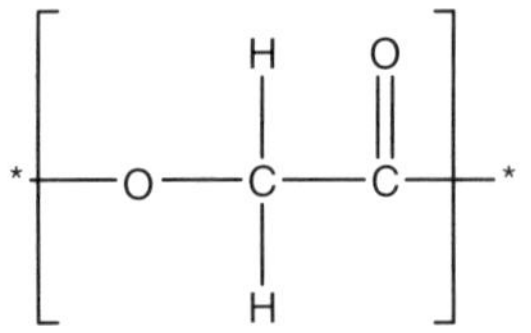

Polyglycolic acid (PGA)

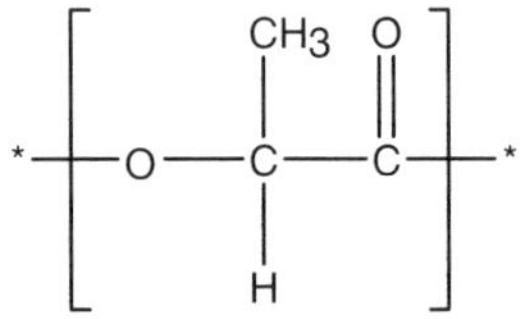

Polylactic acid (PLA)

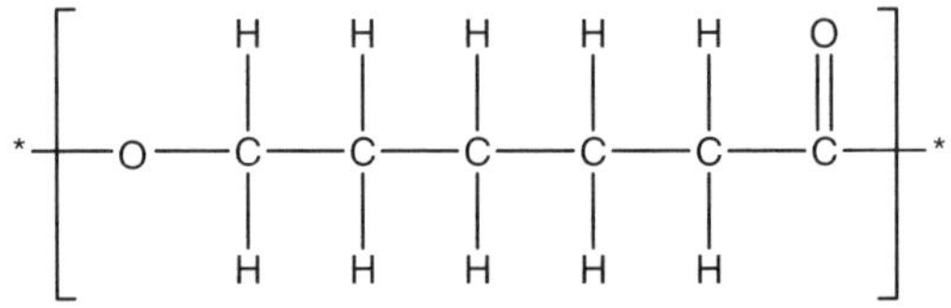

Polycaprolactone (PCL)

1.1 Chemical structure of three members of the poly(α-hydroxy acid) family of polymers.

usually used in drug delivery applications where it is important to have a homogeneous dispersion of the active species within the monophasic matrix.[32] On the other hand, L-PLA is crystalline and is preferred in applications where high mechanical strength and toughness are required such as sutures or orthopaedic devices.

In addition, copolymerisation approaches are used when the homopolymer does not possess all the required physical and chemical properties alone for the intended application. Copolymers of PLA and PGA (PLGA) have been formed in an attempt to synthesise polymers with shorter absorption times than PLA and yet a tough amorphous nature.[7] This has been successful and the ability to tailor the absorption profile of PLA and PGA has rendered the polymers desirable materials for tissue scaffold applications.

Both PLA and PGA have also been used in the past as tissue-engineering scaffolds and orthopaedic devices. Chondrocytes have been found to proliferate and secrete GAG within porous PGA meshes and PLA foams.[33,34]

However, PLA and PGA induce inflammatory responses when implanted in the body for over 12 weeks. This is due to the release of acidic degradation products such as lactic acid and glycolic acid.

Polycaprolactone (PCL) is another polymer that is currently used as a biodegradable tissue scaffold.[6] PCL is an aliphatic polyester that can be degraded by a hydrolytic mechanism under physiological conditions.[35,36] It can also be degraded by enzymatic surface erosion. Low-molecular-weight fragments of PCL are taken up by macrophages and degraded intracellularly. PCL degrades significantly more slowly than PLA or PGA owing to the long methylene backbone (Fig. 1.1) and is used as a long-term implantable contraceptive device, *Capronor*.[36]

PCL exhibits a low melting temperature of approximately 57 °C and a low glass transition temperature Tg of –60 °C, which renders it rubbery at room temperature.[37] PCL therefore has a high permeability to a number of therapeutic drugs, which is useful. PCL also has a high thermal stability (T_d = 350 °C) compared with other polyesters (T_d = 235–255 °C), which enables it to be processed using a variety of routes.[6] Currently, PCL is classified as non-toxic and tissue compatible by the FDA but is not used extensively as a biomaterial. However, its high propensity to form compatible blends with a variety of polymers and monomers may enhance its future biomaterial role.[38–40]

Polymeric hydrogels are often employed in tissue engineering, as they are less invasive than solid polymer constructs. Poly(ethylene glycol) (PEG) has formed the basis for the synthesis of a number of cross-linked hydrogels.[7] By increasing the molecular weight of the PEG central segment, the swollen hydrogel can be varied from a rigid to a highly flexible material. The identity of the bioabsorbable segment also dictates the bioabsorption times. The degradation rate can be varied from days to weeks to months, by the incorporation of glycolate, lactate or trimethylene carbonate, respectively.

Injectable polymers are also typically used, as they are able to fill irregularly shaped defects and to minimise surgical intervention. Ideally, injectable polymers should polymerise *in situ* without a detrimental effect to the surrounding tissue such as an increase in temperature.[41] One polymer, which has been employed in the past, is poly(propylene fumarate), an unsaturated linear polyester that has the appropriate mechanical properties and degrades to non-toxic by-products.

1.3.2 Scaffold morphology

The migration of individual cells within a tissue is critical in the formation of the appropriate architecture of organs.[42] Likewise, cell migration is an important factor in tissue engineering because the ability of the cells to move either in association with the polymer surface or other cells is an essential part of new tissue formation. Therefore, for cells attached to a solid substrate, cell behaviour and function depend on the characteristics of the substrate.

Polymeric matrices are designed to control and guide tissue regeneration to elicit specific cellular interactions and responses. They also serve as scaffolds to support cell transplantation. The goal of morphogenesis is to create an environment where cells are encouraged to form functional tissue structures.[2] The surface chemical characteristics of an implanted device are known, therefore, to exert profound effects on cell attachment, alignment and proliferation.[43]

One of the greatest features of polymeric biomaterials is their scope for modification.[7] Properties of synthetic polymer scaffolds can be altered by varying the functional group, changing the polymer architecture using a linear, branched or comb-shaped polymer or modifying the polymer combination by preparing a physical mixed polymer or a chemically bonded copolymer.[4] This offers fine control over the behaviour of the scaffold when it is implanted *in vivo* in terms of cell–material interaction and scaffold degradation rate.

Most tissue-derived cells are anchorage dependent and require attachment to a solid surface for viability and growth.[6] For this reason, the initial events that occur when a cell approaches a surface are of fundamental interest. In tissue engineering, cell adhesion to a surface is critical because adhesion precedes other events such as cell spreading, migration and differentiated cell function. Therefore, it is recognised that the behaviour of the adhesion and proliferation of different types of cell on polymer materials depend on the surface characteristics such as wettability, chemistry, charge, roughness and rigidity.

It has been found that cell adhesion is maximised on surfaces with intermediate wettability.[44,45] This is because, for most surfaces, cell adhesion requires the presence of serum and because polymers with intermediate contact angle measurements provide an optimum condition for proteins such as fibronectin to adsorb to the surface. As such, cell adhesion is maximised on surfaces with intermediate contact angle values. In the absence of serum, however, adhesion is enhanced on positively charged surfaces.[46] Fibroblast spreading has been correlated with surface free energy but the rate of fibroblast growth on polymer surfaces appears to be relatively independent of surface chemistry.[6]

The microscale texture or roughness of an implanted material can also have a significant effect on the behaviour of cells in the region of the implant.[6] The behaviour of cells cultured on surfaces with grooves or patterns is different from the cellular behaviour observed on a smooth surface. Polydimethylsiloxane (PDMS) surfaces with 4 or 25 μm^2 peaks uniformly distributed on the surface have been found to provide better conditions for fibroblast growth than PDMS surfaces with 100 μm² peaks or 4, 25 or 100 μm² valleys.[47] The grooves or peaks act as anchorage points which the cells are able to attach to and to begin to spread and proliferate.

Polymer surfaces can be made more suitable for cell attachment and growth by surface modification techniques. Polystyrene substrates typically used for tissue culture are often treated by glow discharge or exposure to sulphuric acid to increase the number of charged groups at the surface, which improves attachment and growth of many types of cell.[48] The availability of specific chemical groups on the polymer surface such as hydroxyl groups –OH or surface C–O functionalities are also important factors in modulating the fate of surface-attached cells.[49,50]

Grafting hydrophilic monomers on to the polymeric substrate can change the surface properties of a polymer presented to a cell.[7] Furthermore, grafting results in improving the interfacial chemistry between the polymer and biological fluid. The incorporation of poly(ethylene oxide) (PEO) on to a polymeric substrate creates a surface that is blood compatible by exerting a steric repulsion to proteins and cells that approach the surface. The motion of the PEO chains also creates microflows of water, which prevent plasma protein adsorption. Moreover, PEO significantly decreases bacterial adhesion through steric repulsion.

Adhesion-dependent cell types often exhibit increased longevity and increased cellular function when cultured on extracellular proteins, such as fibronectin and laminin, rather than on virgin plastic ware.[7,50] As such, it is useful to immobilise bioactive molecules or biomimetic species on to polymeric substrate surfaces. This can be achieved if a biomedical polymer possesses reactive functional groups, which enable the conjugation of bioactive species such as peptides, growth factors or enzymes.[14] Covalent attachment of synthetic peptides to poly(ethylene terephthalate) and polytetrafluoroethylene has been found to promote cell adhesion, spreading and focal contact formation on otherwise non-adhesive or weakly adhesive polymers.[6]

However, a number of studies have shown that materials that promote good cell adhesion through appropriate surface chemistry and topography do not necessarily induce cell spreading and migration.[6,51] Similarly, several groups have reported that the surfaces that display the best primary attachment characteristics are not necessarily the substrates on which cell proliferation or differentiation is improved.[51,52] It can be seen, therefore, that cell–substrate interaction is a complex relationship.

1.3.3 Scaffold microstructure

A three-dimensional structure is vital for successful tissue engineering. Chondrocytes attached to flat surfaces are able to spread but adopt a fibroblast-like morphology, which is indicative of a change in phenotype and dedifferentiation.[5] Dedifferentiated cells do not possess the correct mechanical properties and, furthermore, if cells do not express the true chondrocyte phenotype, their ability to regenerate damaged cartilage tissue is impaired. A porous three-dimensional scaffold is therefore required to optimise viable cell growth.

Pore morphology and porosity are important properties that need to be tailored to the type of tissue being regenerated.[53] It has been found that precise geometric parameters are required for the successful regeneration of certain cells. Bony ingrowth predominates in porous structures with pore sizes of approximately 450 μm whereas connective tissue grows preferentially in pores of 100 μm in size or less.[43] Vascular infiltration, however, ideally attaches and grows within pores of approximately 1000 μm. Structures consisting of macropores (150–300 μm) highly interconnected by micropores (less than 50 μm) have been found to be conducive to ingrowth of fibrocartilaginous tissue in polyurethane implants. Therefore, the implant porosity can allow limited tissue ingrowth for stabilisation of implants or provide pathways for tissue regeneration within a biodegradable scaffold or matrix.

The geometry of a scaffold can also impact on the competition between cell adhesion and proliferation, and maintenance of cell phenotypic morphology. It has been found that, on porous polycarbonate (PC) membrane sheets with a small micropore diameter (0.2–1.0 μm), chondrocytes easily adhered, spread and assumed a fibroblast-like morphology.[54] However, on PC membrane sheets with large micropores (3–8.0 μm), cells maintained the round morphology and were indicative of cells with articular cartilage phenotype.

A polymer scaffold must also provide a structure that can maintain the distance between parenchymal cells and permit the diffusion of gas and nutrients. Ideally, the scaffold should allow a supply of nutrients to the cells that matches the removal of their waste products.[55] The success of the approach is also dependent on whether the mass transport between the engineered and surrounding host tissues is sufficient to meet the metabolic requirements of the engineered tissue.[21] Diffusion is sufficient for this purpose when a small number of cells are transplanted on or within the polymeric device or if the metabolic needs of the transplanted cells are very low, such as chondrocyte transplantation.

Furthermore, in order for a tissue to regenerate, a scaffold, needs to create potential space for the cells to grow into. A scaffold, therefore, needs to be a porous structure that enables the ingress of cells into the synthetic support to occur. The scaffold also needs to acts as a vehicle to deliver isolated cells such as chondrocytes or chondroprogenitor cells to voids created by the removal of dysfunctional tissue.[56] As such, the scaffold initially acts as a spacer between damaged ends of cartilage or bone. As the cells proliferate and are able to provide their own structural integrity, the scaffold degrades to create more space for the tissue to develop in to.

1.3.4 Mechanical properties of scaffolds

Initially, polymeric scaffolds need to provide structural integrity. This is because, at the outset, the volume of cells and intercellular material is likely to be considerably less than that in mature tissue. As such, a temporary synthetic support is required to withstand the dynamic *in vivo* stresses that occur whilst the tissue is regenerating. It is therefore desirable to match the mechanical properties of the material with that of the native tissue.

The mechanical properties of the scaffold are imperative for the success of a scaffold in its intended application. Strength is the primary concern in applications such as bone regeneration, whereas pliability is an important consideration when tubular constructs are required for intestine and blood vessel use. Flexibility is also a parameter that can affect the suitability of a scaffold when it is required for skin regeneration, as the polymer matrix needs to be able to adapt to different contours.

The mechanical environment has been found to affect profoundly the development, maintenance and remodelling of tissue *in vivo*. Therefore, mechanical stimulation may be an important determinant of the quality of engineered tissue grown *in vitro*. Typically four different types of mechanical stimulies are presented to cells *in vivo*. Mechanocoupling is the conversion of an applied physical force to secondary forces or physical phenomena detected by the cells.[7] In bone, the application of a primary force has been found to result in deformation of the bone, which in turn deforms bone cells and elicits pressure gradients and interstitial fluid flow. The interstitial fluid flow applies mechanical shear stress to osteoblasts and osteocytes, which promotes osteogenesis.

The second type of mechanical stimulation is mechanotransduction.[7] This is the conversion of either primary or secondary physical stimulus into an electrical, chemical or biochemical response and typically occurs in mechanically activated ion channels and receptors.[7] Owing to the avascular, alymphatic and aneural nature of cartilage, changes in chondrocyte activity are believed to occur by transduction of mechanical events to metabolic events and structural adaptations.[1] As such, mechanical loading or stirring of chondrocytes grown *in vitro* has been found to induce cells to assemble a matrix that is structurally similar to native cartilage.

Signal transduction is a similar type of stimulus to mechanotransduction but involves the conversion of one biochemical signal to another.[7] The fourth stimulus is final cellular response, which completes the conversion from initial stimulus to final tissue level response.[7] The activation of signal transduction pathways regulates cellular activities such as protein synthesis and gene expression, leading to a response on the tissue level.[7] Therefore, by modifying the mechanical or biochemical environment, the development of engineered tissue can be controlled.

The effects of dynamic compression on chondrocyte biosynthesis have been well characterised in cartilage explants and chondrocyte-seeded scaffolds. In explants continuously applied with dynamic compression and dynamic tissue shear, an increase in the synthesis of proteins and proteoglycans was found.[56] Intermittent compressive loading increased proteoglycan synthesis during short-term loading and increased material properties and GAG contents.[7] Loading has been found to enhance the long-term deposition of ECM in cell-seeded constructs during *in vitro* culture. As such, a conduit, which can transmit mechanical forces to the cells during tissue regeneration, would improve engineered tissue functionality.

Bone actively remodels in response to mechanical loading, increasing density and strength in areas exposed to stress whilst losing density in unstimulated regions.[7] It is also well documented that bone mass is rapidly lost under conditions of diminished mechanical loading. Furthermore, a more rapid and complete differentiation of osteoblasts cells cultured in a mechanically active environment has been found compared with culturing in a stationary setting.[7] Therefore, the mechanical environment is a key determinant of bone development.

In vivo arteries are cyclically stretched by the fluctuating blood pressure associated with the cardiac cycle.[7] Therefore, it would be desirable if the developing bioartificial blood vessel was exposed to a similar cyclic strain to preserve the contractile phenotype and also to align the smooth muscle cells in the correct orientation in the vessel wall.

1.3.5 Biodegradation kinetics of scaffolds

The macromolecular structure of the polymer is selected so that the scaffold is completely degraded and eliminated as need for the artificial support diminishes.[53] The degradation rate of the polymer scaffold needs to be tailored to suit the intended application of the synthetic structure.[28,57] It is desirable that the polymer is degradable so that potential long-term biological reactions to the polymer are eliminated. Furthermore, biodegradable polymers may provide an additional benefit to tissue-engineering applications.[6] During polymer degradation, the surface of the polymer is constantly renewed, thereby providing a dynamic substrate for cell attachment and growth.

Biodegradable implants degrade by hydrolysis and/or enzymatic action, forming tissue-compatible metabolites that can be used in the carbohydrate or protein metabolism.[27,28] Eventually, generated breakdown products such as water and carbon dioxide (CO_2) will be excreted in urine or faeces or exhaled. During degradation, the implant will lose its strength gradually and the load on the regenerating tissue will gradually shift from implant to tissue.

Typically, the ester bonds of poly(hydroxy acids) are cleaved by hydrolysis, which results in a decrease in the polymer's molecular weight.[58] This initial degradation occurs until the molecular weight is less than 5000, at which point cellular degradation ensues. The final degradation and resorption of the poly(hydroxy acid) implants involve inflammatory cells such as macrophages and lymphocytes.

It has been asserted that the rate of degradation is governed by water access to the ester bond rather than by the intrinsic rate of ester cleavage. The access of water to the ester bond is determined by the combined effect of a number of polymer characteristics. These include the glass transition temperature of the polymer, the degree of crystallinity, the molecular weight, the hydrophobicity of the monomer and the bulk sample dimensions.[59,60]

PGA is an attractive biodegradable support owing to its relatively fast rate of biodegradation, which frees up the space for the ECM and minimises the host inflammatory response.[1] However, PGA does exhibit relatively low strength, making it impractical for immediate transplantation. PLA is a stronger material but, because of the extra methyl group in the main chain, PLA degrades more slowly. This causes the implant to reside in the wound site for longer and the void is filled with cartilaginous matrix much more slowly. The longer residence time can result in the eliciting of a more severe immune response.[19]

1.3.6 Biocompatibility of scaffolds

The host response to the biomaterial can impact on the immune response towards transplanted cells. The implantation of a biomaterial without transplanted cells initiates a sequence of events similar to a foreign body response.[19] Cellular mechanisms are activated to produce inflammation and healing mechanisms upon implantation. The extent of the pathphysiological response is a measure of the host reaction to the implant.[60] The size, shape and physical properties of the biomaterial have been found to be responsible for the intensity and duration of the inflammatory and wound-healing process.[19]

The sequence of local events following implantation is generally considered as the tissue response continuum with each individual event leading into the next event. Typically, injury or implantation leads to acute inflammation, which proceeds to chronic inflammation.[60] This is followed by granulation tissue formation, then foreign body reaction and finally fibrous encapsulation.

The tissue response to an implanted polymer is usually characterised as occurring in three phases. The first phase (phase I) occurs within the first 2 weeks following implantation and includes the initiation, resolution and organisation of the acute and chronic inflammatory response.[60] This response is generally similar, regardless of the degradation rate of the bioerodible polymer. Within days, monocytes (inflammatory cells) predominate the implantation site and differentiate into macrophages.

The second phase (phase II) is initiated by the predominance of monocytes and macrophages. While the components of the second phase are similar, the duration of their persistence is determined by the degradation rate of the implant. It has been observed that poly(D,L-lactide-co-glycolide) have a 50–60 day phase II response,[61] whereas the more slowly degrading poly(D,L-lactide) has a phase II response of the order of 350–400 days. The degradation rate of the polymer is therefore important and, as the implant degrades, the polymer begins to undergo macrophage phagocytosis and complete degradation.

It has been proposed that the biodegradation process of the scaffold material may modulate the intensity of the tissue response.[19] As biodegradation proceeds, shape, porosity and surface roughness changes ensue; there is a release of polymeric oligomer and monomer degradation products and a formation of particulates. It is the extent and duration of this deviation from the optimal wound-healing condition that determines the biocompatibility of the scaffold material.

As the immune response continues, monocytes migrating into the site of implant differentiate into macrophages, which can coalesce and form foreign body giant cells. These are typically present at the tissue–implant interface. As the tissue response moves into the third phase (phase III), the resident macrophages accelerate the degradation process and the fibrous capsule formed in phase II is also enhanced. More cells begin to migrate into the volume generated by the loss of the implant volume and neovascularisation proceeds.

In order to minimise the foreign body response, precautions can be taken. Autologous cells do not elicit an immune response and they provide active repair process to the joint.[5] As such, donor cells can be incorporated into the scaffold to minimise the risk of inflammation and rejection. Implanted PLGA scaffolds have been found to elicit a moderate, acute and chronic inflammatory response after 14 days' implantation.[62] Unorganised connective tissue with macrophages and foreign body giant cells are seen to surround the implant. However, scaffolds impregnated with osteoblasts exhibited no apparent tissue necrosis or inflammatory response up to 8 weeks post-implantation.

The chosen scaffold must also be selected to integrate easily with the adjacent tissue and to favour new tissue ingrowth such as osteoconduction but to reduce the incidence of a foreign body response.[10] Implanted PLA and PGA solid rods for femoral shaft fracture fixation have been found to elicit a severe foreign body response accompanied by an inflammatory reaction.[27] It is believed that the large volume of material implanted into the wound site and the absence of autologous cells incorporated into the implant contributed to the invasion of multinuclear cells and thick fibrous tissue formation.

It is imperative to minimise the premature loss of implanted cells because of ischaemia and apoptosis by the host, as this is detrimental to the success of the implanted device.[19] Therefore, the addition of growth factors that induce ingrowth of host vessels, use of autologous host cells and polymers with a rapid and yet controllable degradation rates are beneficial to successful tissue engineering.

1.3.7 Scaffold design

The scaffold is designed to mimic the body's own ECM. It provides a porous biocompatible network into which the surrounding tissue is induced and acts as a temporary template for the new tissue's growth and reorganisation.[53] Typical scaffold designs have included meshes, fibres, sponges and foams. These designs are chosen because they promote uniform cell distribution, diffusion of nutrients and the growth of organised cell communities.[63]

To obtain bone cell colonisation and bone tissue formation throughout the entire scaffold, a construct with a morphology similar to that of trabecular bone has been found to be necessary. The successful polymer matrix exhibited a high degree of interconnectivity with an open-pore structure.[64] Interconnectivity is imperative because it enables cells to diffuse through the entire network instead of accumulating at the surface of the scaffold.[53]

Fibrous conduits are commonly used as tissue scaffolds because most types of cell are known to orientate and move rapidly along fibres.[55] This phenomenon is called *contact guidance* and involves cells spanning fibres forming a *sail* structure. Cells are therefore able to use the fibres as a template to form a three-dimensional structure. Fibroblasts have also been found to orientate on grooved surfaces with texture dimensions of 1–8 μm.[65] PGA meshes with fibre diameters comparable with chondrocyte dimensions have also been found to minimise the focal points for cell adhesion and thus to prevent cell flattening.[12]

Fibre meshes and foams are typical scaffold designs because they create three-dimensional environments for cell proliferation and function and provide structural supports for tissue regeneration. When cultured on three-dimensional PGA fibre meshes, chondrocytes proliferated, producing

GAG and collagen and forming structures that were histologically similar to cartilage.[66] The physical dimensions of the polymer fibre influenced growth rate, with slower growth in thicker meshes.[67] Highly porous structures (97%) have also been seen to provide a suitable three-dimensional structure that can be uniformly seeded with chondrocytes at high initial densities.[12] This enables the establishment of cell–cell contacts, which are essential in the initiation of chondrogenesis and cartilage tissue development.

1.4 Fabrication techniques for tissue scaffolds

A number of fabrication techniques are currently employed to manufacture tissue scaffolds. These include fibre extrusion and bonding, template synthesis, use of gases and solvents as porogens, solvent casting, particulate leaching, membrane lamination, melt moulding, temperature-induced phase separation and rapid prototyping.[9,68,69]

Previously, fibres have been used for cell transplantation in the form of tassels or felts.[70] However, these constructs are not structurally stable. To overcome this, fibre bonding has been employed to join fibres physically in a stable structure without changing the chemical composition or shape of the fibres.[7] Typically, PLA is dissolved in methylene chloride and cast over a non-woven mesh of PGA fibres.[6] After the solvent is evaporated, the construct is heated above the melting temperature of PGA to weld the fibres at their cross-points. The PLGA can then be selectively removed by dissolution in methylene chloride. However, ideally, polymeric scaffolds should deliver angiogenic factors directly from the polymer matrices to the transplanted cells.[21] However, a processing technique such as fibre bonding involves high temperatures and organic solvents, which would be expected to damage the active biological agents.

Fibre bonding also does not allow the manufacture of scaffolds with a defined pore size and surface-area-to-volume ratio.[7] Solvent casting and particulate leaching, however, does afford a level of control over the microstructure of the scaffold. A matrix is created by casting a polymer solution over water-soluble particles such as NaCl salt, the solvent is evaporated and the salt is leached out, yielding a porous scaffold.[71] Salt particles of a defined size can be utilised to achieve a highly porous structure with interconnected pores of a controlled pore size.[7] However, the interconnectivity between the pores is low and difficult to control and the pore walls often have an uncontrollable morphology.[71] Furthermore, the solvent required is often organic and can leave toxic residues within the polymeric scaffold.

The chemical and thermal environment that the polymer and biological ingredients are exposed to during processing can drastically decrease the activity of such molecules. As such, supercritical CO_2 is currently being employed as a non-toxic low-temperature solvent–porogen.[69,72,73] Polymer discs or pellets are exposed to high-pressure gas to saturate the polymer. The gas pressure is subsequently reduced, causing nucleation and formation of pores in the polymer matrix from the CO_2 gas. However, the matrices often have a closed-cell morphology and an inhomogeneous distribution of cell sizes. As such, a combination of particulate leaching and supercritical foaming has recently been used to produce an interconnected open-pore structure.[73]

Melt moulding also does not utilise organic solvents or high temperatures and is therefore suitable for the incorporation of bioactive molecules for drug delivery applications.[7] Melt moulding involves loading a Teflon mould with a mixture of PLGA powder and gelatin microspheres of a certain diameter range. The Teflon mould is heated above the T_g of PLGA and pressure is applied to bond it together. The construct is subsequently cooled and the gelatin is leached out by immersion in water. Varying the amount of gelatin added can control the porosity of the construct, and the geometry of the scaffold can be altered by changing the mould dimensions.[6] The pore size of the TEC also correlates to the size of the gelatin microspheres incorporated into the composite. However, the distribution of pores is not easily controlled.

Rapid prototyping, however, is a mechanical processing technique that allows highly complex but reproducible structures to be constructed one layer at a time via computer-aided design (CAD) models and computer-controlled tooling processes (computer-aided manufacture). These include stereolithography, selective laser sintering, ballistic particle manufacture and three-dimensional printing.[7] These processes enable the production of intricate three-dimensional shapes, which can be made by layering with a resolution down to 300 μm. The automated aspect of the fabrication method also makes them desirable, as it is possible to produce three-dimensional shapes that emulate tissue in a repeatable manner.[6]

Fused-deposition modelling (FDM) uses rollers to feed a preformed fibre through a heated nozzle on to a computer-controlled table.[18] Previously, FDM has utilised PCL but the processing route requires preformed fibres with specific dimensions and material properties. FDM therefore has quite a narrow processing window, which could restrict its future use. As such, there is not a single type of processing route that is ideal for scaffold production. The chosen fabrication method depends on TEC requirements in terms of both the cellular behaviour and the chosen polymeric material.

1.5 Supercritical fluid processing

A novel technique, which has been developed as an alternative to conventional manufacturing routes, is supercritical fluid (SCF) processing. An SCF

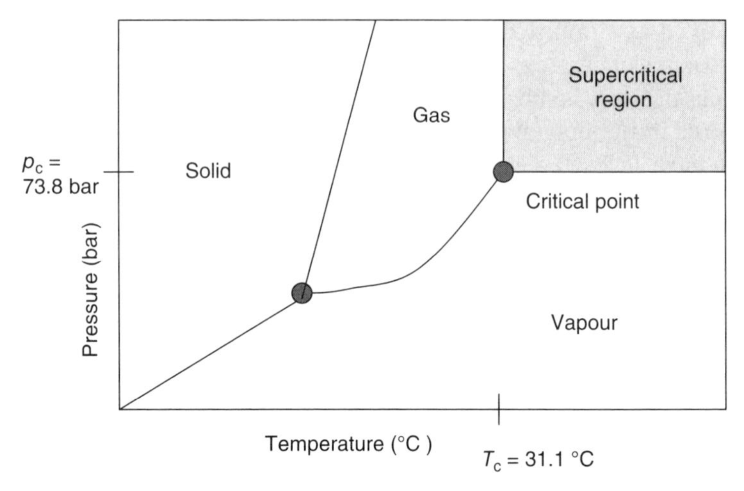

1.2 Phase diagram of CO_2.

is described as any substance, the temperature and pressure of which are higher than their critical values, and which has a density close to or higher than its critical density.[74,75] As can be seen in Fig. 1.2, SCFs combine liquid and gas properties to create a unique solvent. SCFs have liquid-like densities, which allows for solvent power of orders of magnitude higher than gases, while gas-like viscosities lead to higher rate of diffusion.[76,77] In addition, SCFs are highly compressible and the density and solvent properties can be *tuned* over a wide range by varying the pressure.[72]

The use of SCFs is particularly important when the effective viscosity of the bulk polymer is high. This is because it has been shown that high viscosity is a major obstacle to conventional processing of high-molecular-weight polymers.[78] Usually this can be rectified by raising the processing temperature; however, this can be costly as it requires high energy consumption and may lead to thermal degradation. SCFs are therefore employed to plasticize the polymer effectively. The SCF acts as a solvent, which reduces the chain–chain interactions and increases the interchain distance, thereby acting as a molecular lubricant.[79]

Because of their unique characteristics, a potential application for SCF solvents is as a medium from which to nucleate solid materials and this was presented by Hannay and Hogarth[80] as early as 1879. They proposed that a solid with no measurable gaseous pressure can be dissolved in a gas but, when the solid is precipitated by suddenly reducing the pressure, it is crystalline. In addition, they stated that the solid can be brought down as a *snow* or as a *frost*, which is thought to refer to the different morphologies and size distribution that ensue because of changes in the rate of pressure release.

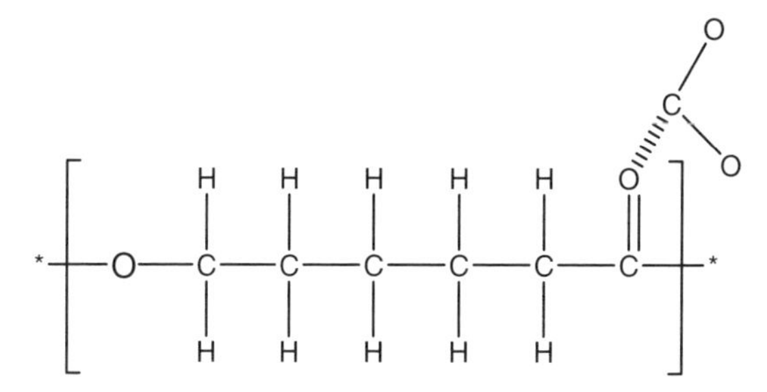

1.3 Lewis acid–base type of interaction between CO_2 and the polymer functional group.

This concept has been recently developed to produce microcellular polymers from SCFs.[72,81] Supercritical carbon dioxide ($scCO_2$) is commonly used as a foaming agent for non-reactive processing of polymeric foams, which can subsequently be used as tissue scaffolds in medical applications. Goel and Beckman[76] have developed an approach whereby a polymer is saturated with $scCO_2$ at moderately elevated temperatures followed by rapid depressurisation at constant temperature.[76] As the gas diffuses into the polymer matrix, a polymer–gas solution is formed. The pressures and temperatures needed to dissolve a polymer in $scCO_2$ depend on the intermolecular forces between solvent–solvent, solvent–polymer segment, and polymer segment–segment pairs in solution, and on the free volume difference between the polymer and CO_2.[72]

Carbon dioxide has a low dielectric constant (1.01–1.67) and its polarisability (27.6×10^{-25} cm^3) is close to that of gases such as methane and is therefore classified as a weak solvent.[72] Owing to the structural symmetry, CO_2 does not have a dipole moment, but it does have a substantial quadrupole moment that operates over a much shorter distance scale than dipolar interactions.[77] CO_2 is a dense solvent at modest temperatures and pressures and under these conditions the quadrupolar interactions are magnified. However, the dipolar interactions still outweigh the quadrupolar interactions, which means that CO_2 is a weak solvent for non-polar polymers. Despite this, Kazarian[79] has shown that CO_2 can participate in Lewis acid–base type of interactions with polymers containing electron-donating groups such as carbonyls as seen in Fig. 1.3.

Interactions between CO_2 and polymer functional groups such as carbonyl groups reduce chain–chain interactions and increase the mobility of polymer segments.[79] This chain motion has been observed when poly(methyl methacrylate) (PMMA) is heated to 40 °C and subjected to CO_2 at a pressure of 100 bar.[75] In the absence of CO_2, mobility of the ester group is only observed when PMMA is heated above its T_g (105 °C). This demonstrates how $scCO_2$ mimics the effect of heating the polymer and enables glassy polymers to be processed at much lower temperatures.

The next processing stage is when the polymer–gas solution is subject to a thermodynamic instability to nucleate microcells. This is based on the classic theory of nucleation as described by Zeldovich in 1943.[76,81,82] Nucleation is achieved by lowering the solubility of the solution by controlling the temperature and/or pressure. The system will then seek a state of lower free energy, which results in the clustering of gas molecules in the form of cell nuclei. The formation of cell nuclei provides a relatively small mean free distance for the gas molecules in solution to diffuse through before reaching a cell nucleus. As the gas diffuses into the cells, the free energy of the system is lowered. The cell nucleation process is very important as it governs the cell morphology of the material and, to a large extent, the properties of the tissue scaffold.

One way of inducing pore formation and growth is by supersaturation, which is caused by a sudden pressure drop from the equilibrium solution state. Quick reduction in the pressure at a constant temperature both generates the pores and drives the system towards vitrification, freezing in the microstructure. Consequently, as the pressure is suddenly reduced from the equilibrium state, thermodynamic fluctuations give rise to clusters of gas molecules and these clusters grow or decay depending upon whether their size is greater or less than the critical size.[82] The critical cluster is one for which the free energy of the cluster formation is a maximum. This phenomenon of the appearance of supercritical clusters is known as nucleation.

Nucleation is a rate process and the nuclei grow by diffusion of the gas from the polymer matrix. The process continues until the pressure is reduced to a point where the polymer solidifies, trapping the microcellular structure. The more rapidly the pressure drops, the greater is the number of cells that would be nucleated because a greater thermodynamic instability would be induced. It is therefore possible to maintain specific melt temperature profiles, melt pressure profiles and vent times to produce a foam with the desired microstructure.

Once the cells have nucleated, they continue to grow as available gas diffuses into the cells. The cells grow and reduce the total polymer density as the gas molecules diffuse into the nucleated cells from the polymer matrix. As the CO_2 diffuses from the polymer–gas mixture, the polymer begins to crystallise because of the reduced diluent concentration in the matrix. Thus, growth of the nuclei continues until sufficient gas has left the sample to crystallise the polymer, then the pore growth due to gas expansion will be curtailed. It has been observed that the foam structure only appears at the end of the reaction when the pressure has dropped to below 65 bar.[83] The mechanism for the formation of pores in polymer foams is therefore solely due to the pressure quenching.

SCF foaming of polymers can be performed on both amorphous and semicrystalline polymers. The mechanism for production of glassy polymeric foams using $scCO_2$ is fairly well understood. It is assumed that polymer segments remain relatively immobile below their glass transition temperature T_g, under normal conditions.[84–86] However, when $scCO_2$ is introduced, the T_g value of the amorphous polymer is reduced and this is usually called plasticisation.[79] Plasticisation occurs when CO_2 molecules penetrate the polymer matrix and interact with the basic sites on the polymer molecule. These sites are typically functional groups such as carbonyl groups and result in reduced chain–chain interactions and an increase in mobility of polymer segments. This enables processing to be carried out at lower temperatures but, when CO_2 diffuses out of the polymer–gas mixture, the T_g value of the polymer rises again because of reduced solvent concentration in the system.[87] At this point the polymer vitrifies and the microstructure is frozen into the polymer.

Processing of semicrystalline polymers using $scCO_2$ is less well documented. It is assumed that the melting point of semicrystalline polymers is depressed by the addition of high-pressure gases such as $scCO_2$.[88] This is a similar concept to the plasticisation of glassy polymers and $scCO_2$ is thought to penetrate preferentially the amorphous phase of semicrystalline polymers because of the increased gas dissolution.[21,89] This plasticisation of the amorphous region increases the mobility of the polymer chains and enables them to rearrange into a more ordered configuration. This induces crystallisation and concomitant changes in morphology. It is therefore believed that SCF technology provides the ability to control polymeric foam characteristics such as pore size and degree of crystallinity to produce a tissue scaffold with the appropriate properties for tissue regeneration.

1.6 Future trends

Owing to the stringent requirements of tissue engineering, a number of key characteristics need to be met by the polymer. The chosen polymer must provide a biocompatible and biodegradable matrix with interconnected pores to ensure that the body tolerates the conduit and also promotes nutrient and cellular diffusion. Furthermore, the scaffold initially needs to provide mechanical stability and to act as a template to guide three-dimensional tissue growth. As such, the scaffold must possess a desirable surface chemistry to enhance cell attachment and growth, as well as a suitable architecture to recruit reparative cells in an organised manner. Consequently, there are a number of challenges that need to be addressed as tissue engineering advances.

Integration of biomaterials within the body has been a long-standing problem in medicine. If there is a lack of integration, the function and longevity of the implant will suffer. In order to overcome the problems associated with rejection of polymeric implants, prevascularisation has been investigated. During recent development of a bioartificial pancreas, prevascularisation was believed to improve the supply of nutrients and oxygen to islets.[90] There was also no observation of a foreign body response. Further work is required to confirm the efficacy of this approach but the initial findings are promising.

Scaffolds provide the temporary structural framework for tissue-forming cells and, consequently, need to provide a suitable architecture to the cells to promote three-dimensional growth. Recent advances in processing techniques such as electrospinning and tissue printing offer promise for cell-based regeneration therapies that are repeatable and robust.[91] In addition, advances in computerised design packages will offer greater control and repeatability over processing, which will be beneficial to tissue engineering. Nanotechnology and microfabrication also show much promise for well-controlled processing on the microlevel and nanolevel.[92]

Another important characteristic of polymer scaffolds is surface chemistry. The scaffold must present a surface to the cell that will promote tissue regeneration. Intelligent biomaterials that encourage cohesive integration of cells with the implant have been proposed. Work is being carried out on chemical modification of polymer surfaces such as grafting PEO segments on to existing polymer surfaces, which has enhanced protein adsorption.[92] The inclusion of ionisable side groups have also been found to respond to changes in pH and these polymers are termed environmentally responsive biomaterials. This is an exciting area of research that should enhance cell adhesion and improve the success of tissue regeneration. Furthermore, the ability to attract endogenous stem cells by using trophic and growth factors tagged to the scaffold or repair site is another possibility. By manipulating the natural regenerative capacities of the host by addition of growth or guidance factors, reconstruction can be enhanced.[93] Work is evolving rapidly on this concept and will greatly improve the success of TECs.

Repair to damaged neural cells is a specific medical area that presents a challenge to the field of issue engineering. Neural cells are cells with a complex architecture, which rely on their intrinsic genetic programme, the extracellular environment and integration with synaptic connections to function correctly.[93] A strategy that has been devised to deliver neural cells to a local site of action is to encapsulate cells in a polymeric vehicle to protect their genetic integrity. However, this requires effective immunoisolation of the tissue that is to be transplanted, in addition to an appropriate polymer that will allow protection but also delivery and growth of the cells. This can prove problematic and encapsulation does not always enable integration with the host synaptic connections. A further limitation of neural cell regeneration is geometric constraints that may restrict intracerebral implants for more localised delivery of a neuroactive factor. As such, additional research is required to optimise neuroactive component polymeric delivery systems.[93]

Enhanced knowledge of stem cells and widespread suffering from arthritis have provided the driving force for investigation into stem-cell-based composite tissue constructs.[92] Mesenchymal stems cells have the ability to differentiate into multiple tissue-forming cell linkages such as osteoblasts and chondrocytes and have instigated recent work on stem-cell-based *in vivo* reconstruction of multiple tissue constructs such as fibro-osseous grafts. This has begun to offer clues to the replacement of complex anatomical linkages such as synovial joint condoyle. However, when developing a composite osteochondral construct for bone and cartilage, there are contrasting needs that present problems when choosing the scaffold material. The opposing requirements for a multicomponent polymeric system, which is intended to be composed of bone and cartilage, is an area that is important to resolve as tissue engineering advances into joint replacement.

1.7 References

1 Heath C A and Magari S R, 'Mini review: mechanical factors affecting cartilage regeneration *in vitro*', *Biotechnol Bioeng*, 1996 **50** 430–437.
2 Langer R, 'Biomaterials and biomedical engineering', *Chem Eng Sci*, 1995 **50** 4109–4121.
3 Bonassar L J and Vacanti C A, 'Tissue engineering: the first decade and beyond', *J Cell Biochem Suppl*, 1998 **30–31** 297–303.
4 Marler J J, Upton J, Langer R and Vacanti J P, 'Transplantation of cells in matrices for tissue regeneration', *Adv Drug Deliv Rev*, 1998 **33** 165–182.
5 Brodkin K R, Garcia A J and Levenston M E, 'Chondrocyte phenotypes on different extra cellular matrix monolayers', *Biomaterials*, 2004 **25** 5929–5938.
6 Lanza R P, Langer R and Vacanti J, *Principles of Tissue Engineering*, 2nd edition, San Diego, California, Academic Press, 2000.
7 Patrick Jr C W P, Mikos A G and McIntire L V (Eds), *Frontiers in Tissue Engineering*, Oxford, Pergamon, 1998.
8 Bhardwaj T, Pilliar R M, Grynpas M D and Kandel R A, 'Effect of material geometry on cartilagenous tissue formation *in vitro*', *J Biomed Mater Res*, 2001 **57** 190–199.
9 Woodfield T B F, Malda J, de Wijn J, Peters F, Riesle J and van Blitterswijk C A, 'Design of porous scaffolds for cartilage tissue engineering using a three dimensional fiber-deposition technique', *Biomaterials*, 2004 **25** 4149–4161.
10 Cancedda R, Dozin B, Giannoni P and Quarto R, 'Tissue engineering and cell therapy of cartilage and bone', *Matrix Biol*, 2003 **22** 81–91.
11 Jakob M, Demarteau O, Schafer D, Hinterman B, Heberer D M and Martinw I, 'Specific growth factors during the expansion and redifferentiation of adult human articular chondrocytes enhance chondrogenesis and cartilaginous tissue formation *in vitro*', *J Cell Biochem*, 2001 **81** 368–377.

12 Martin I, Vunjak-Novakovic G, Yang J, Langer R and Freed L E, 'Mammalian chondrocytes expanded in the presence of fibroblast growth factor 2 maintain the ability to differentiate and regenerate three dimensional cartilaginous tissue', *Exp Cell Res*, 1999 **253** 681–688.
13 Li W, Danielson K G, Alexander P G and Tuan R S, 'Biological response of chondrocytes cultured in three dimensional nanofibrous poly(caprolactone) scaffolds', *J Biomed Mater Res, Part A*, 2003 **67A** 1105–1114.
14 Yang X B, Roach H I, Clarke N M P, Howdle S M, Quirk K M, Shakesheff K M and Oreffo R O C, 'Human osteoprogenitor growth and differentiation on synthetic biodegradable structures after surface modification', *Bone*, 2001 **29** 523–531.
15 Rohner D, Hutmacher D W, Cheng T K, Oberholzer M and Hammer B, '*In vivo* efficacy of bone marrow coated polycaprolactone scaffolds for the reconstruction of orbital defects in the pig', *J Biomed Mater Res, Part B: Appl Biomater*, 2003 **66B** 574–580.
16 Demetriou A A, Reisner A, Sanchez J, Levenson S M, Moscioni A D and Chowdhury J R, 'Transplantation of microcarrier-attached hepatocytes into 90% partially hepatectomized rats', *Hepatology*, 1988 **8** 1006–1009.
17 Yannas I V, Burke J F, Orgill D P and Skrabut E M, 'Wound tissue can utilize a polymeric template to synthesise a functional extension of skin', *Science*, 1982 **215** 174–176.
18 Hutmacher D W, Schantz T, Zein I, Ng K W, Teoh S H and Tan K C, 'Mechanical properties and cell cultural response of polycaprolactone scaffolds designed and fabricated via fused deposition modeling', *J Biomed Mater Res*, 2001 **55** 203–216.
19 Babensee J E, Anderson J M, McIntire L V and Mikos A G, 'Host response to tissue engineered devices', *Adv Drug Deliv Rev*, 1998 **33** 111–139.
20 Shanmugasundaram N, Ravichandran P, Neelakanta Reddy P, Ramamurty N, Pal S and Panduranga Rao K, 'Collagen–chitosan polymeric scaffolds in the *in vitro* culture off human epidermoid carcinoma cells', *Biomaterials*, 2001 **22** 1943–1951.
21 Sheridan M H, Shea L D, Peters M C and Mooney D J, 'Bioabsorbable polymer scaffolds for tissue engineering capable of sustained growth factor delivery', *J Control Release*, 2000 **64** 91–102.
22 Gugala Z and Gogolewski S, '*In vitro* growth and activity of primary chondrocytes on a resorbable polylactide three dimensional scaffold', *J Biomed Mater Res*, 2000 **49** 183–191.
23 Miller A and Stegmann R (Eds), *Healon (Sodium Hyaluronate): A Guide to its Use in Ophthalmic Surgery*, New York, Wiley, 1983.
24 Sung K C and Topp E M, 'Swelling properties of hyaluronic acid ester membranes', *J Membr Sci*, 1984 **92** 157–167.
25 Taravel M N and Domard A, 'Relation between the physicochemical characteristics of collagen and its interactions with chitosan: I', *Biomaterials*, 1993 **14** 930–938.
26 Partridge K, Yang X, Clarke N M P, Okubo Y, Bessho K, Sebald W, Howdle S M, Shakesheff K M and Oreffo R O, 'Adenoviral BMP-2 gene transfer in mesenchymal stem cells: *in vitro* and *in vivo* bone formation on biodegradable polymer scaffolds', *Biochem Biophys Res Commun*, 2002 **292** 144–152.

27 van der Elst M, Klein C P A T, de Blieck-Hogervorst J M, Patka P and Haarman H J Th M, 'Bone tissue response to biodegradable polymers used for intra-medullary fracture fixation: a long term *in vivo* study in sheep femora', *Biomaterials*, 1999 **20** 121–128.
28 Jeong S I, Kim B, Kang S W, Kwon J H, Lee Y M, Kim S H and Kim Y H, '*In vivo* biocompatibility and degradation behaviour of elastic poly(L-lactide-co-ε-caprolactone) scaffolds', *Biomaterials*, 2004 **25** 5939–5946.
29 Li S, 'Hydrolytic degradation characteristics of aliphatic polyesters derived from lactic and glycolic acids', *J Biomed Mater Res*, 1999 **48** 342–353.
30 Reed A M and Gilding D K, 'Biodegradable polymers for use in surgery – poly(glycolic)/poly(lactic acid) homo and copolymers: 2. *In vitro* degradation', *Polymer*, 1981 **22** 494–498.
31 Mochizuki M and Hirami M, 'Structural effects on the biodegradation of aliphatic polyesters', *Polym Adv Technol*, 1997 **8** 203–209.
32 Leenslag J W, Pennings A J, Bos R R M, Rozema F R and Boering G, 'Resorbable materials of poly(L-lactide). VI. Plates and screws for internal fracture fixation', *Biomaterials*, 1987 **8** 70–73.
33 Freed L E, Marquis J C, Nohria A, Emmanual J, Mikos A G and Langer R, 'Neocartilage formation *in vitro* and *in vivo* using cells cultured on synthetic biodegradable polymers', *J Biomed Mater Res*, 1993 **27** 11–23.
34 Karjalainen T, Hiljanen-Vainio M, Malin M and Seppala J, 'Biodegradable lactone copolymers. III. Mechanical properties of ε-caprolactone and lactide copolymers after hydrolysis *in vitro*', *J Appl Polym Sci*, 1996 **59** 1299–1304.
35 Pitt G G, Gratzl M M, Kimmel G L, Surles J and Sohindler A, 'Aliphatic polyesters II. The degradation of poly(DL-lactide), poly(ε-caprolactone), and their copolymers *in vivo*', *Biomaterials*, 1981 **2** 215–220.
36 Chasin M and Langer R, *Biodegradable Polymers as Drug Delivery Vehicles*, New York, Marcel Dekker, 1990.
37 Corden T J, Jones I A, Rudd C D, Christian P and Downes S, 'Initial development into a novel technique for manufacturing a long fibre thermoplastic bio-absorbable composite: *in-situ* polymerisation of poly-ε-caprolactone', *Composites: Part A*, 1999 **30** 737–745.
38 Dell'Erba R, Groeninckx G, Maglio G, Malinconico M and Migliozzi A, 'Immiscible polymer blends of semicrystalline biocompatible components: thermal properties and phase morphology analysis of PLLA/PCL blends', *Polymer*, 2001 **42** 7821–7830.
39 Gan Z, Liang Q, Zhang J and Jing X, 'Enzymatic degradation of poly(ε-caprolactone) film in phosphate buffer solution containing lipases', *Polym Degrad Stab*, 1997 **56** 209–213.
40 Kweon H, Yoo M K, Park I K, Kimm T H, Lee H C, Lee H, Oh J, Akaike T and Cho C, 'A novel degradable polycaprolactone networks for tissue engineering', *Biomaterials*, 2003 **24** 801–808.
41 Peter S J, Miller M J, Yasko A W, Yaszemski M J and Mikos A G, 'Polymer concepts in tissue engineering', *J Biomed Mater Res* (*Appl Biomater*), 1998 **43** 422–427.
42 Trinkhaus J P, *Cells into Organs: the Forces that Shape the Embryo*, Englewood Cliffs, New Jersey, Prentice-Hall, 1984.

43 Ikada Y, 'Surface modification of polymers for medical applications', *Biomaterials*, 1994 **15** 725–736.
44 Tamada Y and Ikada Y, 'Fibroblast growth on polymer surfaces and biosynthesis of collagen', *J Biomed Mater Res*, 1994 **28** 783–789.
45 van Wacham P B, Hogt A H, Beugeling T, Feijen J, Bantjes A, Detmers J P and van Aken W G, 'Adhesion of cultured human endothelial cells onto methacrylate polymers with varying surface wettability and charge', *Biomaterials*, 1987 **8** 323–328.
46 Schmidt J A and von Recum A F, 'Texturing of polymer surfaces at the cellular level', *Biomaterials*, 1992 **12** 385–389.
47 Amstein C and Hartman P, 'Adaptation of plastic surfaces for tissue culture by glow discharge', *J Clin Microbiol*, 1975 **2** 46–55.
48 Curtis A S G, Forrester J V, McInnes C and Lawrie F, 'Adhesion of cells to polystyrene surfaces', *J Cell Biol*, 1983 **97** 1500–1506.
49 Chinn J A, Horbett T A, Ratner B D, Schway M B, Hoque Y and Hauschka SD, 'Enhancement of serum fibronectin adsorption and the clonal plating efficiencies of Swiss mouse 3T3 fibroblasts and MM14 mouse myoblast cells on polymer substrates modified by radiofrequency plasma depostion', *J Colloid Interface Sci*, 1989 **127** 67–87.
50 Hubbell J A, 'Biomaterials in tissue engineering', *Biotechnology*, 1995 **13** 565–576.
51 Kirkpatrick C J and Dekker A, 'Quantitative evaluation of cell interactions with biomaterials *in vitro*', *Adv Biomater*, 1992 **10** 31–41.
52 Conley-Wake M, Gupta P K and Mikos A G, 'Fabrication of pliable biodegradable polymer foams to engineer soft tissues', *Cell Transplant*, 1996 **5** 465–473.
53 Coombes A G A, Rizzi S C, Williamson M, Barralet J E, Downes S and Wallace W A, 'Precipitation casting of polycaprolactone for applications in tissue engineering and drug delivery', *Biomaterials*, 2004 **25** 315–325.
54 Lee S J, Lee Y M, Han C W, Lee H B and Khang G, 'Response of human chondrocytes on polymer surfaces with different micropore sizes for tissue engineered cartilage', *J Appl Polym Sci*, 2004 **92** 2784–2790.
55 Curtis A and Riehle M, 'Tissue engineering: the biophysical background', *Phys Med Biol*, 2001 **46** R47–R65.
56 Kisiday J D, Jin M, DiMicco M A, Kurz B and Grodzinsky A J, 'Effects of dynamic compressive loading on chondrocyte biosynthesis in self-assembling peptide scaffolds', *J Biomech*, 2004 **37** 595–604.
57 Gomes M E, Ribeiro A S, Malafaya P B, Reis R L and Cunha A M, 'A new approach based on injection moulding to produce biodegradable starch-based polymeric scaffolds: morphology, mechanical and degradation behaviour', *Biomaterials*, 2001 **22** 883–889.
58 Vert M and Li S M, 'Bioresorbability and biocompatibility of aliphatic polyesters', *J Mater Sci: Mater Med*, 1992 **3** 432–446.
59 Cho K, Lee J and Kwon K, 'Hydrolytic degradation behaviour of poly(butylene succinate)s with different crystalline morphologies', *J Appl Polym Sci*, 2001 **79** 1025–1033.
60 Anderson J M and Shive M S, 'Biodegradation and biocompatibility of PLA and PLGA microspheres', *Advd Drug Deliv Rev*, 1997 **28** 5–24.

61 Visscher G E, Robison R L, Maulding H V, Fong J W, Pearson J E and Argentieri G J, 'Biodegradation of and tissue reaction to 50:50 poly(DL-lactide) microcapsules', *J Biomed Mater Res*, 1986 **20** 667–676.
62 Burdick J A, Padera R F, Huang J V and Anseth K S, 'An investigation of the cytotoxicity and histocompatibility of in situ forming lactic acid based orthopaedic biomaterials', *J Biomed Mater Res* (*Appl Biomater*), 2002 **63** 484–491.
63 Freed L E and Vunjak-Novakovic G, 'Culture of organized cell communities', *Advd Drug Deliv Rev*, 1998 **33** 15–30.
64 Holy C E, Shoichet M S and Davies J E, 'Engineering three dimensional bone tissue *in vitro* using biodegradable scaffolds: investigating initial cell seeding density and culture period', *J Biomed Mater Res*, 2000 **51** 376–382.
65 Dunn G A and Brown A F, 'Alignment of fibroblasts on grooved surfaces described by a simple geometric transformation', *J Cell Sci*, 1986 **83** 313–340.
66 Puelacher W C, Mooney D, Langer R, Upton J, Vacanti J and Vacanti C A, 'Design of nasoseptal cartilage replacements synthesized from biodegradable polymers and chondrocytes', *Biomaterials*, 1994 **15** 774–776.
67 Freed L E, Vunjak-Novakovic G and Langer R, 'Cultivation of cell–polymer cartilage implants in bioreactors', *J Cell Biochem*, 1993 **51** 257–264.
68 Barry J J A, Gidda H S, Scotchford C A and Howdle S M, 'Porous methacrylate scaffolds: supercritical fluid fabrication and in vitro chondrocyte responses', *Biomaterials*, 2004 **25** 3559–3568.
69 Hutmacher D W, 'Scaffolds in tissue engineering bone and cartilage', *Biomaterials*, 2000 **21** 2529–2543.
70 Cima L G, Ingber D E, Vacanti J P and Langer R, 'Hepatocyte culture on biodegradable polymeric substrates', *Biotechnol Bioeng*, 1991 **38** 145–158.
71 Chen V J and Ma P X, 'Nano-fibrous poly(L-lactic acid) scaffolds with interconnected spherical macropores', *Biomaterials*, 2004 **25** 2065–2073.
72 Cooper A I, 'Polymer synthesis and processing using supercritical carbon dioxide', *J Mater Chem*, 2000 **10** 207–234.
73 Quirk R A, France R M, Shakesheff K M and Howdle S M, 'Supercritical fluid technologies and tissue engineering scaffolds', *Curr Opin Solid State Mater Sci*, 2004 313–321.
74 Darr J A and Poliakoff M, 'New directions in inorganic and metal–organic coordination chemistry in supercritical fluids', *Chem Rev*, 1999 **99** 495–541.
75 Penninger J M L, Radosz M, McHugh M A and Krukonis V J (Eds), *Process Technologies Proceedings 3 – Supercritical Fluid Technology*, Amsterdam, Elsevier, 1985.
76 Goel S K and Beckman E J, 'Generation of microcellular polymeric foams using supercritical carbon dioxide. I: effect of pressure and temperature on nucleation', *Polym Eng Sci*, 1994 **34** 1137–1147.
77 Sun Y (Eds), *Supercritical Fluid Technology in Materials Science and Engineering – Syntheses, Properties and Applications*, New York, Marcel Dekker, 2002.
78 Woods H M, Silva M M C G, Nouvel C, Shakesheff K M and Howdle S M, 'Materials processing in supercritical carbon dioxide: surfactants, polymers and biomaterials', *J Mater Chem*, 2004 **14** 1663–1678.
79 Kazarian S G, 'Polymer processing with supercritical fluids', *Polym Sci Ser C*, 2000 **42** 78–101.

80 Hannay J B and Hogarth J, 'On the solubility of solids in gases', *Proc R Soc*, 1879 **29** 324–326.
81 Park C B, Baldwin D F and Suh N P, 'Effect of pressure drop rate on cell nucleation in continuous processing of microcellular polymers', *Polym Eng Sci*, 1995 **35** 432–440.
82 Shafi M A, Joshi K and Flumerfelt R W, 'Bubble size distributions in freely expanded polymer foams', *Chem Eng Sci*, 1997 **52** 635–644.
83 Parks K L and Beckman E J, 'Generation of microcellular polyurethane foams via polymerization in carbon dioxide. II: foam formation and characterization', *Polym Eng Sci*, 1996 **36** 2417–2431.
84 DiMarzio E A and Gibbs J H, 'Molecular interpretation of glass transition temperature by plasticizers', *J Polym Sci, Part A: Gen Pap*, 1963 **1** 1417–1428.
85 Kalospiros N S and Paulaitis M E, 'Molecular thermodynamic model for solvent induced glass transitions in polymer supercritical fluid systems', *Chem Eng Sci*, 1994 **49** 659–668.
86 Chow T S, 'Molecular interpretation of the glass transition temperature of polymer–diluent systems', *Macromolecules*, 1980 **13** 362–364.
87 Goel S K and Beckman E J, 'Generation of microcellular polymeric foams using supercritical carbon dioxide. II: cell growth and skin formation', *Polym Eng Sci*, 1994 **34** 1148–1156.
88 McHugh M A and Yogan T J, 'A study of three-phase solid–liquid–gas equilibria from three carbon dioxide–solid hydrocarbon systems, two ethane–hydrocarbon solid systems, and two ethylene–hydrogen solid systems', *J Chem Eng Data*, 1984 **29** 112–115.
89 Kazarian S G and Martirosyan G G, 'Spectroscopy of polymer/drug formulations processed with supercritical fluids: *in situ* ATR-IR and Raman study of impregnation of ibuprofen into PVP', *Int J Pharm*, 2002 **232** 81–90.
90 Silva A I, Norton de Matos A, Brons G and Mateus M, 'An overview on the development of a bioartificial pancreas as a treatment of insulin-dependent diabetes mellitus', *Med Res Rev*, 2006 **26** 181–222.
91 Rahaman M N and Mao J J, 'Stem cell based composite tissue constructs for regenerative medicine', *Biotechnol Bioeng*, 2005 **91** 261–284.
92 Langer R and Peppas N A, 'Advances in biomaterials, drug delivery and bionanotechnology', *AIChE J: Bioeng, Food Nat Prod*, 2003 **49** 2990–3006.
93 Bellamkonda R and Aebischer P, 'Review: tissue engineering in the nervous system', *Biotechnol Bioeng*, 1994 **43** 543–554.

2
Introduction to polymeric drug delivery systems

K HARRISON, GlaxoSmithKline R&D Ltd, UK

2.1 Introduction: controlled drug release

Polymeric delivery systems are mainly used to achieve either temporal or spatial control of drug delivery.[1] Essentially, polymeric vehicles enable drugs to be delivered over an extended period of time and to the local site of action. They are designed to enhance drug safety and efficacy, and to improve patient compliance. The use of polymers is designed to maintain therapeutic levels of the drug, to reduce the side-effect profile, to decrease the amount of drug molecule and the dosage frequency, and to facilitate the delivery of drugs with short *in vivo* half-lives.[2]

Controlled-release drug delivery systems function by enabling the drug molecule's inherent kinetic properties to be manipulated by the property of the polymeric vehicle.[3] Controlled-release devices allow potent drugs with short half-lives to be administered with minimal fluctuations over an extended period of time and with a potentially lower incidence of toxicity.[4] Ultimately, sustained-action dosage forms improve therapeutic management through assuring a uniform plasma concentration of drug at a steady state. Ideally, the device should offer slow first-order or slow zero-order absorption of the drug from the gastrointestinal tract.

If the blood drug level profiles of sustained-release dosage forms are compared with the administration of conventional and controlled dosage forms, the profiles in Fig 2.1 are obtained. The conventional tablet or capsule provides a single and transient burst of drug. Furthermore, a pharmacological response is only observed if the amount of drug is above the minimum effective concentration.[3] Sustained-release formulations reduce the burst effect but the plasma concentrations are not maintained for as long as controlled-release systems and gradually begin to deplete. Controlled-release systems, however, reduce fluctuations in plasma drug levels by slowing down the absorption rate owing to a slower drug release rate and result in an effective pharmacological response.

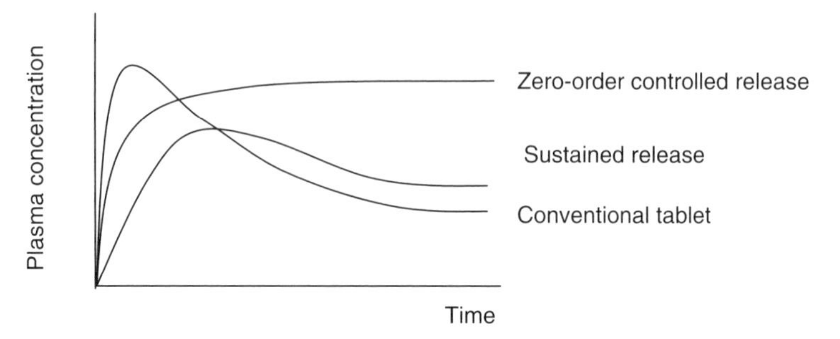

2.1 Plasma drug concentration profiles for conventional tablet, sustained-release and zero-order controlled-release formulations.

An understanding of the drug and polymer characteristics is essential to the success of the drug delivery device. By altering the properties of the polymer, the release rate of the drug can also be controlled. In addition, the environment in which the device is to function impacts on the choice of polymer, drug and device design. A multifaceted approach is therefore crucial for successful drug delivery from polymeric systems.

2.1.1 Conventional film coatings

Conventional dosage forms are typically drug dispersed through soluble excipients. The drug is rapidly liberated from its dosage form and quickly builds up to a high concentration.[5] The concentration falls exponentially until the next dose is administered. Consequently, there is an undulating concentration pattern of the drug in the plasma and tissue and the optimal therapeutic level is only present briefly. Conventional dosage forms, unlike controlled-release systems, do not control the rate of drug release.[6]

A conventional film coating is utilised to improve product appearance, to improve handling and to prevent dusting.[7] In addition, a film coating is used to mask unpleasant taste and odour and to improve product stability.[8] However, film coats are not typically applied to modify the drug-release characteristics. This can often cause conventional dosage forms to exhibit fluctuating drug levels, insufficient influence on the mechanism of the disease and inconvenient dosing regimens.[5]

Typically, cellulose derivatives are chosen to act as film coats, with the most common polymer being hydroxypropyl methylcellulose (HPMC). HPMC provides aqueously soluble films which can also be coloured by the use of pigments. It also affords easy processing because of its non-tacky nature. However, HPMC has a very high tensile strength and a very low elongation value.[8] Consequently, a large force can be applied to the film before it breaks, but the film lengthens only a small amount before the break occurs. This can present problems if the film is required to coat difficult tablet cores such as vitamins and monogrammed tablets.

In order to modify the characteristics of the polymer, plasticisers are added to improve flexibility.[8] HPMC can also be blended with hydroxypropylcellulose, which has a lower tensile strength and much higher elongation value. A blend of the two grades can eliminate the bridging observed in monogrammed tablets, improve film adherence to tablet substrates and also reduce the incidence of cracking at tablet edges.[8] A conventional coat, however, will not control the rate of drug release from the core.

2.1.2 Functional polymers

Functional polymers are designed to modify the pharmaceutical function of the dosage form and to control the release of the active ingredient.[7] The majority of controlled-release dosage forms can be categorised as matrix, reservoir or osmotic systems.[9] In matrix systems, the drug is embedded in the polymer matrix and release takes place by partitioning of the drug into the matrix and the release medium.[10] It may be characterised as a mass transport phenomenon. In contrast, reservoir systems have a drug core surrounded by a rate-controlling membrane such as enterically coated products and implants. Factors such as pH and presence of food affect the drug release rate from reservoir devices. An increase in hydrostatic pressure drives osmotic devices, forcing the drug solution or suspension out of the device through a small delivery port.[11] Drug release is independent of pH and it is possible to modulate the release characteristics by optimising the properties of the drug and polymer coat.

2.2 Mechanisms of action for controlled drug release

The most important attribute of a controlled-release device is the ability to maintain a constant rate of drug delivery. The duration must also be compatible with the physiological constraints and the route of administration.[12] As such, numerous devices have been developed, which function via various mechanisms of action to achieve the desired rate of drug release. Three common mechanisms of action, namely diffusion, osmotic effects and erosion, are outlined below.

2.2.1 Diffusion

Polymer films that use a diffusion mechanism permit the entry of aqueous fluids from the gastrointestinal (GI) tract into the tablet core. Dissolution of the drug ensues, which is followed by diffusion of the drug solution through the polymeric membrane into the body.[12] The rate of drug diffusion can be determined by the physicochemical properties of the drug and the membrane itself.[7] The properties of the polymer membrane can be altered by the choice of polymer, the molecular weight of the polymer and the inclusion of plasticisers. All these factors can alter the structure of the film and the drug can diffuse through a network of pores and channels within the membrane, thus facilitating the release process.

If the chosen polymer membrane is hydrophilic, the rate of absorption of liquid is very high and the dosage swells. Consequently, as the dosage form swells, there is an associated increase in diffusivity, which enhances the rate of drug release.[5] Conversely, if the polymer is hydrophobic and swelling is negligible, the diffusion of the drug out of the polymer matrix is much slower.

Diffusion-controlled devices tend to be divided into two main types: monolithic devices and reservoir devices.[3] Monolithic devices consist of the active pharmaceutical ingredient (API) intimately mixed in the rate-controlling polymer either through dispersion in the polymer or through dissolution of the API in the polymer. Although API release from a monolithic device does not typically proceed by zero-order kinetics, it is one of the simplest and most convenient methods of obtaining prolonged release.[3] An example of this mechanism is used with transdermal therapeutic systems (TTSs). The TTS delivers the drug systemically into the circulatory system of the patient through the skin. The rate of drug delivery is governed by the diffusion gradient between the system and the skin. The drug is uniformly distributed through the polymer matrix and begins to permeate through the skin as soon as the TTS is placed on the skin.[13] Fentanyl is delivered via a TTS to relieve pain in cancer patients.[14]

A further use of the diffusion mechanism is in reservoir devices. Reservoir devices consist of the API contained in a core that is surrounded by a rate-controlling membrane. Transport of the API held in the core, through the surrounding polymer film, occurs by dissolution at the film interface. The properties of the boundary film can be used to vary the release mechanism. In certain applications, it is desirable to use a dense membrane with a microporous hydrophobic structure.[3] The pores connect the two sides of the membrane and enable the API to diffuse in liquid carriers through the porous channels. However, if the API has low aqueous solubility, then diffusion will be slowed and may even stop. Conversely, if a membrane with known permeability is used and infinite sink conditions are obtained, then the rate of active release will be constant and nearly zero-order kinetics can be achieved. An example of a successful reservoir system is Alza Progestasert®, which contains the steroid progesterone in a core surrounded by an ethylene–vinyl acetate copolymer.[15] This successfully maintains a relatively constant release rate of progesterone for a number of years.

There is, however, a disadvantage to reservoir systems and that is the propensity for dose dumping.[12] *Dose dumping* is a phenomenon whereby a relatively large quantity of API is rapidly released, introducing potentially toxic levels of the drug into the systemic circulation.[3] Bursting effects can occur when the API saturates the membrane surrounding the core during storage. Once the device is placed in an aqueous media, the active ingredient will rapidly desorb from the membrane causing a bursting effect and a rapid dose dump. The magnitude of the burst is determined by the diffusion coefficient of the active agent in the membrane, the membrane thickness and the length of storage time.

2.2.2 Osmotic effects

Osmotic drug delivery systems suitable for oral administration typically consist of a compressed tablet core that is coated with a semipermeable membrane coating.[11] Most osmotic devices use relatively water-permeable materials such as cellulosic polymers, particularly cellulose acetate (CA).[9,16] Cellulosic membranes generally exhibit a water permeability range between 1×10^{-5} and 1×10^{-7} cm^3 cm/cm^2 h atm. The permeability of CA films can be tailored by adjusting the degree of acetylation; as the acetyl content increases, the permeability decreases.[9] Ethyl cellulose is also widely used as a membrane for oral osmotic systems. The water permeability of pure ethyl cellulose is low but is enhanced by the incorporation of water-soluble additives such as HPMC.

Upon immersion in aqueous media, the hydrostatic pressure inside the tablet will build up because of the selective ingress of water across the semipermeable membrane.[7] To ensure that the coating is able to resist the pressure within the device, the thickness of the membrane is usually between 200 and 300 μm.[9] The membrane is non-extensible and the increase in volume caused by the imbibition of water raises the hydrostatic pressure.[16] Drug dissolution ensues in isolation from the GI environment. The pressure is relieved by a flow of saturated solution out of the device through a small orifice.[12]

Once the internal osmotic pressure has risen sufficiently and the drug solution or suspension is being expelled at a predetermined rate through a delivery orifice, the process continues until the entire solid drug has been removed and a solution-filled shell remains. Initially, 60–80% of drug is released at a zero-order rate.[9] The residual dissolved drug continues to be delivered but at a depleted rate until the osmotic pressures inside and outside the tablet are equal.[16]

The impetus to draw water into the device is the difference between the osmotic pressures of the outside environment and the drug solution. The osmotic pressure of the drug solution needs to be relatively high to overcome the osmotic pressure of the body.[16] Consequently, the system often contains additional osmotically active materials such as sugars or salts within the core as the API may not always be soluble in water to the extent of being able to exert adequate osmotic pressure to drive the device. The drug composition may also contain solubilisers such as buffering agents which solubilise the drug by maintaining a pH microenvironment that aids in drug dissolution and absorption.[11]

Osmotic drug delivery systems release drug at a rate that is independent of the pH and hydrodynamics of the external dissolution medium. The system is also applicable to drugs with a broad range of aqueous solubilities.[11] Consequently, the drug can either be released as a solution or as a suspension. However, if the drug is released as a suspension, it must dissolve *in vivo* before it becomes systemically available.

2.2.3 Polymer erosion

Biodegradable polymers are used to reduce the need for additional surgical intervention required to remove non-biodegradable matrices. Biodegradation designates the process of polymer chain cleavage, which leads to a loss in molecular weight.[17] Degradation induces the subsequent erosion of the material which is defined by a mass loss. For polymers, biodegradation occurs by two main mechanisms: surface or bulk erosion. Surface or heterogeneous erosion occurs when the rate of erosion exceeds the rate of water permeation into the bulk of the polymer.[1] Bulk or homogeneous erosion occurs when water molecules permeate into the bulk polymer at a faster rate than erosion.

Drug release from biodegradable polymers can occur via three main mechanisms. The first mechanism entails the active agent covalently attached to the polymer backbone, often called a pendant chain system.[12] As the backbone cleaves, there is a concomitant release of API at a controlled rate.[3] The second mechanism occurs when API is contained within a core surrounded by the biodegradable shell. The rate of biodegradation of the polymer shell governs the rate of drug release and, as the shell will eventually degrade entirely, surgical removal of the drug-depleted device is unnecessary. In the final mechanism, the drug is homogeneously dispersed in the polymer, and drug release is controlled by diffusion, by a combination of diffusion and erosion or by erosion alone.[3]

Numerous biodegradable polymers have been synthesised to deliver drugs, cells and enzymes. The properties of these polymers can be modified by incorporating a variety of labile groups such as esters, anhydride and urethane in their backbone.[1] Polyester-based polymers are one of the most widely used systems, particularly poly(lactic acid) (PLA), poly(glycolic acid) (PGA) and their copolymers poly(lactic-acid-co-glycolic acid) (PLGA).[18] The biodegradation kinetics can be altered by tuning the proportion of PLA and PGA in the copolymer and altering the molecular weight of the polymer.[1,19] For PLGA microspheres, low molecular weight and high glycolic acid content resulted in a faster release. However, PLGA suffers from an increase in local acidity during degradation, which can cause irritation and can also be detrimental to the stability of protein drugs.[20]

Polyesters degrade by water penetration into the device, which results in the breakage of ester bonds via random hydrolytic ester cleavage.[17] Although this can be tailored to a certain extent by the degree of crystallinity, copolymer ratio and polydispersity, polyesters tend to degrade over a long period of time. This can be disadvantageous when the drug needs to be released for only a few days or weeks and, consequently, polyorthoesters (POEs) have become more prominent. POE contain an orthoester linkage which is acid labile and the rate of hydrolysis is accelerated in acidic environments.[17] Conversely, the rate of hydrolysis can also be decreased with an increase in pH. As such, the rate of drug release for POEs can vary from a few days to several months and so has a wide range of applications.

Oral dosage forms that rely on the degradation of the polymer matrix also depend on the transit time of the dosage form through the GI tract.[3] Following food intake, the stomach is in the fed state in which liquids and digested material are readily emptied. As such, the gastric residence time of slowly eroding dosage form may vary greatly depending on the state of the stomach, either fed or fasted, and the dosage form will be able to degrade to a greater or lesser extent. In addition, the pH of the stomach varies greatly depending on the fed or fasted state and this can also affect the rate of degradation of the polymer matrix.

2.3 Examples of controlled-release delivery systems

2.3.1 Modified release

A variety of dosage forms utilise the concept of modified release; the release kinetics of the drug are governed by the properties of the polymeric matrix the API is contained within.[15] Typically, the active ingredient is dispersed in particulate form throughout the polymer matrix, which is either hydrophilic or lipophilic in nature. This principle is used for the contraceptive vaginal ring. A silicone elastomer ring designed to fit around the cervix contains a dispersion of the contraceptive steroid medroxyprogesterone acetate. The steroid is released slowly via diffusion achieving a steady level of plasma progestin and a prolonged period of contraception.[12,15]

Membrane diffusion-controlled devices are also commonly used in pharmaceuticals. The membrane acts as an interphase that separates two phases and restricts the transport of compounds between the phases. The simplest design involves a synthetic polymer membrane such as a polyethylene film and the permeant passes through by simple diffusion. More complex systems involve the use of microporous systems in which the permeant material must diffuse through liquid-filled pores within the membrane. If a membrane is biodegradable, the release of drug will depend on the rate of diffusion of the drug through the membrane and the rate of dissolution of the membrane.[15]

Hydrogels are a further example of modified release devices. Hydrogels are a cross-linked network of hydrophilic polymers, which have the ability to absorb large amounts of water and swell, whilst maintaining their three-dimensional structure.[21] A typical hydrogel membrane usually consists of either a solid core of drug or a cross-linked hydrogel matrix containing dissolved or dispersed drug with a surrounding rate-controlling hydrogel membrane.[12] Hydrogels are glassy in their dehydrated state; however, on coming into contact with an aqueous environment, water penetrates into the free spaces on the surface between the macromolecular chains.[21]

When sufficient water has entered the matrix, the glass transition temperature T_g of the polymer drops to the environmental temperature. The presence of water causes the development of stresses that are accommodated by an increase in the radius of gyration and end-to-end distance of polymer molecules. This is seen macroscopically as swelling.[21] As the swelling occurs, there is a concomitant increase in dissolution of the core and drug is released through the swollen flexible regions.[12]

In addition to the mechanism of controlled release, which is attributed to the properties of the matrix and the drug, systems have also been designed that can be manipulated by remote control such as ultrasound, ion exchange control and a magnetic field.[22] This is desirable as drug release is mediated by a factor that does not change with time and is independent of the pharmacological effect of the device.[15] Consequently, zero-order release kinetics should be attainable. However, these are less prevalent and are typically in the development stage.

2.3.2 Enteric coated products

Enteric coated products are designed to remain intact in the stomach and then to release the API in the upper intestine; as such, they are termed delayed-release dosage forms.[23,24] The rationale for using enteric coatings is to prevent damage from being caused to the API by gastric enzymes or by the acidity of the gastric fluid, to reduce the incidence of nausea caused by irritation of the gastric mucosa, to deliver the drug to the local site of action in the mucosa and at the highest possible concentration and to provide a delayed-release profile.[7]

Since drugs must be in solution before they can be absorbed, compounds with very low aqueous solubility often suffer oral bioavailability problems because of limited GI transit time of the undissolved drug particles and limited solubility at the absorption site.[3] Consequently, the drug delivery system needs to be capable of retaining the drug in the stomach and gradually releasing it into the small intestine.

The polymers that are typically used to achieve this delayed-release profile are anionic polymethacrylates such as Eudragit®, cellulose-based polymers or poly(vinyl acetate phthalate) (PVAP). The release profile is facilitated by the pH-dependent solubility of the polymeric acidic functional groups.[24] For example, the aqueous acrylic dispersion Eudragit® L30-D55, is an anionic copolymer based on methacrylic acid and ethyl acrylate, with free carboxyl groups in the ratio 1 : 1 with the ester group. The carboxylic groups only begin to ionize in aqueous media at pH 5.5 and above, rendering the polymer resistant to acidic media but soluble in intestinal fluid.[12]

The rate of drug release from enteric coated products tends to be controlled by the polymer characteristics and its mechanism of drug release.[24] The drug can be released through flaws or cracks in the matrix, by transport of the drug through media filled pores in the coat, by transport through the swollen film or by transport due to the permeability of the API through a non-porous coat. The desired release rate can therefore be attained by tailoring the polymer characteristics.

2.3.3 Microspheres

Microspheres involve a drug encapsulated in a polymer matrix, which is released at a relatively slow rate over a prolonged period of time.[4] Consequently, in comparison with conventional dosage forms, microspheres afford less frequent drug administration; therefore an increase in patient compliance is often noted. In addition, the polymer matrix provides protection to the API and enables molecules that have been difficult to administer previously, such as nucleic acids, to be delivered to the site of action in high local concentrations. Also, since the drug is loaded inside the microsphere, the API is kept separate from other microspheres. Consequently, multiple drugs can be administered in a single injection, which owing to compatibility issues may not have otherwise been possible.[25]

Microspheres can be ingested or injected and offer a number of advantages over conventional oral drug administration.[25] The drug is encapsulated in either a slowly degrading matrix or a diffusion-controlled matrix, which enables the drug to travel through the pores formed during sphere hardening.[6] Drug release rates can be manipulated through the choice of polymer matrix and its associated chemical and physical properties. Block copolymers with a varying number of hydrophilic regions can control the rate of drug release. The greater the number of hydrophilic regions, the faster is the ingress of solvent and the more rapid is the rate of drug release.[4]

However, copolymerisation can also lead to an initial burst during which a significant fraction (typically between 5% and 50%) of the encapsulated compound is released. This is undesirable as the drug is not available for prolonged release and the large burst may result in toxicity.[26]

A further primary determinant of drug release rate is particle size. Larger spheres tend to release encapsulated compounds more slowly and for longer than smaller microspheres. In a previous study, the initial release rate of both rhodamine and piroxicam was found to decrease with increasing sphere diameter.[4] This has been attributed to the decrease in surface-area-to-volume ratio with increasing particle size. This enables the desired release profile to be achieved relatively easily by manipulation of the spray process.

The ability to tailor the drug release rate can also be achieved by mixing microspheres of different characteristics.[25] For example, Ravivarapu *et al.*[27] mixed microspheres fabricated from low-molecular-weight PLGA with microspheres consisting of a high-molecular-weight formulation.[27] The low-molecular-weight polymer resulted in porous microspheres, which released the drug rapidly. However, the high-molecular-weight microspheres were dense and produced a slower sigmoidal release profile. By combining the two formulations, the release rate could be tailored and was a combination of the two formulations. However, microencapsulation can result in lowering bioavailability of the drug and, consequently, careful control of the polymeric film needs to be carried out. If the polymer layer is too thick, the drug is unable to cross the boundary and will not become available for circulation.[10] Consequently, the drug will not be absorbed and perform the necessary function.

Microencapsulated dosage forms will often reduce fluctuations in the blood levels but, when compared with the native drug, may have lower peak plasma levels of the drug. In a study which compared conventional aspirin with microencapsulated aspirin, conventional aspirin was more immediately available and showed nearly twofold peak plasma levels compared with the sustained-release formulation.[28] However, aspirin was maintained at a higher level for the sustained-release tablet and, in terms of bioavailability, both dosage forms were equivalent. As such, the microencapsulated dosage form would require less frequent administration and the steady release profile may result in a reduced level of toxicity and adverse effects from the drug.

There are a number of successful examples of the use of microspheres. Aspirin tablets have been formulated with microencapsulated acetylsalicylic acid, provide a sustained release of the API and are tolerated much better by the GI tract than are conventional aspirin tablets.[28] The bitter taste of the API can also be successfully masked by utilising a microencapsulation process and this was achieved for Tylenol®. In addition, greater tolerability of a dosage form can be attained when microspheres are incorporated. For example, microencapsulated acetylsalicylic acid incorporated into a suppository resulted in a much lower incidence of irritation of the rectal mucosa than from a conventional suppository.[28]

2.3.4 Implants

Over recent years, novel delivery systems such as implants have impacted cancer treatment dramatically. Many cancer drugs have short *in vivo* half-lives and polymer delivery systems afford suitable protection to enable the drugs to be delivered at a controlled rate and duration.[14] Cancer drugs can also cause toxicity; therefore the ability to deliver locally rather than systemically can improve both the safety and the efficacy of cancer chemotherapy. Polyanhydride wafers such as polyanhydride 20:80 poly[(1,3,bis-*p*-carboxyphenoxypropane)-co-(sebacic anhydride)] have been used to deliver chemotherapeutic drugs such as carmustine locally to treat brain cancer.[18,29,30] The wafer is placed at the surface of the tumour resection site and the drug is slowly released for approximately 3 weeks, destroying the remaining tumour. The comonomer ratio can also be varied to produce erosion profiles that range from days to years which is very beneficial.[30]

Another use of implants is in the controlled release of contraceptive steroids.[3,12] A solid drug in micronised form is homogeneously dispersed through the polymer matrix made from a bioerodable or biodegradable polymer. The polymer is moulded into a pellet or bead-shaped implant. The controlled release of the embedded drug particles is made possible by a combination of polymer erosion via hydrolysis and diffusion through the eroded polymer matrix. The rate of drug release is determined by the hydrolysis rate of the polymer, the molecular weight and the drug loading.[3] Contraceptive steroids such as levonorgestrel are embedded in biodegradable POEs and, as the polymer is hydrolysed, the steroid is released into the circulatory system.

A limitation that is often seen with implants is an inflammatory response to the implant.[3] In an attempt to minimise this, the implant should have the minimum surface area by design and a very smooth surface finish. In addition, the implant should have a similar structure to the tissue that it is being implanted into. A further factor that also needs to be considered with implants is the loss in mechanical properties that will ensue as the polymer degrades. As chain cleavage occurs, the tensile strength of the implant will decrease and the integrity of the implant may be compromised. Consequently, the implant may not perform optimally.

A recent advancement in the field of implants is injectable *in situ* setting semisolid drug depots.[26] The depots are typically made from biodegradable polymers, which can be injected via a syringe into the body and, once injected, form a semisolid structure. These have many advantages particularly in cancer treatment. Taxol®-loaded polymeric implants have been used to treat brain tumour resection sites in rats.[31] However, to circumvent the need for invasive procedures, a thermoplastic triblock polymer injectable system has been investigated.[32] This system released Taxol® for longer than 60 days and reduced side effects due to local delivery. There are inherent disadvantages with the proposed injection system, however. The polymer is required to be in the molten state during injection and this can be very painful for a patient during administration. In addition, the drug release is often slower than would be ideal and, consequently, this method of administration is still in development.

2.4 Commonly used polymers for drug delivery systems

A large number of polymers are used in drug delivery systems to accommodate the vast array of designs, drug interactions and release profiles that are required. The following section is therefore by no means a conclusive list of polymers but may serve as a guide to some of the more commonly used polymers and the rationale behind their use.

Synthetic polymers are typically used in drug delivery systems because of the fine control over their inherent properties that is possible. Methacrylate ester copolymers are often used as they are insoluble over the entire physiological pH range. However, they are able to swell and become permeable to water and dissolved substances; so they are often used in modified release applications that rely on diffusion.[7] The addition of hydrophilic materials such as soluble cellulose ethers can render the polymer more soluble and, consequently, the drug release profile can be manipulated.

Cellulose acetate phthalate (CAP) is one of the most widely used synthetic polymers and has its use in enteric coated products. The polymer consists of a free hydroxyl group contributed by each glucose unit of the cellulose chain; approximately half are acylated and one quarter esterified with one of the two carboxylic groups of the phthalate moiety. The second carboxylic acid group is free to form salts and serves as the basis of its enteric character.[7] The carboxylic group only ionises in aqueous environments with a pH above 5.5. This renders CAP resistant to acidic media such as those in the stomach but soluble in gastric fluids.[12]

PVAP is prepared from esterification of partially hydrolysed poly(vinyl acetate) with phthalic anhydride.[33] It is typically used as a coating ingredient for solid oral dosage forms and is available commercially as an aqueous dispersible form (Sureteric) for water-based spraying.[7] Because of the spraying application, a specification is often placed on the viscosity of the polymer as this can impact the surface finish of the coat. The characteristics can also be manipulated by phthalyl content, which is commonly between 60% and 70% and has been found to affect the pH at which tablets coated with PVAP disintegrate.[7]

Osmotic devices require a semipermeable polymer membrane, i.e. a polymer that is permeable to water but impermeable to solutes.[9] Typically cellulose acetate (CA) is used. CA films are insoluble and yet semipermeable. The extent of permeability can be altered by changing the degree of acetylation. As the acetyl content increases, there is a concomitant decrease in permeability. Furthermore, the permeability of CA can be improved by incorporation of hydrophilic flux enhancers or plasticisers.[9] The addition of a hydrophilic plasticiser (PEG-200) was found to increase release of nifedipine from an osmotic pump.[34]

Synthetic degradable polyesters are commonly used in drug delivery and the most common are derived from three monomers: lactide, glycolide and caprolactone.[18] The rate of degradation ranges from days to years and is affected by crystallinity, molecular weight and monomer hydrophobicity. This is because, by varying these physical properties, access of water to the ester bond is affected and, consequently, degradation rate is manipulated.[17] The acidic by-products of degradation of polyesters have been implicated in a number of adverse tissue reactions and, consequently, a number of other biodegradable polymers have been explored.

Polyanhydrides are often used in drug delivery systems as they are biodegradable and biocompatible.[18,25] Polyanhydrides are usually hydrides of aliphatic and aromatic dicarboxylic acids which have hydrophobic regions separated by relatively hydrophilic acid anhydride bonds. The anhydrides are hydrolysed under physiological conditions, which results in polymer degradation.[25] However, owing to the hydrophobic regions, the degradation is restricted to the surface as the water cannot penetrate the bulk of the polymer. This leads to a better controlled erosion process and, subsequently, drug release is often more sustained.[17,30]

Polyorthoesters have also been explored as controlled delivery devices.[17] An advantage of POE devices is that the orthoester linkages are acid labile and consequently the degradation rate of the device can be modulated by pH. By lowering the pH, the rate of hydrolysis is accelerated, whereas an increase in pH lowers the hydrolysis rate. The degradation time of POEs can therefore vary from a few days to several months. However, because POEs are hydrophobic, the amount of water available to react with the hydrolytically labile orthoester linkages is limited.[35] Consequently, under physiological conditions the polymer is very stable.

Natural polymers have also been used in drug delivery systems as they offer excellent biocompatibility; however, naturally derived polymers often suffer from batch-to-batch variability.[1] Hydroxypropylcellulose is a non-ionic water-soluble cellulose ether. The molecular substitution of hydroxypropylcellulose is fixed; however, the molecular weight is varied by controlling the degree of polymerisation of the cellulose backbone.[8] As the degree of polymerisation increases, the viscosity of the polymer increases. This variation enables hydroxypropylcellulose to be employed for a range of purposes including use as a binder, as a sustained-release matrix and also as a film coating.

Hydroxyethylcellulose is also a non-ionic water-soluble polymer derived from cellulose, which can be tailored to a desirable viscosity by altering the molar substitution and degree of substitution.[8] Hydroxyethylcellulose is used as a thickening agent, as a bioadhesive material and as a film coating agent. Hydroxypropyl methylcellulose (HPMC) is a partly *O*-methylated and *O*-(2-hydroxypropylated) cellulose that is available in various viscosity grades. High-viscosity grades can be used to retard the release of water-soluble drugs from the matrix, whereas low-viscosity HPMC can enhance drug release.[8,36]

HPMC is widely used in pharmaceutical formulations as a tablet binder, film coating and controlled-release matrix.[8] HPMC acts as a controlled-release matrix by creating a sharp concentration gradient at the polymer–water interface.[36] This results in water imbibation into the matrix. The water acts as a plasticiser and reduces the T_g of the HPMC. Consequently, the polymer chains are more flexible and the polymer begins to swell. The drug also begins to dissolve and diffuse through the swollen matrix. The chain length and degree of substitution can be altered to vary the time that the polymer itself takes to dissolve.[36]

Guar gum is a natural non-ionic polysaccharide obtained from the ground endosperm of the guar plant, which is grown in climates such as those in India and Pakistan.[8,37] Guar gum is a galactomannan which is able to disperse and swell in cold and hot water to form a viscous sol or gel. The hydration rate and optimum viscosity are strongly affected by the galactomannan content, the molecular weight and its particle size distribution. Guar gum is typically used as a binder and thickening and stabilising agent in topical products.[8]

Gelatin is a commonly used natural polymer, which is derived from collagen.[38] It is a biodegradable and biocompatible polymer, which has been utilised as a microsphere.[19] Gelatin can be produced via two different routes; the alkaline process (known as *liming*) targets the amide groups of asparagine and glutamine and hydrolyses them into carboxyl groups, whereas the acidic process does little to affect the amide groups. Gelatin processed via the alkaline route possesses a greater proportion of carboxyl groups, rendering it more negatively charged than the acidic processed gelatin. This is important as it determines which therapeutic agents can be incorporated successfully into gelatin and subsequently remain protected from degradation and release over an extended time period.[38]

As can be seen, a wide variety of polymers can be used as drug delivery vehicles and the release properties can be tailored by manipulating the physicochemical characteristics of the polymer.[10] The properties of the polymer need to complement the chosen API and enable interaction as well as functioning effectively in the environment that the delivery system is intended for.

2.5 Polymer characteristics and properties

As described in the previous section, a wide variety of polymers are employed as drug delivery vehicles. The controlling effect of a chosen polymer on drug release depends on the physicochemical properties of the polymer.[10] A number of polymer characteristics are important in determining the behaviour of the drug delivery system and the ensuing release of the active ingredient.

The molecular weight is an important consideration when choosing a polymer as it impacts on the properties of the polymeric drug delivery system. As the molecular weight of the polymer increases, the magnitudes of the mechanical properties also rise.[3] Polymers with high-molecular-weight chains can often be tougher than low-molecular-weight polymers owing to the increased entanglements between chains. In addition, entanglements can prevent the ingress of aqueous media into the bulk; consequently, dissolution of the drug is retarded and drug release is significantly slower.[10,39]

The degradation behaviour of polymers is typically affected by the molecular weight.[6] Polymer chains undergo scission until the molecular weight has been reduced to a critical value whereby oligomers are able to diffuse out of the bulk.[39] This leads to significant degradation, and pores are created. The pores imbibe water and promote drug release. As such, if the initial molecular weight of the polymer is high, the degradation process will be slower, as it will take longer to reach the critical reduction in molecular weight, which instigates drug release. Conversely, if the initial molecular weight is low (approximately 4000 g/mol), drug release occurs immediately, implying that the polymer is solubilised immediately.[39]

The degree of crystallinity is another property that is an important determinant in the function of the polymeric drug delivery device. Polymers that have regular structures and are able to achieve a regular packing organisation of chains are described as crystalline.[40,41] The close packing of polymer chains enhances the intermolecular interactions and the polymer is tougher and stiffer than its amorphous counterpart. Furthermore, crystalline regions are impermeable to diffusing molecules and thus an enhancement in crystallinity often results in a decrease in permeability.[12] Consequently, crystalline regions are essentially impermeable to water so that the rate of hydrolysis in crystalline regions is significantly reduced.[3] This enables the properties of the polymer to be manipulated by varying the degree of crystallinity.[6]

The glass transition temperature T_g of a polymer can define how the polymer behaves at a given temperature. At low temperatures, amorphous polymers exist in the glassy state where no large-scale molecular motion can occur. Glassy polymers are typically hard and brittle in nature and, consequently, drug diffusion coefficients will be low at temperatures below T_g.[36] As the temperature is elevated, polymers undergo a transition denoted as the glass transition temperature where the polymer changes from glassy to rubbery. As a result of this transition, the polymer undergoes an abrupt change in properties such as flexibility, permeability and expansion.[12] Consequently, knowledge of T_g and whether the device will be functioning above or below T_g is imperative when designing a controlled-release device.

Viscosity is an important parameter, particularly if the polymer solution is to be sprayed on to the dosage form.[7] An optimal viscosity is required to attain a suitable surface finish and to prevent the solids from precipitating out of the suspension. HPMC-based systems are often used to coat solid oral dosage forms and, at a viscosity of 5 mPa s, a solid concentration of approximately 15% w/w can be attained. However, if the viscosity is increased to 50 mPa s, only 5% w/w solids concentration can be achieved. The lower-viscosity system is therefore advantageous as it permits a greater solids content and a lower solvent concentration which in turn reduces the processing time as less time is required to remove the solvent during the coating process.[7] However, if the viscosity is reduced too much, the resulting polymer film will suffer from poor film strength owing to the low-molecular-weight composition.

When a polymer is placed in an aqueous environment, it will gradually absorb water and the amount of water is determined by the polymer structure. This is of considerable importance as controlled-release devices will invariably function within an aqueous milieu.[3] According to the nature of the polymer–water interaction, the polymer can be classified into one of four groups. Hydrophobic polymers are essentially water impermeable and, when placed in an aqueous environment, will absorb very little water. This impermeability is attributed to the polymer chain stiffness, the high degree of crystallinity and the presence of hydrophobic groups such as C–F bonds. Hydrophilic polymers typically absorb more than 5 wt% water and, as with hydrophobic polymers, this is related to the polymer's properties. The chain flexibility, the absence of crystallinity and the presence of groups such as amino, carboxyl and hydroxyl all aid water absorption.[3] In addition, varying levels of hydrophilicity can be achieved by copolymerisation of two monomers with different degrees of hydrophilicity such as hydroxyethyl methacrylate and methyl methacrylate.

The third class of polymers are freely soluble in water, even though they are of high molecular weight. Typical polymers include poly(vinyl alcohol), poly(acrylic acid) and poly(ethylene oxide).[3] The fourth type of classification is highly hydrophilic or water-soluble polymers that have been cross-linked by means of covalent bonds. The presence of covalent bonds renders the polymer unable to dissolve in the water but enables greater uptake of water and hence the polymer swells. This gives it characteristics that cannot be obtained by using hydrophilic linear polymers.

Porosity can influence the rate of transport of a solute through the polymer. Porous controlled-release systems contain pores large enough to enable diffusion of the drug to occur via liquid carriers that have filled the pores.[12] However, if the pores are below 200–500 Å in size, diffusion may be hindered. Porosity is also important in degradable polymer systems. Pores enable aqueous media to ingress into the polymer structure and initiate both polymer degradation and subsequent dissolution of the active ingredient.[39] The drug solution can then be released into the systemic circulation. This will occur more rapidly if the structure is porous compared with a dense non-porous polymer matrix.[6]

Tackiness is a property that, if not controlled adequately, can lead to processing difficulties. Tack is related to the forces that are required to separate two surfaces joined by a thin film of the solution.[7] If the film solution is too tacky, the surfaces of adjacent film-coated dosage forms will adhere to one another. When separated, the dosage forms will often have defects such as picking, which can compromise the integrity of the film and result in undesirable release profiles or unstable dosage forms. An optimum level of tack therefore needs to be attained so that the film will adhere to the tablet core but not to other tablet coats.

Blending and copolymerisation can offer a tailored drug release profile which is an intermediate of the two constituent parts.[1,6] Microspheres composed of a random copolymer of 1,6-bis(*p*-carboxyphenoxy)hexane (CPH) and sebacic acid (SA) have been utilised to manipulate the drug release profile.[25] CPH is aromatic and degrades over approximately 1 year, whereas SA is aliphatic and degrades in a few days. Consequently, by optimising the ratio of the copolymer the degradation rate can be tailored to the desired duration.

Incompatible monomers can also be blended to achieve polymers with microphase-separated environments. The two distinct domains can subsequently affect the release profile of the active ingredient. If a strongly hydrophobic monomer is blended with a hydrophilic monomer, the hydrophilic monomer will release rapidly, leaving behind a porous structure. The porous structure will be primarily composed of the remaining hydrophobic monomer. Therefore, the drug release occurs in a two-step process and does not correlate with the total polymer degradation but with the individual monomer release.[30] In addition, the domains within copolymers and blends may interact differently with the incorporated drug. A model drug *p*-nitroaniline (PNA) has been observed to be highly compatible with CPH but less compatible with SA within a CPH–SA copolymer system. This led to the initial release of drug-deficient SA domains followed by PNA-rich CPH domains.[30]

2.5.1 Mechanical properties

Film coats are required to provide physical protection for the dosage form.[7] During the rigours of the coating process, the film needs to provide mechanical strength to protect the tablet from undue attrition. The coating must also remain intact, be durable and be resistant to chipping and cracking during handling. The mechanical properties of the films can often be attributed to the molecular weight of the polymer. It has been found that HPMC with a molecular weight of 33 000 exhibits greater toughness than HPMC with a molecular weight of 20 000.[42] The long (high-molecular-weight) chains result in an increase in entanglements that create a tougher and more rigid structure.

The mechanical properties of the polymer are also influenced by the proportion or soft and hard segments in blends and copolymers. Shellac has been mixed with single esters, which function as soft resins.[42] The soft resin plasticises the shellac and results in a more flexible polymer. Furthermore, if polar groups are incorporated into the polymer structure, they promote intermolecular interaction through hydrogen bonding. This leads to the formation of a highly structured matrix, which is rigid and has a high tensile strength.[42]

Mechanical properties are particularly important for implantable delivery devices. The implant needs to retain its mechanical integrity, whilst it delivers the drug and then to degrade to non-toxic by-products. If low-molecular-weight PGA is used as a three-dimensional drug-releasing scaffold, the polymer loses integrity over a few hours.[39] Consequently, the structure cannot function effectively over a sustained period. The degradation rate of the polymer therefore needs to match the desired release duration of the drug so that a controlled rate of drug release is achieved and the device does not dose dump as the polymer degrades.

Mechanical properties are also important for rupturable dosage forms.[43] An outer polymer coating is required to imbibe water and to rupture after a time lag. Besides water permeability, the mechanical properties are therefore important. It has been found that, if the polymer coat is too flexible, e.g. Eudragit RS, the capsules will only rupture slightly with very small cracks.[43] Complete rupture will not occur and no significant drug release will be attained. However, if less flexible and more brittle polymers such as ethyl cellulose or cellulose acetate propionate are used, rupture is complete and drug release is achieved.

2.5.2 Processing parameters

Simple diffusion-controlled dosage forms can be fabricated by compressing the drug with a slowly dissolving carrier.[3] The rate of drug availability is controlled by the rate of penetration of the dissolution fluid into the matrix. This can be controlled by the porosity of the matrix, which in turn can be altered by the compression force that is applied during manufacture. The greater the compression force, the greater is the adhesion forces between the polymeric units and the denser and less porous the matrix will be. In addition, the presence of hydrophobic additives can be added to decrease the effective porosity by limiting the number of pores that can be penetrated by eluting fluid.[3]

Another processing route is film coating. This requires a film coating suspension to be formulated with the appropriate density, surface tension and viscosity.[7] The physical properties of the suspension control the wetting, spreading and adhesion of the droplets on to the solid dosage form. For example, if the concentration of HPMC is doubled from 6 to 12% w/w, a nearly tenfold increase in viscosity is observed. This is due to the large hydrodynamic volume of the randomly coiled polymer chains and their associated hydrogen-bonded water molecules that resist flow and result in high viscosity values.[7] If the viscosity is too high, the film will spread poorly and may lead to an uneven surface finish.

Once an optimum coating suspension has been formulated, the uncoated solid dosage forms are placed inside a cylindrical drum such as an Accelacota unit. The unit has a horizontal rotating cylindrical drum with a perforated curved inner surface. The ends of the drum are conically shaped so that the tablets in the drum are turned over and mixed laterally. There are baffles to aid mixing and hot air enters the drum as the tablets are tumbled. As the tablets are continuously tumbled, the coating fluid is sprayed into the drum at a defined temperature, speed and pressure. The film-coated tablets are then retrieved.

Film coating is also used with osmotically controlled devices. The device is formed by compressing a drug with a suitable osmotic pressure into a tablet.[16] This can often present problems as the components of osmotic devices tend to have poor flow and compression properties.[11] A semipermeable membrane is then applied to the tablet core. The coat, typically CA, is applied using a solvent-based process to ensure a smooth surface finish. The coating membrane is rigid and non-swelling so as to maintain the integrity of the system during drug release. Consequently, when the delivery orifice is drilled into each system by laser or by a high-speed mechanical drill, care must be taken not to damage the coat.[3,9] Although the processing steps are complex, osmotic devices have been successfully used in many commercial products.[11]

Monolithic systems are commonly utilised for the controlled release of contraceptive steroids. PLA has been typically used for the sustained release of progesterone and β-oestradiol. Devices are fabricated by dissolving the drug and the polymer in dichloromethane.[2,12] The solvent is evaporated under reduced pressure and the solid residue is melt pressed into the desired shape. In this procedure, the polymer residue is placed in the lower half of a heated mould.[3] The mould is closed and air, and excess polymer, are forced out. The mould is cooled and the appropriately shaped polymeric device is removed.

Reservoir systems are typically water-insoluble polymeric materials encasing a core of drug. The chosen polymeric membrane, such as chitosan, is attached to a backing membrane with a non-removable adhesive, thereby creating an empty reservoir.[44,45] A small circular hole is made in the backing membrane. A separate polymeric sheet with a circular hole in it is aligned with the chitosan membrane; so the reservoir coincides with the circular hole. The device is pressed and left to dry overnight. A thin layer of pressure-sensitive adhesive is applied to the releasing face of the device to secure the device to the skin. The drug formulation is injected through the opening at the backing to the reservoir and sealed with an adhesive patch. The transdermal delivery system can then be placed on the skin for the controlled release of the active ingredient into the skin.

Micronised drug particles or ultrafine drug droplets incorporated in capsules of a few microns in size are termed microspheres. Microspheres can be fabricated by solidification of emulsion (coacervation), solvent evaporation or solvent extraction.[19] Typical solvent evaporation is carried out in oil-in-water or oil-in-oil emulsions, whose inner oil phase is composed of drug, polymer and solvent.[25] A polymer in water is emulsified by sonication into an organic phase. The polymeric particles are chemically cross-linked or hardened by heat treatment and the residual organic phase is removed. Water-soluble drug molecules can be incorporated into the microspheres by including them in the polymer solution. Up to 10% w/w drug can sometimes be trapped in the microspheres by this approach. The diameter of the microsphere can be affected by various processing parameters such as the stir rate, the concentration of additives and the internal phase volume.

Microspheres are also fabricated by coacervation. This refers to a four-stage process, which transfers macromolecules with film properties from a solvated state (stage 1) via an intermediate phase, the coacervation phase (stage 2), into a phase in which there is a film around each drug particle (stage 3); finally the polymer film solidifies and encases the drug (stage 4).[28] Stage 1 is a two-phase system, which involves the drug dissolved in the solvated film-forming material. Stage 2 is a three-phase system involving the external phase of the solvated polymer, the dissolved drug and a new phase called the coacervation phase. This is an enrichment of polymer droplets in the solvent and occurs as a result of changes in pH, temperature or ionic strength variations. During phase 3, a continuous polymer film begins to encase each particle. By enriching the coacervate, a transition from the sol state into the gel state takes place and the three-phase system returns to a binary system. Finally in stage 4 the polymer solidifies and enables the microspheres to be formulated into dosage forms such as capsules, granules and suspensions.[28]

Microencapsulation can also be performed using an atomisation procedure.[28] The micronised or nanomilled drug suspension is atomised in an outer aqueous phase or a fine drug emulsion in an aqueous system containing reactive monomers or precondensates. Under the influence of heat during spraying the film-forming materials polymerise or polycondense. In conjunction, the aqueous phase evaporates and an enrichment of the film-forming monomers or polycondensates takes place at the surface of the drug. The polymer solidifies and forms a network around the drug particles, and microspheres are formed.

2.6 Future trends

Polymeric drug delivery is a constantly evolving field of therapeutics and, consequently, new technologies and enhanced modes of action are continuously emerging. A major advancement in the future will be the development of a continuous glucose sensor to treat diabetes.[1] The sensor would ideally be sensitive to small changes in glucose, remain in contact with either blood or bodily fluid and respond rapidly and reliably to any fluctuations in blood glucose levels.[12] This could be in the form of a hydrogel that is able to respond to the local environment such as a change in pH induced by an enzymatic reaction which occurs only in the presence of a substrate such as glucose.[18,22] This would then be regulated by a release of insulin from the hydrogel system.

A future development that is important is the ability to deliver nucleic acids particularly to single tissue or cells. Consequently, an approach is required that results in stable gene expression and targeted administration to the binding site. Attempts have been made in the past that have utilised positively charged polymers such as polylysine to complex negatively charged deoxyribonucleic acid (DNA) in a stable configuration.[18] However, this is potentially toxic and immunogenic. As such, additional work is required to identify new polymers with suitable ligands for the DNA to complex with.

Although vast improvements in cancer treatment have been made, undesirable interactions between drug and delivery vehicles still exist.[14]

An advancement that would alter cancer treatment dramatically would be a device that could be regulated to release drugs at any time, pattern or rate. This may enable combination therapies to be administered, which initially release angiogenisis inhibitors to attack the tumour cell followed by chemotherapeutic drugs to destroy the remaining tumour.[46] The device would then maintain the patient on antiangiogenic therapy long term.

The administration of drugs to the central nervous system (CNS) is a significant challenge as many drugs will not cross the blood–brain barrier (BBB).[2] This can be bypassed by injection of microspheres into a specific region of the brain, enabling sustained delivery to the CNS. However, encapsulating the required drug is often technically challenging and microspheres also have a tendency to release a drug rapidly in a burst effect. This is undesirable as potent levels of a drug within the CNS can be reached. Consequently, new methods that produce a more linear release of a drug to the CNS and yet still bypass the BBB are required.

2.7 References

1 Pillai O and Panchagnula R, 'Polymers in drug delivery', *Curr Opin Chem Biol*, 2001 **5** 447–451.
2 Whittlesey K J and Shea L D, 'Delivery systems for small molecule drugs, proteins and DNA: the neuroscience/biomaterial interface', *Exp Neurol*, 2004 **190** 1–16.
3 Robinson J R and Lee V H L, *Controlled Drug Delivery – Fundamentals and Applications*, 2nd edition, New York, Marcel Dekker, 1987.
4 Berkland C, King M, Cox A, Kim K K and Pack D W, 'Precise control of PLG microsphere size provides enhanced control of drug release rate', *J Control Release*, 2002 **82** 137–147.
5 Ainaoui A and Vergnaud J M, 'Effect of the nature of the polymer and of the process of drug release (diffusion or erosion) for oral dosage forms', *Comput Theor Polym Sci*, 2002 **10** 383–390.
6 Frieberg S and Zhu X X, 'Polymer microspheres for controlled drug release', *Int J Pharm*, 2004 **19** 282–287.
7 Cole G, Hogan J and Aulton M, *Pharmaceutical Coating Technology*, London, Taylor & Francis, 1995.
8 Guo J, Skinner G W, Harcum W W and Barnum P E, 'Pharmaceutical applications of naturally occurring water-soluble polymers', *Pharm Sci Technol Today*, 1998 **6** 254–261.
9 Verma R K, Krishna D M and Garg S, 'Formulation aspects in the development of osmotically controlled oral drug delivery systems', *J Control Release*, 2002 **79** 7–27.
10 Efentakis M and Politis S, 'Comparative evaluation of various structures in polymer controlled drug delivery systems and the effect of their morphology and characteristics on drug release', *Eur Polym J*, 2006 **42** 1183–1195.

11 Thombre A G, Appel L E, Chidlaw M B, Daugherity P D, Dumont F, Evans L A F and Sutton S C, 'Osmotic drug delivery using swellable core technology', *J Controlled Release*, 2004 **94** 75–89.
12 Ranade V V and Hollinger M A, *Drug Delivery Systems – Pharmacology and Toxicology*, 2nd edition, Boca Raton, Florida, Taylor & Francis Routledge, 2004.
13 Ouriemchi E M and Vergnaud J M, 'Processes of drug transfer with three different polymeric systems with transdermal drug delivery', *Comput Theor Polym Sci*, 2000 **10** 391–401.
14 Moses M A, Brem H and Langer R, 'Advancing the field of drug delivery: taking aim at cancer', *Cancer Cells*, 2003 **4** 337–341.
15 Duncan R and Seymour L W, *Controlled Release Technologies – A survey of Research and Commercial Applications*, Oxford, Elsevier Advanced Technology, 1989.
16 Santus G and Baker R W, 'Osmotic drug delivery: a review of the patent literature', *J Control Release*, 1995 **35** 1–121.
17 Winzenburg G, Schmidt C, Fuchs S and Kissel T, 'Biodegradable polymers and their potential use in parenteral veterinary drug delivery systems', *Advd Drug Deliv Rev*, 2004 **56** 1453–1466.
18 Griffith L G, 'Polymeric biomaterials', *Acta Mater*, 2000 **48** 263–277.
19 Kawaguchi H, 'Functional polymer microspheres', *Prog Polym Sci*, 2000 **25** 1171–1210.
20 Fu K, Griebenow K, Hsieh L, Kilbanov A M and Langer R, 'FTIR characterization of the secondary structure of protein encapsulation within PLGA microspheres', *J Control Release*, 1999 **58** 357–366.
21 Gupta P, Vermani K and Garg S, 'Hydrogels: from controlled release to pH-responsive drug delivery', *Drug Discov Today*, 2002 **7** 569–579.
22 Sherhen S and West J, 'Implantable, polymeric systems for modulated drug delivery', *Advd Drug Deliv Rev*, 2002 **54** 1225–1235.
23 Cole E T, Scott R A, Connor A L, Wilding I R, Petereit H, Schminke C, Beckert T and Cade D, 'Enteric coated HPMC capsules designed to achieve intestinal targeting', *Int J Pharm*, 2002 **231** 83–95.
24 Bruce L D, Petereit H, Beckert T and McGinity J W, 'Properties of enteric coated sodium valproate pellets', *Int J Pharm*, 2003 **264** 85–96.
25 Kipper M J, Shen E, Determan A and Narasimhan B, 'Design of an injectable system based on bioerodible polyanhydride microspheres for sustained drug delivery', *Biomaterials*, 2002 **23** 4405–4412.
26 Hatefi A and Amsden B, 'Biodegradable injectable *in situ* forming drug delivery systems', *J Controlled Release*, 2002 **80** 9–28.
27 Raivivarapu H B, Burton K and De Luca P P, 'Polymer and microsphere blending to alter the release of a peptide from PLGA microspheres', *Eur J Pharm Biopharm*, 2000 **50** 263–270.
28 Nixon J R, *Drugs and the Pharmaceutical Sciences*, Vol. 3 – *Microencapsulation*, New York, Marcel Dekker, 1976.
29 Brem H Langer R, 'Polymer based drug delivery to the brain', *Sci Med*, 1996 **3** 52–61.
30 Shen E, Kipper M J, Dziadul B, Lim M and Narasimhan B, 'Mechanistic relationships between polymer microstructure and drug release kinetics in bioerodible polyanhydrides', *J Controlled Release*, 2002 **82** 115–125.

31 Walter K A, Cahan M A, Gur A, Tyler B, Hilton J, Colvin O M, Burger P C, Domb A and Brem H, 'Interstitial Taxol delivered from a biodegradable polymer implant against experimental malignant glioma', *Cancer Res*, 1994 **54** 2207–2212.
32 Zhang X, Jackson J K, Wong W, Min W, Cruz T, Hunter W L and Burt H M, 'Development of biodegradable polymeric paste formulations for taxol: an *in vivo* and *in vitro* study', *Int J Pharm*, 1996 **137** 199–208.
33 Schoneker D R, DeMerlis C C and Borzelleca J F, 'Evaluation of the toxicity of polyvinylacetate phthalate in experimental animals', *Food Chem Toxicol*, 2003 **41** 405–413.
34 Liu J and Williams R O, 'Long term stability of heat–humidity cured cellulose acetate phthalate coated beads', *Eur J Pharm Biopharm*, 2002 **53** 167–173.
35 Heller J, Barr J, Ng S Y, Abdellauoi K S and Gurny R, 'Poly(ortho esters): synthesis, characterization, properties and uses', *Advd Drug Deliv Rev*, 2002 **54** 1015–1019.
36 Siepmann J and Peppas N A, 'Modeling of drug release from delivery systems based on hydroxypropyl methylcellulose', *Advd Drug Deliv Rev*, 2001 **48** 139–157.
37 Wang J, Somasundaran P and Nagaraj D R, 'Adsorption mechanism of guar gum at solid–liquid interfaces', *Miner Eng*, 2005 **18** 77–81.
38 Young S, Wong M, Tabata Y and Mikos A G, 'Gelatin as a delivery vehicle for the controlled release of bioactive molecules', *J Control Release*, 2005 **109** 256–274.
39 Braunecker J, Baba M, Milroy G E and Cameron R E, 'The effects of molecular weight and porosity on the degradation and drug release from polyglycolide', *Int J Pharm*, 2004 **282** 19–34.
40 Young R J and Lovell P A, *Introduction to Polymers*, London, Chapman & Hall, 1991.
41 Cowie J M G, *Polymers: Chemistry and Physics of Modern Materials*, 2nd edition, Glasgow, Blackie, 1991.
42 Limmatvapirat S, Limmatvapirat C, Luangtana-anan M, Nunthanid J, Oguchi T, Tozuka Y, Yamamoto K and Puttipipatkhachorn S, 'Modification of physicochemical and mechanical properties of shellac by partial hydrolysis', *Int J Pharm*, 2004 **278** 41–49.
43 Bussemer T and Bodmeier R, 'Formulation parameters affecting the performance of coated gelatin capsules with pulsatile release profiles', *Int J Pharm*, 2003 **267** 59–68.
44 Thacharodi D and Panduranga Rao K, 'Development and *in vitro* evaluation of chitosan-based transdermal drug delivery systems for the controlled delivery of propranolo-hydrochloride', *Biomaterials*, 1995 **16** 145–148.
45 Thacharodi D and Panduranga Rao K, 'Rate-controlling biopolymer membranes as transdermal delivery systems for nifedipine: development and *in vitro* evaluations', *Biomaterials*, 1996 **17** 1307–1311.
46 Jain R K, 'Normalizing the tumour vasculature with anti-angiogenic therapy: a new paradigm for combination therapy', *Nat Med*, 2001 **7** 987–989.

3
Hydrogels in cell encapsulation and tissue engineering

A HILLEL, P SHAH and J ELISSEEFF,
Johns Hopkins University, USA

3.1 Introduction

A hydrogel is a network of hydrophilic polymers that absorbs water or biological fluid but does not dissolve. Hydrogels can be created from a number of water-soluble materials and commonly include synthetic polymers, proteins and natural molecules. The three-dimensional (3D) structure of hydrogels is a result of polymer cross-linking that forms an insoluble structure within the fluid environment. The high water content and elasticity create a resemblance to biological tissue, creating extensive biomedical applications. A few scientists have even hypothesized that a primitive hydrogel may have provided the environment responsible for assembly of the first cell (Trevors and Pollack, 2005).

Wichterle and Lim invented the synthetic hydrogel in 1954 with the goal of designing the ideal biocompatible substance (see Wichterle and Lim, 1960). Hydrolytically stable molecular chains of 2-hydroxyethyl methacrylate (HEMA) were interconnected by a succession of chemical bonds to form a uniform molecular structure (Wichterle, 1978). Wichterle (1978) achieved four criteria with the design.

1 Preventing component release.
2 Creating a stable chemical and biochemical structure.
3 Having a high permeability for nutrients and waste.
4 Assuming physical characteristics similar to natural living tissue.

The water content and mechanical properties of hydrogels are similar to those of human tissue and yield many biomedical applications. The first biomedical use for synthetic hydrogels was as an orbital implant in 1954. Subsequently, Wichterle designed soft contact lenses from hydrogels in 1961 (see Wichterle, 1978). Since then, hydrogel biomedical applications have included wound dressings, drug delivery systems, hemodialysis systems, artificial skin and tissue engineering (Moise *et al.*, 1977; Corkhill *et al.*, 1989; Murphy *et al.*, 1992; Peppas *et al.*, 2000; Bouhadir *et al.*, 2001; Nguyen and

West, 2002; Nuttleman *et al.*, 2002; Flynn *et al.*, 2003; Wang *et al.*, 2003; Brown *et al.*, 2005; Levesque *et al.*, 2005; Li *et al.*, 2006; Varghese and Elisseeff, 2006). The structural similarity of hydrogels to that of the human extracellular matrix (ECM) creates promising applications as a scaffold material for cell-based tissue engineering (Varghese and Elisseeff, 2006).

Tissue engineering is a multidisciplinary field that applies the principles of engineering, life sciences, cell and molecular biology toward the development of biological substitutes to restore, maintain and improve tissue function (Mooney and Mikos, 1999). Three general components are involved in tissue engineering.

1 Reparative cells that can form a functional matrix.
2 An appropriate scaffold for transplantation and support.
3 Bioactive molecules, such as cytokines and growth factors that will support and choreograph formation of the desired tissue (Sharma and Elisseeff, 2004).

These three components may be used individually or in combination to regenerate organs or tissue.

Wichterle's four criteria for hydrogel design parallel scaffold principles for cell-based tissue engineering. Scaffolds must be biocompatible and adapt their shape and structure to integrate with the target tissue. Hydrogels maintain close contact with tissues with negligible adhesion and provoke minimal immune response (Sawhney *et al.*, 1994). Furthermore, scaffolds should be able to encase cells and to promote proliferation without injuring cells or permitting component extravasation. Importantly, scaffolds should be porous to allow the diffusion of nutrients and metabolites between cells and the local environment (Peppas *et al.*, 2000; Varghese and Elisseeff, 2006). Hydrogels have two additional advantages for tissue engineering. Firstly, as a potential minimally invasive application, they solidify *in situ* within a defect site in the body, thereby avoiding open surgery for implantation (Anseth *et al.*, 2002). Hydrogels may be cross-linked under relatively mild conditions such that encapsulated cells survive the physical or chemical change causing gelation (Elisseeff *et al.*, 2000; Wang *et al.*, 2003). Secondly, scaffolds should be biodegradable as the cellular component proliferates into functional tissue, a characteristic that some hydrogels demonstrate (Anseth *et al.*, 2002). Scaffold degradation increases temporal and spatial control of the engineered construct (Anseth *et al.*, 2002).

3.2 Structure and properties of a cross-linked hydrogel

The function of a hydrogel is, in large part, dependent on its cross-linked structure. The degree of cross-linking may be measured by the average molecular weight of the polymer chain between cross-links. Cross-linking density directly effects other fundamental properties of hydrogels such as swelling, mechanical strength and elasticity, permeability and even diffusion (Lowman and Peppas, 1999; Peppas *et al.*, 2000). These properties, which may be calculated experimentally or theoretically, contribute to the understanding of hydrogel structure.

3.2.1 Definition

Hydrogels are hydrophilic cross-linked polymers that are able to swell in water and form an insoluble 3D network. The insoluble state and 3D structure result from polymer cross-linking. The network remains at equilibrium in an aqueous environment owing to the balance of elastic forces of the cross-linked polymer with osmotic forces of the liquid (Fig. 3.1). The chemical composition and molecular weight determine cross-linking density, which in turn influences the swelling that determines gel porosity (Rosenblatt *et al.*, 1994; Peppas *et al.*, 2000). Furthermore, it is cross-linking that is responsible for the behavior of hydrogels as a solid, instead of a liquid, allowing an elastic response to stress (Gehrke *et al.*, 1997).

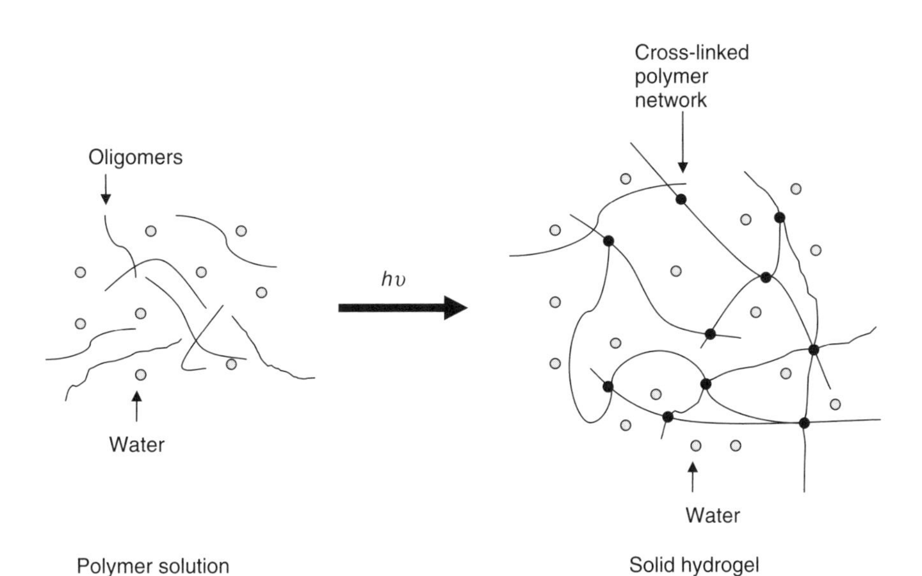

3.1 Schematic diagram of the hydrogel liquid–gel transition by photopolymerization. The cross-linked network may be created through physical cross-linking, covalent bonds or ionic bonds (Varghese and Elisseeff, 2006).

3.2.2 Characterization

Swelling

Hydrogel swelling, or the amount of water absorbed, helps to define the physical properties of hydrogels. Swelling is strongly dependent on the chemical structure of the polymer and inversely related to the degree of cross-linking density. Flory and Rehner (1943) first correlated the cross-link density to polymer swelling in 1943 to quantify the characteristics of rubber. In the Flory-Rehner (1943) model, the degree of swelling is in equilibrium between the elastic forces of the polymer and the thermodynamic force because of polymer and solvent mixing. In 1977, Peppas and Merrill (1977) modified the Flory–Rehner theory to apply to the production of hydrogels from polymer solutions. Owing to elastic forces, the presence of water modifies the change in the chemical potential within the system (Peppas and Mirrill, 1977; Peppas *et al.*, 2000). The chemical structure affects swelling due to the presence of chemical groups within hydrogels. For example, hydrogels with hydrophilic groups swell more than hydrophobic groups, which do not expand in the presence of water (Peppas *et al.*, 2000). For the class of smart hydrogels, whose volume changes are dependent on environmental conditions, swelling may also be dependent on pH, temperature or radiation (Lowman and Peppas, 1999).

Equilibrium swelling may be determined experimentally or be theoretically calculated. Accurate measurement of equilibrium swelling assists in the calculation of cross-linking density, mesh size and diffusion coefficients. Experimental methods to measure hydrogel swelling include gravimetric measurement following fluid immersion, use of dedicated instruments to measure dimensional change, and absorbance measurement of dextran dye excluded from the solid phase (Noomrio *et al.*, 2005). Measurement of swelling at equilibrium is an established standard; however, some stimuli-responsive applications, such as controlled drug release, benefit from dynamic measurement (Traitel *et al.*, 2003).

Elasticity

Swollen hydrogels conform to stress with elastic behavior, which includes elastic stretching and its reciprocal, compression. Elasticity, similar to swelling, is dependent on and may be calculated from a known cross-link density. A high cross-linking density results in greater mechanical strength, as well as decreased elasticity and swelling. For some hydrogels, greatly increasing the degree of cross-linking results in a brittle gel (Peppas *et al.*, 2000). Therefore, the optimal degree of hydrogel cross-linking density balances elasticity with desired strength (Peppas *et al.*, 2000). In synthesizing a new hydrogel macromer, poly(6-aminohexyl propylene phosphate), Li *et al.*

(2006) enhanced cross-linking by increasing acrylate contents to improve mechanical strength and to decrease the gel swelling ratio. Similarly, Kim *et al.* (2004) demonstrated greater mechanical strength with increased cross-linking of silk fibroin due to higher gelation temperatures and higher fibroin concentration.

Permeability

Hydrogel porosity ξ, or mesh size, is a structural property that estimates the length between successive cross-links in a hydrogel. Porosity is a function of cross-linking density, monomer composition and monomer concentration (Lowman and Peppas, 1999). In a 1998 study of poly(ethylene glycol) diacrylate (PEGDA), Cruise *et al.* (1998) showed significant changes in porosity characteristics when altering the molecular weight of the polymer and more modest changes in pore size with modifications in PEGDA concentration. Given an inert network and uniform changes in porosity, mesh size increases with greater swelling and decreases with decreased swelling (Gehrke *et al.*, 1997). Kim *et al.* (2004) demonstrated a similar relationship in experiments with silk hydrogels, showing a decrease in pore size with an increase in fibroin cross-linking. Direct measurements of permeability include electron microscopy or quasi-elastic laser-light scattering (Stock and Ray, 1985). Alternatively, indirect methods may yield additional calculations such as mercury porosimetry, rubber elasticity measurements and equilibrium swelling experiments (Canal and Peppas, 1989; Mikos *et al.*, 1993; Lowman and Peppas, 1997, 1999).

Diffusion

The rate of solute diffusion is important to determine drug release or transport of nutrients and waste in cell-based tissue engineering. Diffusion of nutrients, waste or other solutes is dependent on a multitude of factors, including network morphology, polymer composition, water content, solute and polymer concentration, gel swelling and degradation (Lowman and Peppas, 1999). These fundamental factors may combine to create chemical or frictional effects that slow solute diffusion. A chemical effect describes the attractive force between solute and hydrogel matrix while physical size exclusion represents the principal frictional effect on diffusion through a hydrogel (Gehrke *et al.*, 1997).

3.3 Methods to form a hydrogel

Polymer cross-linking represents the fundamental factor in the hydrogel structure. It affects hydrogel formation, shape, size and degradation. For successful biomedical use, control over cross-linking is imperative. This section will review the different types of hydrogel cross-linking: covalent, ionic and physical interactions (Hennink and van Nostrum, 2002). Furthermore, it will address specific hydrogel materials that exhibit each type of cross-linking interaction with a focus on applications for tissue engineering. Finally, biomimetic hydrogels will be discussed – an area with great promise in biomedical engineering.

3.3.1 Covalent cross-linking

Covalent cross-linking may be initiated by radical polymerization, although cross-linking may occur through addition reactions, condensation reactions, high-energy irradiation (gamma and electron beam radiation) and enzyme catalyzation (Hennink and van Nostrum, 2002). Before radical polymerization begins, polymers usually require modification through the addition of polymerizable units. For example, in poly(ethylene glycol) (PEG), acrylate is added to functional groups to promote covalent linkages within the polymer (West and Hubbell, 1995). Radical polymerization of the acrylate groups may then be initiated by light, thermal initiation systems or redox catalysts (Nguyen and West, 2002; Shung *et al.*, 2003). Once cross-linking is induced, the process cannot be altered or stopped (Elisseeff *et al.*, 2005).

Photopolymerization involves the conversion of liquid polymer solutions that form a gel in the presence of a photoinitiator catalyst and light (Hennink and van Nostrum, 2002). Photopolymerization is an ideal method for clinical implantation because it enhances spatial (3D) and temporal (quick on- and -off) control (Williams *et al.*, 2003). Hydrogels may be injected, shaped and solidified *in situ* (Elisseeff *et al.*, 2000). This approach is compatible with minimally invasive techniques and may be applied in craniofacial applications with transdermal photopolymerization or arthroscopic procedures using a fiber-optic light source (Anseth *et al.*, 2002, Williams *et al.*, 2003).

Two covalently linked hydrogels used in tissue engineering are PEG and hyaluronic acid (HA), a glycosaminoglycan found in the ECM. Modifying the gels with bioactive molecules and/or chemical cross-link groups enhances their utility as scaffolds by improving biochemical functionality and mechanical stability as well as slowing degradation (Segura *et al.*, 2005). The Poly(ethylene glycol) acrylate (PEGA) molecules undergo radical polymerization and form a chemically cross-linked hydrogel (Sawhney *et al.*, 1993; Martens *et al.*, 2003). HA requires structural modification of its functional side groups to allow for a radical cross-linking reaction (Baier Leach *et al.*, 2002). Baier Leach *et al.* reacted methacrylate groups with HA to create a radical photopolymerizable hydrogel. Shu *et al.* (2004b) synthesized thiolated HA and then conjugated it to PEG for the benefit of *in-situ* injection, cell encapsulation and proliferation. PEG and HA may be further modified for specific tissue-engineering purposes. Hern and Hubbell (1998) first modified PEGA with the adhesive peptide arginyl–glycyl–aspartic acid (RGD) to enhance cell adhesion and to promote tissue spreading. In separate experiments, PEG methacrylate has been modified with phosphoester and RGD to enhance bone engineering (Burdick and Anseth 2002; Wang *et al.*, 2005). Additionally, HA has been copolymerized with PEGDA + RGD to support cell attachment and proliferation as well as to improve cartilage repair (Park *et al.*, 2003; Shu *et al.*, 2004a).

3.3.2 Ionic cross-linking

A second type of hydrogel cross-linking occurs by ionic interactions. Alginate, a naturally polysaccharide found in algae, commonly forms a hydrogel by ionic bonds in the presence of divalent or multivalent cations (Lee *et al.*, 2000b). In a reaction that occurs at room temperature and physiological pH, calcium ions interact with alginate to create ionic bridges between polymer chains (Drury *et al.*, 2004). Ionic interactions are weaker than covalent cross-linking, and alginate gels undergo rapid dissolution of cross-linking in physiological solution, an environment where biomedical hydrogels are expected to function. LeRoux *et al.* (1999) demonstrated greater than 60% decrease in mechanical strength after exposure for 15 h to sodium chloride solution. The mechanism responsible for cross-link degradation is divalent ions exchanged for monovalent sodium cations (Lee *et al.*, 2000b). One example of a synthetic polymer that forms a hydrogel by ionic interactions with cations is poly [di(carboxylatophenoxy)phosphazene] (Andrianov *et al.*, 1994).

3.3.3 Physical cross-linking

Some cross-linking agents adversely affect cells or proteins encapsulated in gels and have to be removed before application of the gel (Hennink and van Nostrum, 2002). To avoid potentially toxic metabolites, scientists have investigated physically cross-linking hydrogels. Hydrogen bonding, hydrophobic interactions and van der Waals forces are the primary interactions responsible for physical cross-linking. Ionic cross-linking, considered by some to be a physical interaction, was discussed in the previous section. While each individual physical bond is relatively weak, the combination of interactions creates a strong bond (Zhang, 2002). Zhang (2002) described molecular self-assembly as molecular building blocks undergoing a series of steps to spontaneously form a stable and defined network. Cross-link dissolution is prevented by the physical interaction between polymer chains (Hennink and van Nostrum, 2002). While much of Zhang's research focuses on proteins, the principles of self-assembling peptides may be extended to synthetic polymers and natural molecules. This will be described in greater detail in a later section of this chapter. Pluronics® is another example of physical cross-linking where its amphiphilic copolymers, poly(ethylene oxide) (PEO) and poly(propylene oxide), cross-link by hydrophobic interactions in aqueous solution in response to temperature (Kabanov *et al.*, 2002).

Physical cross-linking of bioactive factors is one of the methods used to create biomimetic hydrogels. Growth factors remain active after encapsulation to enhance the proliferation and differentiation of encapsulated cells or to improve local tissue regeneration (Lee *et al.*, 2000a; Burdick *et al.*, 2002b). Growth factors that have been entrapped in hydrogels include bone morphogenetic protein-2 (BMP-2), fibroblast growth factor, vascular endothelial growth factor (VEGF), insulin-like growth factor 1 (IGF-1) and transforming growth factor β (TGF-β), amongst others (Peters *et al.*, 1998; Yamamoto *et al.*, 1998; Tabata *et al.*, 1999; Elisseeff *et al.*, 2001; Lutolf *et al.*, 2003). The examples in the following paragraph illustrate the effect of biomimetic hydrogels on three different tissues.

Lee *et al.* (2000a) studied neoangiogenesis resulting from VEGF incorporated in an alginate hydrogel and implanted in severe combined immunodeficient and non-obese diabetic mice. The results demonstrated enhanced vascularity by histological analysis with VEGF hydrogels when compared with hydrogels without VEGF. When the concentration of VEGF release from the hydrogel was increased, it resulted in a statistically significant increase in vascularization. To improve cartilage formation, Elisseeff *et al.* (2001) incorporated IGF-1 and transforming growth factor β1 (TGF-β1) in poly (ethylene oxide) dimethylacrylate hydrogels with bovine chondrocytes. The hydrogels containing IGF-1 and TGF-β1 demonstrated a significant increase in glycosaminoglycan (GAG) production over hydrogels with one or without any of the growth factors. In an innovative trial, Lutolf *et al.* (2003) cross-linked substrates for matrix metalloprotease (MMP) and RGD into PEG-based hydrogels together with BMP-2 to enhance the healing of rat calvarial defects. The MMP substrates triggered MMP-mediated degradation of the ECM and allowed for cell invasion and matrix remodeling. The BMP-2 release subsequently enhanced bone healing. These results demonstrated that inducing matrix degradation and local cell adhesion combined with growth factor release significantly improved local bone growth by histological and radiological analysis.

3.4 Application to cell encapsulation and tissue engineering

This section will discuss *in vitro* and *in vivo* applications of hydrogels in cartilage tissue engineering. Following a review of the key factors needed to combine living cells with hydrogel polymers, the experimental uses for

Table 3.1 Natural and synthetic polymers commonly used in the synthesis of hydrogels (Peppas *et al.*, 2000; Varghese and Elisseeff, 2006)

Natural hydrogels	Synthetic polymers
Hyaluronic acid (HA)	Hydroxyethyl methacrylate (HEMA)
Chondroitin sulfate	Methoxyethyl methacrylate (MEMA)
Matrigel	*N*-vinyl-2-pyrrolidone (NVP)
Alginate	*N*-isopropyl Aam (NIPAAm)
Collagen	Acrylic Acid (AA)
Fibrin	Poly(ethylene glycol) acrylate (PEGA)
Chitosan	Poly(ethylene oxide) diacrylate (poly(ethylene glycol) diacrylate (PEGDA))
Silk	Poly(vinyl alcohol) (PVA)
Gelatin	Poly(fumarates)
Agarose	
Dextran	

hydrogels will be addressed. Cell encapsulation within hydrogels provides a unique method to study cartilage tissue engineering. The section will conclude with a summary of commonly used materials for both natural and synthetic hydrogels (Table 3.1).

3.4.1 Requirements of encapsulation

The requirements for cell encapsulation using hydrogels differ for *in vitro* studies and *in vivo* applications. The prospective hydrogel must meet certain minimum criteria to be considered suitable for *in vitro* culture: an ability to support cellular proliferation and phenotype, sufficient porosity to allow for the desired cell density as well as nutrient and waste transport, and a lack of toxicity arising from the material itself, its preparation and/or its breakdown. *In vivo* applications additionally require the following.

1 An absence of toxic materials and breakdown products that could injure the host organism or individual cells.
2 Minimal inflammatory or immunogenic response to the implanted material.
3 Sufficient structural integrity for the task (i.e. subcutaneous implants versus articular cartilage repairs).

3.4.2 Applications of hydrogel cell encapsulation

In vitro *applications*

Hydrogel scaffolds play several important roles in *in vitro* tissue-engineering research. For example, hydrogels are used to form a controlled extracellular environment for the study of 3D cell–cell and cell–ECM interactions. The design and synthesis of engineered tissues with specific properties require detailed knowledge of the interactions of cells with other cells, bioactive factors and their microenvironment. It has been observed that certain cell types (e.g. chondrocytes) will dedifferentiate in two-dimensional culture (von der Mark *et al*., 1977; Benya and Shaffer, 1982), whereas maintenance of their phenotype is supported in 3D culture (Homicz *et al*., 2003). In fact, there is interest in 3D culture of harvested human chondrocytes for use in autologous chondrocyte transplantation to prevent or reverse dedifferentiation due to monolayer expansion (Homicz *et al*., 2003).

Hydrogels have also been modified with bioactive factors and cell adhesion peptides to improve tissue generation. Several groups have reported enhanced proliferation of cells encapsulated within scaffolds modified with the RGD cell adhesion peptide (Rowley *et al*., 1999; Alsberg *et al*., 2001, 2002; Hsu *et al*., 2004). Lee *et al.* (2004a) incorporated TGF-β1 into a chitosan scaffold in which chondrocytes were cultured. The chondrocytes cultured in scaffolds containing TGF-β1 exhibited significantly greater proliferation and GAG and type II collagen production than did chondrocytes cultured in control scaffolds lacking TGF-β1.

The microstructure of the scaffold has also been shown to have an effect on cultured cells. Hydrogels synthesized from self-assembling synthetic oligopeptides exhibit a fibrillar microstructure approximately three orders of magnitude smaller than synthetic polymer hydrogels such as PEO, poly(lactic acid) (PLA) and poly(glycolic acid) (PGA) and more closely resembles the scale of native ECM (Kisiday *et al*., 2002). Kisiday *et al.* (2002) cultured chondrocytes in a synthetic peptide-based hydrogel (KLD-12), comparing their proliferation, matrix secretion and mechanical properties with conventional chondrocyte-agarose scaffolds. Chondrocytes cultured in the peptide hydrogel proliferated significantly more than those cultured in the agarose scaffold, although their mechanical properties, histological appearance and biochemical compositions were similar.

In vivo *applications*

Hydrogel scaffolds are also used extensively for *in vivo* tissue-engineering research. They are most commonly used as a vehicle for cells and/or bioactive factors, the ultimate goal of which is to support the growth and development of healthy tissue as well as its integration into surrounding tissue. In this setting, the scaffold must be biocompatible with the host tissue, without releasing toxic materials or inciting a marked inflammatory response. In addition, the scaffold must have sufficient strength and resilience to function where it is implanted without premature breakdown. The current *in vivo* use of hydrogels in cartilage engineering involves implantation of a hydrogel scaffold (usually subcutaneously) in order to determine the ability to generate a tissue that resembles cartilage (Fig. 3.2). Alternatively a cartilage defect may be created followed by application of

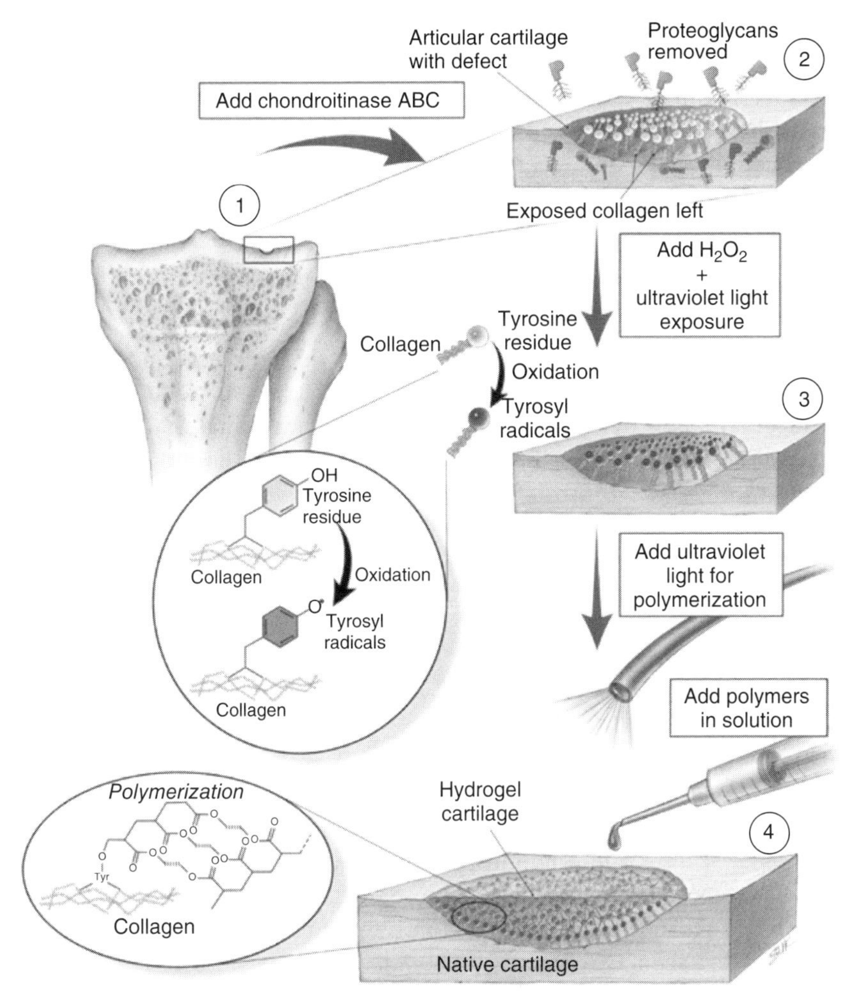

3.2 Schematic illustration for the strategy of hydrogel–cartilage integration by tissue-initiated photopolymerization. Individual steps of the process are as follows: step ①, clearance of the proteoglycans in cartilage by chondroitinase to expose the collagen network; step ②, *in situ* generation of tyrosyl radicals by photo-oxidation of tyrosine residues on collagen with H_2O_2 under low intensity ultraviolet irradiation; step ③, introduction of a macromer solution and *in situ* photogelation via tyrosyl radical initiation and ultraviolet excitation (Wang *et al.*, 2004). (Reprinted with permission from Wiley Interscience ©).

a hydrogel–chondrocyte scaffold to assess healing. Several groups have demonstrated *in vivo* secretion of cartilaginous matrix using chondrocytes encapsulated in hydrogels derived from fibrin (Westreich *et al.*, 2004; Xu *et al.*, 2004, 2005); agarose (Diduch *et al.*, 2000), alginate (Paige *et al.*, 1996; Alsberg *et al.*, 2003; Chang *et al.*, 2003; Kamil *et al.*, 2004), chitosan (Chenite *et al.*, 2000; Hoemann *et al.*, 2005), HA (Dausse *et al.*, 2003; Hsu *et al.*, 2004; Nettles *et al.*, 2004), and synthetic polymers such as PLA, PGA and PEO (Elisseeff *et al.*, 1999b; Mercier *et al.*, 2004; Alhadlaq and Muo, 2005). Again, it is difficult to draw broad conclusions about the suitability of various hydrogels for tissue engineering, owing to the wide variability in experimental design and technique. The use of hydrogels to support chondrocyte growth and matrix production is well established. Current efforts are focusing on bringing hydrogels closer to clinical applications.

3.4.3 Cartilage tissue engineering using hydrogels

The following is a brief overview of recent work on natural and synthetic hydrogels in cartilage tissue engineering. What follows is a description of the most common hydrogels in use, as well as novel materials and techniques that show promise for clinical application of tissue engineering. Examples of *in vitro* and *in vivo* applications will be provided, and the advantages and disadvantages of each material will be discussed. A comprehensive description of every hydrogel in use is beyond the scope of this chapter.

Natural hydrogels

Fibrin

Enzymatic cleavage of soluble fibrinogen, a blood plasma protein, by thrombin yields fibrin which undergoes spontaneous polymerization under physiological conditions (Frenkel and Di Cesare, 2004). The result is a soft gel capable of supporting chondrocyte growth and function. Xu *et al.* (2005) described the generation of a flexible ear-shaped construct using swine auricular chondrocytes encapsulated in a fibrin construct, which was then laminated between two sheets of lyophilized swine perichondium. This construct was then implanted into nude mice, subjected to gross mechanical manipulation after 6 weeks (while still implanted) and explanted after 12 weeks for histological analysis. Control constructs were generated without the perichondrium layer. The experimental and control constructs were similar in gross and histological appearance, with well-formed cartilaginous tissue. The experimental constructs were significantly more flexible than the controls, and much more closely approximated the properties of native ear cartilage. It was noted, however, that fibrin-based hydrogels demonstrated inconsistent support of cartilage growth in immunocompetent organisms.

In a separate experiment, Westreich *et al.* (2004) demonstrated consistent successful autotransplantation of rabbit auricular chondrocytes encapsulated in Tisseel, a commercially available human fibrin preparation. Constructs were prepared with and without IGF-1 and/or basic fibroblast growth factor. The constructs were implanted subcutaneously, harvested after 3 months and analyzed for chondrocyte viability, matrix production, necrosis, inflammation and angiogenesis. Of note, 85% of constructs prepared without a growth factor formed cartilage-like tissue, compared with only 28% of those with a growth factor. This experiment showed that cartilage could be formed with a reasonable success rate using a fibrin scaffold. The advantage of fibrin is that it is readily available as a commercial product that many surgeons have already used clinically. However, it is mechanically weak when first formed and thus unlikely to be suitable for high-load-bearing applications.

Chitosan

Chitosan is a polysaccharide derived from chitin (found in arthropod exoskeletons) that has been partially or fully deacetylated (Chenite *et al.*, 2000). It is a cationic polymer composed of linear chains of β-linked D-glucosamine residues. Alkalinization of an aqueous solution of chitosan to a pH greater than 6.2 results in the precipitation of a hydrogel due to ionic forces (Hoemann *et al.*, 2005). Chenite *et al.* (2000) described mixing chitosan with glycerol phosphate to synthesize a hydrogel that is liquid at room temperature and physiological pH, but which gels at body temperature. Chondrocytes were mixed with the thermogelling chitosan and cultured *in vitro* or implanted subcutaneously in nude mice. The subcutaneous implants were explanted after 4 weeks and subjected to histological analysis for matrix production using Von Kossa and toluidine blue staining. *In vitro* constructs were analyzed for chondrocyte viability using live–dead staining. Maintenance of chondrocyte viability and phenotype, as well as matrix production was observed. Hoemann *et al.* (2005) used thermogelling chitosan to encapsulate chondrocytes for *in vitro* culture as well as implantation into rabbit knee articular defects. The constructs were observed to still be in place after 1 week in a fully mobile load-bearing rabbit joint, although the time period was insufficient for significant neocartilage formation.

Chitosan represents a promising scaffold for cartilage tissue engineering. Its chemical composition directly affects its properties *in vivo*. As the degree of deacetylation of chitosan increases, its residence time *in vivo* increases and the inflammatory reaction that it incites decreases (Chenite, 2000). As a polycationic molecule, chitosan naturally adheres to biological tissues, which usually have a net negative surface charge. This may explain its retention in rabbit articular defects despite free joint mobility (Hoemann *et al.*, 2005), and despite chitosan's initial lack of mechanical strength. In addition, chitosan preparations do not rely on potentially toxic cross-linking agents or organic solvents, thus minimizing toxicity to encapsulated cells or the host in which it is implanted (Chenite *et al.*, 2000).

Alginate

Alginates are polysaccharides derived from seaweed, consisting of a family of linear mannuronate–guluronate copolymers that differ in their sequence and specific composition (Rowley *et al.*, 1999). Addition of a divalent cation such as calcium results in the polymerization of alginate to form an insoluble hydrogel. The polymerization of alginate is mediated by ionic forces and is completely reversible by chelating the divalent cation used for polymerization (Paige *et al.*, 1996). Alginate hydrogels have been used to encapsulate chondrocytes and for growth factor delivery (Suzuki *et al.*, 2000).

Support of chondrocyte growth and matrix secretion during 3D culture in alginate is well documented (Paige *et al.*, 1996; Rowley *et al.*, 1999; Kamil *et al.*, 2004; Chia *et al.*, 2005). Chia *et al.* (2005) cultured human nasal septal chondrocytes in alginate and compared them with controls in monolayer culture. The outcomes studied were proliferation, collagen synthesis and GAG synthesis. Chondrocytes cultured in alginate proliferated less than those in monolayer but produced significantly more GAG and type II collagen. In comparison, chondrocytes in monolayer culture demonstrated greater type I collagen synthesis and minimal GAG secretion.

Alginate hydrogels are useful for cartilage tissue engineering, because of their lack of toxicity, their ease of handling and their minimal inflammatory response (Kamil *et al.*, 2004). As with most hydrogels, their mechanical strength is sufficient for non-load-bearing applications, or for implantation after *in vitro* or *in vivo* culture for several weeks, but their initial fragility is a problem for high-stress environments such as weight-bearing joints. One interesting application of alginate is in the promotion of chondrocyte phenotype and enhanced function during *in vitro* culture. Following culture, the hydrogel is dissolved with a chelating agent and the expanded chondrocytes are recovered for use, e.g. in autologous chondrocyte transplantation (Diduch *et al.*, 2000; Homicz *et al.*, 2003). Other investigators have studied modifications of alginate in order to control more precisely its mechanical properties and degradation rate. Strategies have involved altering the molecular weight of the polymer chains that make up the hydrogel, the use of partial oxidation to form hydrolyzable points in the polysaccharide chain, and the functionalization of residues along the polysaccharide chain in order to make use of covalent cross-linking with more predictable mechanical and degradation characteristics (Kong *et al.*, 2004; Lee *et al.*, 2001, 2004b; Boontheekul *et al.*, 2005).

Homicz *et al.* (2003) studied the redifferentiation of human nasal septal chondrocytes in three culture systems: alginate, PGA fibre and a high-density monolayer. Chondrocytes were subjected to initial monolayer expansion prior to seeding in each of these three systems. The chondrocytes were noted to have an elongated fibroblastic morphology after initial expansion. Outcome measures included morphological analysis, morphological quantification of proliferation, and GAG synthesis. It was observed that chondrocytes regained their native morphology in alginate culture and produced large quantities of GAG, although their proliferation was significantly less than that observed in a high-density monolayer. In contrast, chondrocytes proliferated in a high-density monolayer, but the total GAG content and GAG per cell were significantly less than that produced by chondrocytes culture in alginate.

Hyaluronan

Hyaluronan (i.e. HA) is a polysaccharide that is naturally found in cartilage ECM and in synovial fluid. Hyaluronan injection has been used to treat the symptoms of osteoarthritis, and hyaluronan has been shown to have a stimulatory effect on chondrocyte matrix secretion (Akmal *et al.*, 2005). Hyalograft C, a commercially available tissue-engineered graft composed of autologous chondrocytes seeded on to a preformed nonwoven HA scaffold, has been in clinical use since 1999 in Europe for the treatment of full-thickness osteochondral defects (Marcacci *et al.*, 2005). Nettles *et al.* (2004) recently described the synthesis of methacrylate-modified hyaluronan which, when mixed with a photoinitiator, is capable of photo-cross-linking *in situ* to form a stable hydrogel. This hydrogel was similar to others in terms of mechanical properties and supported chondrocyte growth and matrix secretion *in vitro*. It was also noted that application of photo-cross-linked hyaluronan to a rabbit knee osteochondral defect, without cells or growth factors, led to infiltration of surrounding cells into the hydrogel and new tissue formation by 2 weeks. This neocartilage was well integrated with surrounding tissue but was fibrocartilaginous in nature. The properties of hyaluronan hydrogels may be easily modified by altering the amount of hyaluronan, the degree of modification (i.e. methacrylation), the degree of cross-linking, the chemical nature of the modifying entity (Nettles *et al.*, 2004), as well as by adding specific functional moieties such as RGD-containing cell adhesion peptides and growth factors (Hsu *et al.*, 2004). Further study will be necessary to determine the suitability of hyaluronan hydrogels for various potential clinical applications.

Synthetic polymers

Poly(ethylene oxide)

PEO is a synthetic polymer used in cartilage tissue engineering. The low-molecular-weight form of PEO is known as PEG. It may be modified to yield a photo-cross-linkable polymer that forms a solid hydrogel on exposure to light. This photopolymer can be used to encapsulate chondrocytes and growth factors for tissue-engineering applications (Elisseeff *et al.*, 1999a, 1999b). There is substantial interest in photopolymerizing polymers for tissue engineering because they lend themselves to minimally invasive applications and they offer the ability to control precisely the formation of engineered tissues (Elisseeff *et al.*, 1999a, 1999b).

It has been observed that altering the cross-linking density of the polymerized hydrogel has a profound impact on chondrocyte proliferation and matrix synthesis. Bryant *et al.* (2004) encapsulated chondrocytes in PEG hydrogels with two different cross-linking densities (10% and 20%) of poly(ethylene glycol) dimethylacrylate (PEGDM), under free-swelling and dynamic loading conditions. Outcome measures were proliferation and GAG synthesis. It was shown that higher cross-linking densities were associated with lower proliferation and GAG synthesis. In addition, dynamic loading (0–15% compression at 1 Hz) resulted in significantly lower proliferation compared with free-swelling controls, and significantly lower GAG synthesis in the 20% PEGDM hydrogel.

Alterations in hydrogel degradation rate also appear to have a significant effect on the structure of engineered tissue. Bryant *et al.* (2003) generated a hydrogel composed of a copolymer of degradable PLA-*b*-PEG-*b*-PLA and nondegradable PEGDM. Varying the ratio of the degradable and nondegradable components generated hydrogels with a range of degradation profiles. It was observed that total deoxyribonucleic acid (DNA) content after *in vitro* culture for 6 weeks in the hydrogels with 75–85% degradable copolymer was nearly twice that in the hydrogels with 50% degradable polymer. Furthermore, the total collagen content in the 85% hydrogel was significantly higher than that in the 50% gel. Interestingly, the degradation of the hydrogels had a significant influence on the distribution of secreted matrix components. The gels with higher degradable cross-links showed type II collagen throughout the gel, while type II collagen was confined to the pericellular region in the 50% gels.

Our group and others have studied the construction of osteochondral engineered tissues by generating bilayered constructs using sequential photopolymerization (Alhadlaq and Mao, 2003, 2005). A refinement of this technique involves the use of 3D photolithography. This technique, described by Liu and Bhatia (2002), involves using a printed mask to photopolymerize selectively a PEGDA solution containing fluorescent-stained cells within a specially constructed chamber. By utilizing different masks in sequence, a complex, fine-resolution and spatially organized structure containing discrete cell populations was generated. This highlights the potential of photo-cross-linkable polymers to be used to engineer complex structures that may more closely approximate native tissues.

Poly(vinyl alcohol)

Poly(vinyl alcohol) (PVA) is synthesized from poly(vinyl acetate) by hydrolysis, alcoholysis or aminolysis (Lee and Mooney, 2001). It forms hydrogels by covalent cross-linking in the presence of glutaraldehyde in an acid environment (Nuttelman *et al.*, 2001). Once polymerized, it is essentially non-degradable *in vivo*, although a photopolymerizable degradable PVA-based hydrogel has been described (Nuttelman *et al.*, 2002). The primary advantage of PVA is that it forms a relatively strong, elastic and flexible hydrogel that has abundant functional sites for the attachment of peptides, growth factors and adhesion molecules. For example, Nuttelman *et al.* (2001) synthesized a PVA hydrogel covalently modified with fibronectin and studied fibroblast attachment and proliferation on this matrix. Fibroblast attachment was significantly enhanced on the modified PVA hydrogel compared with unmodified PVA, and proliferation was greater than that observed on tissue-culture polystyrene. However, the polymerization of PVA requires reagents and conditions that are not suitable for *in situ* applications.

Synthetic self-assembling peptides

A novel class of synthetic peptides spontaneously assembles to form hydrogels based on changes in pH and/or ionic strength. These peptides are characterized by a self-complementary structure of regularly alternating units of positively and negatively charged residues separated by hydrophobic residues (Holmes, 2002). These peptides self-assemble under specific conditions of pH and ionic strength to form β-sheet structures that then aggregate to form a hydrogel composed of interweaving nanofibers (Kisiday *et al.*, 2002). The unique feature of these hydrogels is their fibrillar microstructure, which is approximately three orders of magnitude smaller than that of other polymer hydrogels (Holmes, 2002). Kisiday *et al.* (2002) encapsulated chondrocytes in a peptide-based hydrogel for 3D *in vitro* culture. Maintenance of chondrocyte phenotype and matrix secretion was observed as for other hydrogels, but the proliferation of chondrocytes cultured in the peptide hydrogel was significantly higher than in agarose (Kisiday *et al.*, 2002, 2004). Peptide hydrogels offer nearly unlimited design potential because of the ability to vary the sequence and composition of the component peptides. In addition, functional domains such as the RGD cell adhesion motif may be easily incorporated into the peptide (Holmes, 2002).

3.5 Future trends

At this point, the ability of a wide variety of materials to support the growth and function of chondrocytes and chondrogenic capable stem cells is well documented. Hydrogels, in particular, offer the potential for minimally invasive applications using materials with proven biocompatibility and little or no toxicity and immunogenic potential. As discussed earlier in this chapter a promising technology includes self-assembling hydrogels. Self-assembling hydrogels allow for increased control over *in situ* polymerization and are suitable for minimally invasive applications that will probably speed their translation into clinical use. In addition, the fibrillar microstructure of self-assembling hydrogels has the potential to better mimic the structure of native cartilage ECM, thereby enhancing tissue-engineered cartilage.

Biomimetic hydrogels have great potential for *in vivo* applications of tissue engineering. Growth factors and other bioactive molecules that are regularly added to media to enhance *in vitro* chondrogenic differentiation are now added to hydrogel for local delivery with *in vivo* implants. Greater control over the release of growth factors when needed by encapsulated cells should significantly improve cartilage tissue production.

As a class, hydrogels suffer from poor mechanical strength, particularly immediately after encapsulation and in the setting of high-stress environments. Since there is such a large range of hydrogels that can potentially be used in tissue-engineering applications, and those hydrogels may be further customized by the addition of structural and functional modifications, a hit-or-miss approach to material selection and design is unlikely to yield optimal results with an acceptable expenditure of time or resources. A rational design approach to material engineering, in terms of both the mechanical properties and the ability to support cell growth and function, is probably required. Thorough and systematic materials testing, possibly making use of the tools of high-throughput materials analysis, will reveal trends in hydrogel parameters that may then be used to focus efforts to optimize these materials (Abramson *et al.*, 2005; Anderson *et al.*, 2005). An integral part of this effort will be correlating the microstructural, biochemical, histological and mechanical properties of hydrogels and the tissues engineered from them.

An emerging trend in cartilage engineering is the awareness of the effects of dynamic stresses on engineered and native tissues. As the ultrastructural features of a given hydrogel affect how it reacts to and transmits stresses to the cells that reside within it, detailed study of the structural and mechanical properties and how they affect cellular growth and function will become more important.

Finally, there is a need for further studies of tissue-engineered cartilage in large-animal models. The current focus on *in vitro* and small-animal *in vivo* studies is appropriate for answering fundamental questions regarding the properties of engineered tissues, but translation to large-animal models will be critical for clinical translation. As certain tissue-engineering techniques come closer to clinical application, there will be a need for *in vivo* testing that more closely approximates the conditions and stresses that will be encountered by engineered tissues implanted in humans.

3.6 Sources of further information and advice

Lowman and Peppas (1999) provided an excellent summary of hydrogels in their book. They described the structure and properties, classification and applications of hydrogels.

Varghese and Elisseeff (2006) have reviewed natural and synthetic hydrogels and their applications to musculoskeletal tissue engineering. They addressed current applications in regenerative medicine including biomimetic hydrogels containing bioactive factors and hydrogels as scaffolds for mesenchymal and embryonic stem cells to create biological implants.

Drury and Mooney (2003) have reviewed hydrogel materials and hydrogel design variables in applications for space-filling defect sites and for delivery of bioactive molecules and cells.

Tirelli *et al.* (2002), in a review article, described their laboratory's research into augmenting PEG with other polymers and varying end groups for specific hydrogel functionalization.

Peter *et al.* (1998) discussed the applications of hydrogels in skeletal tissue engineering and their complementary role with current surgical therapies. The review focuses on bone tissue engineering using biodegradable hydrogels.

The Society for Biomaterials is a professional society that promotes advances in biomaterials research and development. Their website www.biomaterials.org provides links to special interest groups including one dedicated to tissue engineering.

The Materials Research Society is a professional organization of materials researchers that promotes the advancement of interdisciplinary materials research. The society hosts semiannual meetings and monthly bulletins including hydrogels and tissue engineering. More information may be found on their website www.mrs.org.

3.7 References

Abramson S D, Alexe G, Hammer P L and Kohn J (2005), 'A computational approach to predicting cell growth on polymeric biomaterials', *J Biomed Mater Res A*, **73**(1) 116–124.

Akmal M, Singh A, Anand A, Kesani A, Aslam N, Goodship A and Bentley G (2005), 'The effects of hyaluronic acid on articular chondrocytes', *J Bone Jt Surg Br*, **87**(8) 1143–1149.

Alhadlaq A and Mao J J (2003), 'Tissue-engineered neogenesis of human-shaped mandibular condyle from rat mesenchymal stem cells', *J Dent Res*, **82**(12) 951–956.

Alhadlaq A and Mao J J (2005), 'Tissue-engineered osteochondral constructs in the shape of an articular condyle', *J Bone Jt Surg Am*, **87**(5) 936–944.

Alsberg E, Anderson K W, Albeiruti A, Franceschi R T and Mooney D J (2001), 'Cell-interactive alginate hydrogels for bone tissue engineering', *J Dent Res*, **80**(11) 2025–2029.

Alsberg E, Anderson K W, Albeiruti A, Rowley J A and Mooney D J (2002), 'Engineering growing tissues', *Proc Natl Acad Sci USA*, **99**(19) 12 025–12 030.

Alsberg E, Kong H J, Hirano Y, Smith M K, Albeiruti A and Mooney D J (2003), 'Regulating bone formation via controlled scaffold degradation', *J Dent Res*, **82**(11) 903–908.

Anderson D G, Putnam D, Lavik E B, Mahmood T A and Langer R (2005), 'Biomaterial microarrays: rapid, microscale screening of polymer–cell interaction', *Biomaterials*, **26**(23) 4892–4897.

Andrianov A K, Payne L G, Visscher K B, Allcock H R and Langer R (1994), 'Hydrolytic degradation of ionically crosslinked polyphosphazene microspheres', *J Appl Polym Sci*, **53**(12) 1573–1578.

Anseth K S, Metters A T, Bryant S J, Martens P J, Elisseeff J H and Bowman C N (2002), '*In situ* forming degradable networks and their application in tissue engineering and drug delivery', *J Control Release*, **78**(1–3) 199–209.

Baier Leach J, Bivens K A, Patrick C W and Schmidt C E (2002), 'Photocrosslinked hyaluronic acid hydrogels: natural, biodegradable tissue engineering scaffolds', *Biotechnol Bioeng*, **82** 578–589.

Benya P D and Shaffer J D (1982), 'Dedifferentiated chondrocytes reexpress the differentiated collagen phenotype when cultured in agarose gels', *Cell*, **30**(1) 215–224.

Boontheekul T, Kong H J and Mooney D J (2005), 'Controlling alginate gel degradation utilizing partial oxidation and bimodal molecular weight distribution', *Biomaterials*, **26**(15) 2455–2465.

Bouhadir K H, Alsberg E and Mooney D J (2001), 'Hydrogels for combination delivery of antineoplastic agents', *Biomaterials*, **22**(19) 2625–2633.

Brown C D, Stayton P S and Hoffman A S (2005), 'Semi-interpenetrating network of poly(ethylene glycol) and poly(D,L-lactide) for the controlled delivery of protein drugs', *J Biomater Sci, Polym Edn*, **16**(2) 189–201.

Bryant S J and Anseth K S (2003), 'Controlling the spatial distribution of ECM components in degradable PEG hydrogels for tissue engineering cartilage', *J Biomed Mater Res A*, **64**(1) 70–79.

Bryant S J, Chowdhury T T, Lee D A, Bader D L and Anseth K S (2004), 'Crosslinking density influences chondrocyte metabolism in dynamically loaded photocrosslinked poly(ethylene glycol) hydrogels', *Ann Biomed Eng*, **32**(3) 407–417.

Burdick J A and Anseth K S (2002a), 'Photoencapsulation of osteoblasts in injectable RGD-modified PEG hydrogels for bone tissue engineering', *Biomaterials*, **23**(22) 4315–4223.

Burdick J A, Mason M N, Hinman A D, Thorne K and Anseth K S (2002), 'Delivery of osteoinductive growth factors from degradable PEG hydrogels influences osteoblast differentiation and mineralization', *J Control Release*, **83**(1) 53–63.

Canal T and Peppas N A (1989), 'Correlation between mesh size and equilibrium degree of swelling of polymeric networks', *J Biomed Mater Res*, **23**(10) 1183–1193.

Chang S C, Tobias G, Roy A K, Vacanti C A and Bonassar L J (2003), 'Tissue engineering of autologous cartilage for craniofacial reconstruction by injection molding', *Plast Reconstr Surg*, **112**(3) 793–799; discussion, 800–791.

Chenite A, Chaput C, Wang D, Combes C, Buschmann M D, Hoemann C D, Leroux J C, Atkinson B L, Binette F and Selmani A (2000), 'Novel injectable neutral solutions of chitosan form biodegradable gels *in situ*', *Biomaterials*, **21**(21) 2155–2161.

Chia S H, Homicz M R, Schumacher B L, Thonar E J M A, Masuda K, Sah R L and Watson D (2005), 'Characterization of human nasal septal chondrocytes cultured in alginate', *J Am Coll of Surgeons*, **200**(5) 691–704.

Corkhill P H, Hamilton C J and Tighe B J (1989), 'Synthetic hydrogels VI: hydrogel composites as wound dressings and implant materials', *Biomaterials*, **10**(1) 3–10.

Cruise G M, Scharp D S and Hubbell J A (1998), 'Characterization of permeability and network structure of interfacially photopolymerized poly(ethylene glycol) diacrylate hydrogels', *Biomaterials*, **19**(14) 1287–1294.

Dausse Y, Grossin L, Miralles G, Pelletier S, Mainard D, Hubert P, Baptiste D, Gillet P, Dellacherie E, Netter P and Payan E (2003), 'Cartilage repair using new polysaccharidic biomaterials: macroscopic, histological and biochemical approaches in a rat model of cartilage defect', *Osteoarthritis Cartilage*, **11**(1) 16–28.

Diduch D R, Jordan L C, Mierisch C M and Balian G (2000), 'Marrow stromal cells embedded in alginate for repair of osteochondral defects', *Arthroscopy*, **16**(6) 571–577.

Drury J L, Dennis R G and Mooney D J (2004), 'The tensile properties of alginate hydrogels', *Biomaterials*, **25**(16) 3187–3199.

Drury J L and Mooney D J (2003), 'Hydrogels for tissue engineering: scaffold design variables and applications', *Biomaterials*, **24**(24) 4337–4351.

Elisseeff J, Anseth K, Sims D, McIntosh W, Randolph M and Langer R (1999a), 'Transdermal photopolymerization for minimally invasive implantation', *Proc Natl Acad Sci USA*, **96**(6) 3104–3107.

Elisseeff J, Anseth K, Sims D, McIntosh W, Randolph M, Yaremchuk M and Langer R (1999b), 'Transdermal photopolymerization of poly(ethylene oxide)-based injectable hydrogels for tissue-engineered cartilage', *Plast Reconstr Surg*, **104**(4) 1014–1022.

Elisseeff J, McIntosh W, Anseth K, Riley S, Ragan P and Langer R (2000), 'Photoencapsulation of chondrocytes in poly(ethylene oxide)-based semi-interpenetrating networks', *J Biomed Mater Res*, **51**(2) 164–171.

Elisseeff J, McIntosh W, Fu K, Blunk B T and Langer R (2001), 'Controlled-release of IGF-I and TGF-beta1 in a photopolymerizing hydrogel for cartilage tissue engineering', *J Orthop Res*, **19**(6) 1098–1104.

Elisseeff J, Puleo C, Yang F and Sharma B (2005), 'Advances in skeletal tissue engineering with hydrogels', *Orthod Craniofac Res*, **8**(3) 150–161.

Flory P J and Rehner J (1943), 'Statistical mechanics of cross-linked polymer networks II. Swelling', *J Chem Phys*, **11**(11) 521–526.

Flynn L, Dalton P D and Shoichet M S (2003), 'Fiber templating of poly(2-hydroxyethyl methacrylate) for neural tissue engineering', *Biomaterials*, **24**(23) 4265–4272.

Frenkel S R and Di Cesare P E (2004), 'Scaffolds for articular cartilage repair', *Ann Biomed Eng*, **32**(1) 26–34.
Gehrke S H, Fisher J P, Palasis M and Lund M E (1997), 'Factors determining hydrogel permeability', *Ann NY Acad Sci*, **831** 179–207.
Hennink W E and van Nostrum C F (2002), 'Novel crosslinking methods to design hydrogels', *Adv Drug Deliv Rev*, **54**(1) 13–36.
Hern D L and Hubbell J A (1998), 'Incorporation of adhesion peptides into nonadhesive hydrogels useful for tissue resurfacing', *J Biomed Mater Res*, **39**(2) 266–276.
Hoemann C D, Sun J, Legare A, McKee M D and Buschmann M D (2005), 'Tissue engineering of cartilage using an injectable and adhesive chitosan-based cell-delivery vehicle', *Osteoarthritis Cartilage*, **13**(4) 318–329.
Holmes T C (2002), 'Novel peptide-based biomaterial scaffolds for tissue engineering', *Trends Biotechnol*, **20**(1) 16–21.
Homicz M R, Chia S H, Schumacher B L, Masuda K, Thonar E J, Sah R L and Watson D (2003), 'Human septal chondrocyte redifferentiation in alginate, polyglycolic acid scaffold, and monolayer culture', *Laryngoscope*, **113**(1) 25–32.
Hsu S-H, Whu S W, Hsieh S-C, Tsai C-L, Chen D C and Tan T-S (2004), 'Evaluation of chitosan–alginate–hyaluronate complexes modified by an RGD-containing protein as tissue-engineering scaffolds for cartilage regeneration', *Artif Organs*, **28**(8) 693–703.
Kabanov A V, Batrakova E V and Alakhov V Y (2002), 'Pluronic block copolymers as novel polymer therapeutics for drug and gene delivery', *J Control Release*, **82**(2–3) 189–212.
Kamil S H, Vacanti M P, Aminuddin B S, Jackson M J, Vacanti C A and Eavey R D (2004), 'Tissue engineering of a human sized and shaped auricle using a mold', *Laryngoscope*, **114**(5) 867–870.
Kim U J, Park J, Li C, Jin H J, Valluzzi R and Kaplan D L (2004), 'Structure and properties of silk hydrogels', *Biomacromolecules*, **5**(3) 786–792.
Kisiday J D, Jin M, DiMicco M A, Kurz B and Grodzinsky A J (2004), 'Effects of dynamic compressive loading on chondrocyte biosynthesis in self-assembling peptide scaffolds', *J Biomech*, **37**(5) 595–604.
Kisiday J, Jin M, Kurz B, Hung H, Semino C, Zhang S and Grodzinsky A J (2002), 'Self-assembling peptide hydrogel fosters chondrocyte extracellular matrix production and cell division: implications for cartilage tissue repair', *Proc Natl Acad Sci USA*, **99**(15) 9996–10 001.
Kong H J, Kaigler D, Kim K and Mooney D J (2004), 'Controlling rigidity and degradation of alginate hydrogels via molecular weight distribution', *Biomacromolecules*, **5**(5) 1720–1727.
Lee J E, Kim S E, Kwon I C, Ahn H J, Cho H, Lee S-H, Kim H J, Seong S C and Lee M C (2004a), 'Effects of a chitosan scaffold containing TGF-beta1 encapsulated chitosan microspheres on in vitro chondrocyte culture', *Artif Organs*, **28**(9) 829–839.
Lee K Y, Bouhadir K H and Mooney D J (2004b), 'Controlled degradation of hydrogels using multi-functional cross-linking molecules', *Biomaterials*, **25**(13) 2461–2466.
Lee K Y and Mooney D J (2001), 'Hydrogels for tissue engineering', *Chem Rev*, **101**(7) 1869–1879.

Lee K Y, Peters M C, Anderson K W and Mooney D J (2000a), 'Controlled growth factor release from synthetic extracellular matrices', *Nature*, **408**(6815) 998–1000.
Lee K Y, Rowley J A, Eiselt P, Moy E M, Bouhadir K H and Mooney D J (2000b), 'Controlling mechanical and swelling properties of alginate hydrogels independently by cross-linker type and cross-linking density', *Macromolecules*, **33**(11) 4291–4294.
LeRoux M A, Guilak F and Setton L A (1999), 'Compressive and shear properties of alginate gel: effects of sodium ions and alginate concentration', *J Biomed Mater Res*, **47**(1) 46–53.
Levesque S G, Lim R M and Shoichet M S (2005), 'Macroporous interconnected dextran scaffolds of controlled porosity for tissue-engineering applications', *Biomaterials*, **26**(35) 7436–7446.
Li Q, Wang J, Shahani S, Sun D D, Sharma B, Elisseeff J H and Leong K W (2006), 'Biodegradable and photocrosslinkable polyphosphoester hydrogel', *Biomaterials*, **27**(7) 1027–1034.
Liu V A and Bhatia S N (2002), 'Three-dimensional photopatterning of hydrogels containing living cells', *Biomed Microdevices*, **4**(4) 257–266.
Lowman A M and Peppas N A (1997), 'Analysis of the complexation/decomplexation phenomena in graft copolymer networks', *Macromolecules*, **30**(17) 4959–4965.
Lowman A M and Peppas N A (1999) 'Hydrogels'. in Mathiowitz E, *Encyclopedia of Controlled Drug Delivery* (Ed E Mathiowitz), New York, Wiley, pp. 397–418.
Lutolf M P, Weber F E, Schmoekel H G, Schense J C, Kohler T, Muller R and Hubbell J A (2003), 'Repair of bone defects using synthetic mimetics of collagenous extracellular matrices', *Nat Biotechnol*, **21**(5) 513–518.
Marcacci M, Berruto M, Brocchetta D, Delcogliano A, Ghinelli D, Gobbi A, Kon E, Pederzini L, Rosa D, Sacchetti G L, Stefani G and Zanasi S (2005), 'Articular cartilage engineering with Hyalograft C: 3-year clinical results', *Clin Orthop Relat Res*, **435** 96–105.
Martens P J, Bryant S J and Anseth K S (2003), 'Tailoring the degradation of hydrogels formed from multivinyl poly(ethylene glycol) and poly(vinyl alcohol) macromers for cartilage tissue engineering', *Biomacromolecules*, **4**(2) 283–292.
Mercier N R, Costantino H R, Tracy M A and Bonassar L J (2004), 'A novel injectable approach for cartilage formation *in vivo* using PLG microspheres', *Ann of Biomed Eng*, **32**(3) 418–429.
Mikos A G, Bao Y, Cima L G, Ingber D E, Vacanti J P and Langer R (1993), 'Preparation of poly(glycolic acid) bonded fiber structures for cell attachment and transplantation', *J Biomed Mater Res*, **27**(2) 183–189.
Moise O, Sideman S, Hoffer E, Rousseau I and Better O S (1977), 'Membrane permeability for inorganic phosphate ion', *J Biomed Mater Res*, **11**(6) 903–913.
Mooney D J and Mikos A G (1999), 'Growing new organs', *Sci Am*, **280**(4), 60–65.
Murphy S M, Hamilton C J, Davies M L and Tighe B J (1992), 'Polymer membranes in clinical sensor applications II: the design and fabrication of permselective hydrogels for electrochemical devices', *Biomaterials*, **13**(14) 979–990.
Nettles D L, Vail T P, Morgan M T, Grinstaff M W and Setton L A (2004), 'Photocrosslinkable hyaluronan as a scaffold for articular cartilage repair', *Ann Biomed Eng*, **32**(3) 391–397.

Nguyen K T and West J L (2002), 'Photopolymerizable hydrogels for tissue engineering applications', *Biomaterials*, **23**(22) 4307–4314.
Noomrio M H, Zhang R, Eisenthal R and Hubble J (2005), 'Characterisation of hydrogel swelling by molecular exclusion', *Biotechnol Lett*, **27**(20) 1587–1590.
Nuttelman C R, Henry S M and Anseth K S (2002), 'Synthesis and characterization of photocrosslinkable, degradable poly(vinyl alcohol)-based tissue engineering scaffolds', *Biomaterials*, **23**(17) 3617–3626.
Nuttelman C R, Mortisen D J, Henry S M and Anseth K S (2001), 'Attachment of fibronectin to poly(vinyl alcohol) hydrogels promotes NIH3T3 cell adhesion, proliferation, and migration', *J Biomed Mater Res*, **57**(2) 217–223.
Paige K T, Cima L G, Yaremchuk M J, Schloo B L, Vacanti J P and Vacanti C A (1996), 'De novo cartilage generation using calcium alginate–chondrocyte constructs', *Plast Reconstr Surg*, **97**(1) 168–178; discussion, 179–180.
Park Y D, Tirelli N and Hubbell J A (2003), 'Photopolymerized hyaluronic acid-based hydrogels and interpenetrating networks', *Biomaterials*, **24**(6) 893–900.
Peppas N A, Bures P, Leobandung W and Ichikawa H (2000), 'Hydrogels in pharmaceutical formulations', *Eur J Pharm Biopharm*, **50**(1) 27–46.
Peppas N A and Merrill E W (1977), 'Crosslinked poly(vinyl alcohol) hydrogels as swollen elastic networks', *J Appl Polym Sci*, **21**(7) 1763–1770.
Peter S J, Miller M J, Yasko A W, Yaszemski M J and Mikos A G (1998), 'Polymer concepts in tissue engineering', *J Biomed Mater Res*, **43**(4) 422–427.
Peters M C, Isenberg B C, Rowley J A and Mooney D J (1998), 'Release from alginate enhances the biological activity of vascular endothelial growth factor', *J Biomater Sci, Polym Edn*, **9**(12) 1267–1278.
Rosenblatt J, Devereux B and Wallace D G (1994), 'Injectable collagen as a pH-sensitive hydrogel', *Biomaterials*, **15**(12) 985–995.
Rowley J A, Madlambayan G and Mooney D J (1999), 'Alginate hydrogels as synthetic extracellular matrix materials', *Biomaterials*, **20**(1) 45–53.
Sawhney A S, Pathak C P and Hubbell J A (1993), 'Interfacial photopolymerization of poly(ethylene glycol)-based hydrogels upon alginate–poly(L-lysine) microcapsules for enhanced biocompatibility', *Biomaterials*, **14**(13) 1008–1016.
Sawhney A S, Pathak C P, van Rensburg J J, Dunn R C and Hubbell J A (1994), 'Optimization of photopolymerized bioerodible hydrogel properties for adhesion prevention', *J Biomed Mater Res*, **28**(7), 831–838.
Segura T, Anderson B C, Chung P H, Webber R E, Shull K R and Shea L D (2005), 'Crosslinked hyaluronic acid hydrogels: a strategy to functionalize and pattern', *Biomaterials*, **26**(4) 359–371.
Sharma B and Elisseeff J H (2004), 'Engineering structurally organized cartilage and bone tissues', *Ann Biomed Eng*, **32**(1) 148–159.
Shu X Z, Ghosh K, Liu Y, Palumbo F S, Luo Y, Clark R A and Prestwich G D (2004a), 'Attachment and spreading of fibroblasts on an RGD peptide-modified injectable hyaluronan hydrogel', *J Biomed Mater Res A*, **68**(2) 365–375.
Shu X Z, Liu Y C, Palumbo F S, Luo Y and Prestwich G D (2004b), '*In situ* crosslinkable hyaluronan hydrogels for tissue engineering', *Biomaterials*, **25**(7–8) 1339–1348.
Shung A K, Behravesh E, Jo S and Mikos A G (2003), 'Crosslinking characteristics of and cell adhesion to an injectable poly(propylene fumarate-co-ethylene

glycol) hydrogel using a water-soluble crosslinking system', *Tissue Eng*, **9**(2) 243–254.

Stock R S and Ray W H (1985), 'Interpretation of photon-correlation spectroscopy data – a comparison of analysis-methods', *J Polym Sci, Polym Phys*, **23**(7) 1393–1447.

Suzuki Y, Tanihara M, Suzuki K, Saitou A, Sufan W and Nishimura Y (2000), 'Alginate hydrogel linked with synthetic oligopeptide derived from BMP-2 allows ectopic osteoinduction *in vivo*', *J Biomed Mater Res*, **50**(3) 405–409.

Tabata Y, Nagano A and Ikada Y (1999), 'Biodegradation of hydrogel carrier incorporating fibroblast growth factor', *Tissue Eng*, **5**(2) 127–138.

Tirelli N, Lutolf M P, Napoli A and Hubbell J A (2002), 'Poly(ethylene glycol) block copolymers', *J Biotechnol*, **90**(1) 3–15.

Traitel T, Kost J and Lapidot S A (2003), 'Modeling ionic hydrogels swelling: characterization of the non-steady state', *Biotechnol Bioeng*, **84**(1) 20–28.

Trevors J T and Pollack G H (2005), 'Hypothesis: the origin of life in a hydrogel environment', *Prog Biophys Mol Biol*, **89**(1) 1–8.

Varghese S and Elisseeff J H (2006), 'Hydrogels for musculoskeletal tissue engineering', *Adv Polym Sci*, **203** 95–144.

von der Mark K, Gauss V, von der Mark H and Muller P (1977), 'Relationship between cell shape and type of collagen synthesised as chondrocytes lose their cartilage phenotype in culture', *Nature*, **267**(5611) 531–532.

Wang D, Williams C G, Li Q, Sharma B and Elisseeff J H (2003), 'Synthesis and characterization of a novel biodegradable phosphate-containing hydrogel', *Biomaterials*, **24**(22) 3969–3980.

Wang D, Williams C G, Yang F, Cher N, Lee H and Elisseeff J H (2005), 'Bioresponsive phophoester hydrogels for bone tissue engineering', *Tissue Eng*, **11**(1–2) 201–213.

Wang D A, Williams C G, Yang F and Elisseeff J H (2004), 'Enhancing the tissue–biomaterial interface: tissue-initiated integration of biomaterials', *Adv Funct Mater* **14** 1152–1159.

West J L and Hubbell J A (1995), 'Photopolymerized hydrogel materials for drug-delivery applications', *Reactive Polym*, **25**(2–3) 139–147.

Westreich R, Kaufman M, Gannon P and Lawson W (2004), 'Validating the subcutaneous model of injectable autologous cartilage using a fibrin glue scaffold', *Laryngoscope*, **114**(12) 2154–2160.

Wichterle O (1978), 'The beginning of the soft lens', in *Soft Contact Lenses: Clinical and Applied Technology* (Ed M Ruben), London, Baillière Tindall, pp. 3–5.

Wichterle O and Lim D (1960), 'Hydrophilic gels for biological use', *Nature*, **185**(4706) 117–118.

Williams C G, Kim T K, Taboas A, Malik A, Manson P and Elisseeff J (2003), '*In vitro* chondrogenesis of bone-marrow derived mesenchymal stem cells in a photopolymerizing hydrogel', *Tissue Eng*, **9**(4) 679–688.

Xu J W, Johnson T S, Motarjem P M, Peretti G M, Randolph M A and Yaremchuk M J (2005), 'Tissue-engineered flexible ear-shaped cartilage', *Plast Reconstr Surg*, **115**(6) 1633–1641.

Xu J W, Zaporojan V, Peretti G M, Roscs R E, Morse K B, Roy A K, Mesa J M, Randolph M A, Bonassar L J and Yaremchuk M J (2004), 'Injectable tissue-engineered cartilage with different chondrocyte sources', *Plast Reconstr Surg*, **113**(5) 1361–1371.

Yamamoto M, Tabata Y and Ikada Y (1998), 'Ectopic bone formation induced by biodegradable hydrogels incorporating bone morphogenetic protein', *J Biomater Sci, Polym Edn*, **9**(5) 439–458.

Zhang S (2002), 'Emerging biological materials through molecular self-assembly', *Biotechnol Adv*, **20**(5–6) 321–339.

4

Biodegradable polymers for drug delivery systems

G S KWON and D Y FURGESON,
University of Wisconsin, USA

4.1 Introduction

The development of numerous biodegradable polymers for drug delivery applications has been significant but difficulties remain for researchers, who hope to produce efficacious drug release profiles, all while avoiding pharmacological or toxicological effects from the base polymer. What have resulted are numerous synthetic alternatives for polymer biomaterials retaining bioactivity *in vivo*; yet, now with advanced recombinant technology, pharmaceutical scientists are now also exploring genetically engineered polymers. A defining therapeutic feature of a biodegradable polymer used in modern drug delivery is facile degradation into oligomers or monomers with concomitant kinetically controlled-drug-release profiles. Biodegradable drug carriers are responsible for delivering drugs and then typically degrading through hydrolysis or common proteases for physiological clearance. However, the use of biodegradable polymers for drug delivery is not widespread, in part because of the fear of systemic retention and inability to clear the polymers from the body – commonly termed the macromolecular syndrome.[1–5] The residence time of polymers within cellular compartments has been an issue of some concern regarding biocompatibility and possible long-term toxicological effects; thus biocompatibility remains a prime concern for sustained-drug-release systems. Therefore, there are numerous drug delivery applications for which biodegradable and biocompatible polymers are intended with the underlying onus of controlled drug release through controlled polymer degradation. This chapter will not be an inclusive list of all biodegradable polymers; however, the intent is to highlight the major species of both synthetic and recombinant systems with detailed design, synthesis, degradation and current status in the literature.

4.2 Synthetic biodegradable block copolymers: polyanhydrides, polyalkylcyanoacrylates, polyphosphazenes and polyphosphoesters

Biodegradable polymers are designed for *in vivo* destruction into biocompatible oligomer or monomer units recognized as common metabolic species for clearance from the body. Moreover, degradation rates and possible side products must be considered for the intended application of the delivery system. The intent of biodegradable polymers is the continued transient breakdown of the polymer preventing long-term residence *in vivo* (common with biostable implants) or intracellular sequestration (macromolecular syndrome). Thus, this section focuses upon the wide range of synthetic polymers appropriate for these designs.

4.2.1 Polyanhydrides

In 1909, Bucher and Slade[6] from Brown University reported the relative ease of terephthalic acid and isophthalic acid anhydride synthesis using high temperatures. From there, the synthesis of polyanhydrides has been shown through a number of different techniques including melt polycondensation,[7] dehydrochlorination,[7] dehydrative coupling,[7] and ring-opening polymerization.[8] For high-molecular-weight polyanhydrides, Domb and Langer[9] used dehydration of diacid monomers to form mixed acetic anhydrides following excess acetic anhydride reflux. Further syntheses of polyanhydrides have resulted in two alternative species with one possessing the anhydride bond in the polymer backbone and the other with the anhydride as a side group (Fig. 4.1).

Polyanhydrides are one of the most highly studied biodegradable polymer classes in the literature, no doubt owing in part to the low cost, ease and control of synthesis with degradation products of acid counterparts. In 1983, Langer's group[10] identified the highly labile anhydride linkage (Fig. 1) for

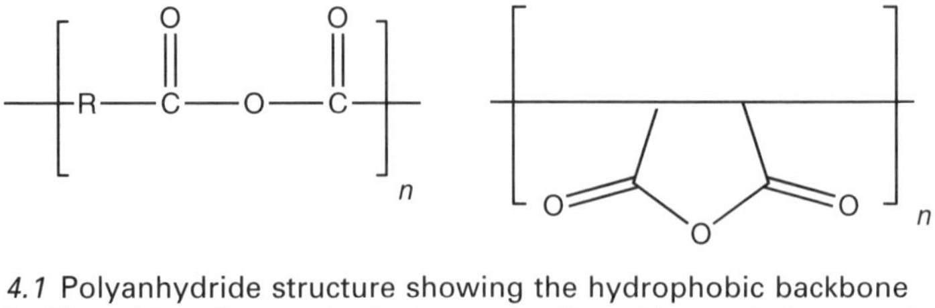

4.1 Polyanhydride structure showing the hydrophobic backbone facilitated by alkane substitution at the R position and the use of the anhydride functional group in the polymer backbone or in a side chain.

hydrolytically biodegradable polymer drug delivery systems by showing zeroth-order release of cholic acid. Subsequent work[11] showed that the degradation rates could be readily controlled by the local hydrophobicity within poly[bis(*p*-carboxyphenoxy) alkane anhydrides] and increasing the pH with biocompatibility studies[12] showing no corneal inflammation over 6 weeks and little subcutaneous inflammation over 6 months. Thus inspired, translation of polyanhydrides to the clinic has produced Gliadel® (polifeprosan 20 carmustine implant), a biodegradable disk containing carmustine indicated for newly diagnosed high-grade malignant gliomas and recurrent glioblastoma multiforme. As an adjunct to surgical resection and radiotherapy, Gliadel® remains the only treatment approved by the Food and Drug Administration for localized biodegradable drug delivery utilizing a biodegradable matrix of 20 : 80 molar ratio poly [(carboxyphenoxy) propane–sebacic anhydride] (Fig. 4.2).[13,14] Block copolymers containing poly(sebacic acid) have also been shown by poly(sebacic acid-co-ricinoleic acid),[15,16] poly(fumaric-co-sebacic anhydride).[17] The backbone of the hydrophobic polyanhydrides precludes rapid degradation of the monolithic matrix by precluding hydration of the inner core; however, surface erosion readily occurs through hydrolytic cleavage of the anhydride bonds. Thus, the degradation rate of polyanhydrides is controlled in large part by monomer composition, especially the hydrophobic R group (Fig. 4.1), illustrated with faster degradation with anhydride bonds between aliphatic rather than aromatic carboxylic acids.[11]

4.2.2 Polyalkylcyanoacrylates

A relative newcomer to polymer-based drug delivery, polyalkylcyanoacrylates (PACAs) emerged through the seminal papers by Speiser's group[18,19] with evolved syntheses through free-radical, anionic or zwitterionic polymerization. Controlled desiccated free-radical or anionic polymerization are most common owing to rapid polymerization kinetics at ambient conditions and with common physiological initiators such as water and amino acids. It is this property that makes PACAs an ideal choice for a tissue binding agent, beyond the scope of this review. Moreover, PACAs have

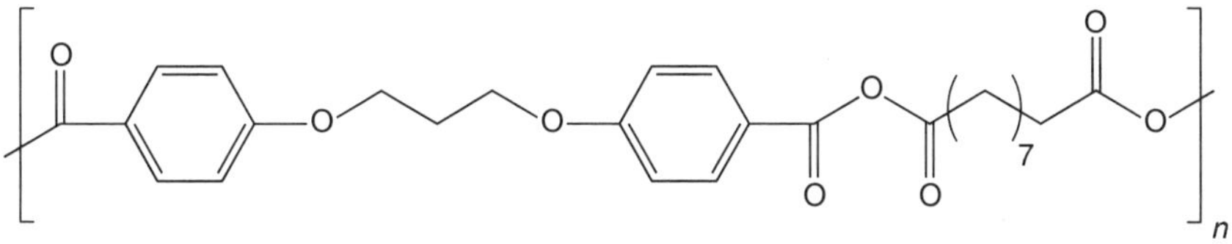

4.2 Poly[(carboxyphenoxy)propane–sebacic acid], the biodegradable polymer matrix found in Gliadel®.

4.3 PACA structure showing the highly activated methylene hydrogen atoms from the neighboring cyano and –COOR groups.

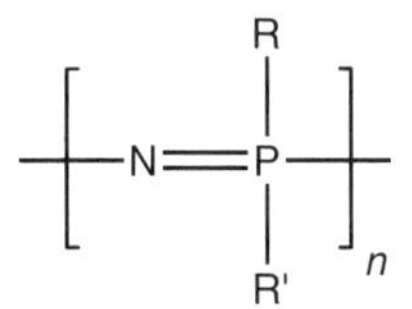

4.4 Polyphosphazene monomer unit.

evolved diverse versatility as drug nanoparticle carriers for indomethacin,[20] gangliosides,[21] oligonucleotides,[22] anti-epileptic medications including Ethosuximide,[23] insulin,[24] saquinavir,[25] hemoglobin[26] and nucleoside analogues against human immonodeficiency virus (HIV).[27] PACAs rely upon hydrolytic cleavage of the carbon–carbon bonds by high inductive activation of the methylene hydrogens by the electron-withdrawing cyano and –COOR groups (Fig. 4.3). The alkyl length of the polymer in effect determines the rate and degree of biodegradation;[28,29] however, lower alkyl derivates such as poly (methyl cyanoacrylate) deleteriously degrades into cyanoacetic and formaldehyde by-products through enzymatic cleavage of the ester function, thereby necessitating the synthesis with higher alkyl derivatives with most alternatives as isobutyl derivates. Translational research into poly(ethylene glycol) (PEG)–PACAs[30,31] and actively targeted PACA systems[32,33] have shown great promise for use *in vivo* such as the recently completed phase I and phase II studies of Doxorubicin Transdrug® for primary liver cancer.

4.2.3 Polyphosphazenes

Initially, the striking difference between polyphosphazenes and other established polymers for drug delivery is the inorganic polymer backbone (Fig. 4.4). Furthermore, the polymer possesses two sites for substitution (R and R′) to afford the polymer alternative degradation kinetics[34,35] and functional groups for drug conjugation and presentation of targeting moieties. The capacity for alternative combinations at these substitution sites grants polyphosphazenes high flexibility for a number of applications. Allcock's group first reported the synthesis of polyphosphazenes in 1965 wherein thermoregulated ring-opening polymerization of hexachlorocyclotriphosphazene resulted in linear high-molecular-weight polydichlorophosphazene. Subsequently, dichlorinated polyphosphazene was duly substituted with alkoyx, aryloxy or amino groups,[36] From this seminal work, typical side-group substitution has been shown with amino acid esters,[34,37–42] aryloxy,[43] poly(*N*-isopropylacrylamide),[44] oligoethyleneglycol,[45] glyceryl,[46] glucosyl,[47] imidazolyl,[48,49] 2-dimethylaminoethanol,[50] 2-dimethylaminoethylamine[50] and lactose[51] derivatives. These homogeneous or heterogeneous side groups control the degradation characteristics of polyphosphazenes through their gross physicochemical properties and the ratios derivatized into the polyphosphazene. Hydrolytically unstable polyphosphazenes result from the choice of side-group substituents, regardless of the biodegradation products produce phosphates, ammonia and the accompanying free side groups.

Polyphosphazenes have been used for controlled release of naproxen,[38,39,49] calcitonin,[52] colchicines,[53] (diamine)platinum,[54] (dach)platinum (II),[55] insulin,[56] other model proteins[57,58] methylprednisolone,[59,60] methotrexate,[61] tacrolimus,[62] tempamine[63] and plasmid decxynbonucleic acid.[50] Studies of blood biocompatibility *in vitro* with polyorganophosphazenes have shown no morphological changes nor aggregation with platelets,[64] good biocompatibility 30 days after transplantation[65] and normal bone histomorphometry;[52] however, numerous studies have demonstrated nonfavorable results with polyorganophosphazene stents producing a histiolymphocytic and fibromuscular reaction.[41,66] The first long-term biocompatibility *in vivo* study with polyphosphazene was reported in 2003 by Huang *et al.*[67] with a porcine coronary stent model, which showed no signs of hyperplasia nor proliferative response after 6 months.

4.2.4 Polyphosphoesters

In the same family as polyphosphazenes, polyphosphoesters (PPEs) are inorganic polymers developed in the early 1970s[68] as analogs of nucleic acids. Further research found synthetic scheme via polycondensation[69–72] and ring-opening polymerization.[73] As Fig. 4.5 shows, PPEs contain two

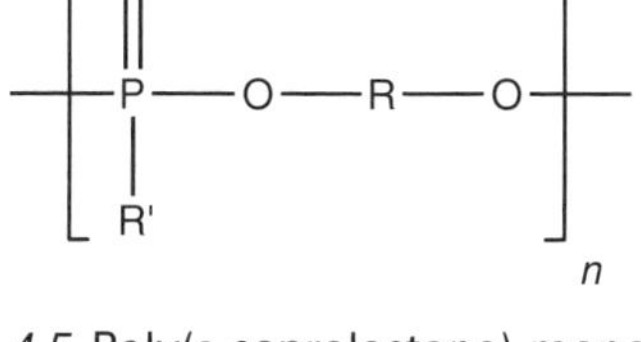

$$\left[-\overset{\displaystyle O}{\overset{\|}{\underset{\displaystyle R'}{\underset{|}{P}}}}-O-R-O- \right]_n$$

4.5 Poly(ε-caprolactone) monomer unit.

substitution sites, R and R′, which subdivide into three PPE families based upon R′ substitution: R′ = H, polyphosphites; R′ = alkyl or aryl group, polyphosphonates; R′ = alkoxy or aryloxy group, polyphosphates. Biodegradation of the phosphate bonds in the PPE backbone by hydrolysis and/or enzymatic cleavage result in phosphate, alcohol and diols. Hence, biodegradation may be controlled by substitution of the R and R′ side groups for homopolymers and the polymer backbone may be altered for block copolymers for alternative physicochemical properties. To date, biocompatibility studies have been quite favorable, showing limited toxicity.[74]

Numerous studies by Leong's group have utilized PPEs for block copolymer design including poly(2-aminoethyl propylene phosphate) (PPE-EA) for gene delivery[74–78] and PPE microspheres for nerve growth factor delivery.[79,80] *In vivo* studies with the Paclimer delivery system, 10% w/w paclitaxel encapsulated in biodegradable polyphosphoester microspheres, with a single intratumoral or intraperitonel injection showed 80% release of the drug after 90 days in a human lung cancer xenograft model. This sustained release showed significant inhibition of nonsmall cell lung cancer nodules with threefold to sixfold longer tumor doubling times compared with free paclitaxel and vehicle controls.[81] Next, Paclimer was evaluated for its ability to cross the blood–brain barrier to treat 9L gliosarcomas with intracranial implants releasing active paclixtaxel. Sustained release of paclitaxel continued for 30 days following intracranial implantation with an approximately twofold increase in the mean survival time against negative controls; however, gross morphology showed favorable biocompatibility properties.[82] A recent translational canine study to evaluate dose escalation and neurotoxicity showed excellent results throughout the 120-day study with no evidence of systemic toxicity, gross morphological or physiological changes with the animals.[83] Two levels of paclitaxel loading, 10% and 40% w/w with the Paclimer vehicle, were studied for locally injected treatment of orthotopic LNCaP tumors. 28 days post-injection the harvested tumors showed significant reduction in tumor growth; moreover, TSU-xenografts treated with adjuvant radiotherapy enhanced tumor growth inhibition, indicating retention of the synergistic properties of paclitaxel with radiation.[84] Paclimer is currently in phase I clinical trials for sustained-release therapy for ovarient or primary peritoneal carcinomas.[85] While this study was discontinued before the maximum tolerated dose was defined, paclitaxel levels were maintained over the 8-week therapy window with plasma concentrations well below toxic levels.[85]

4.3 Biodegradable polyesters for drug delivery

Polyesters represent perhaps the largest family of biodegradable polymers including aliphatic polyesters such as poly(glycolic acid) (PGA), poly(lactic acid) (PLA), poly(lactide-co-glycolide) (PLGA), polydioxanone, polyglyconate, polycaprolactone, and BAK, a polyesteramide manufactured by Bayer AG.[86] Table 4.1 lists the major biodegradable polyesters in drug delivery. Polyesters are the reactive products of polyhydric alcohols and polybasic organic acids described as early as the 1920s and 1930s,[87,88] but low molecular weights and poor hydrolytic stability disallowed proper use in reasonable applications. In the presence of water, any polyester is

Table 4.1 Biodegradable polyesters

Polymer	Monomer unit
BAK	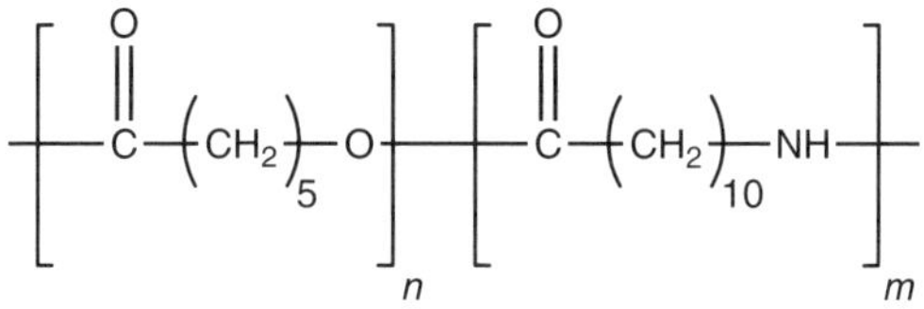 $\left[-C(=O)-(CH_2)_5-O-\right]_n\left[-C(=O)-(CH_2)_{10}-NH-\right]_m$
Poly[α-(4-aminobutyl)-L-glycolic acid] (PAGA)	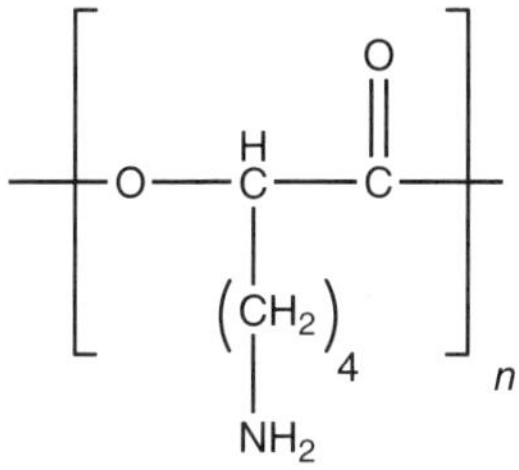 $\left[-O-CH((CH_2)_4NH_2)-C(=O)-\right]_n$
Poly(3-hydroxybutyrate)	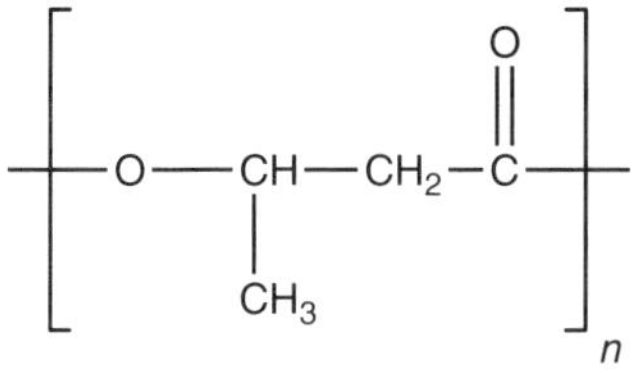 $\left[-O-CH(CH_3)-CH_2-C(=O)-\right]_n$
Poly(3-hydroxyvalerate)	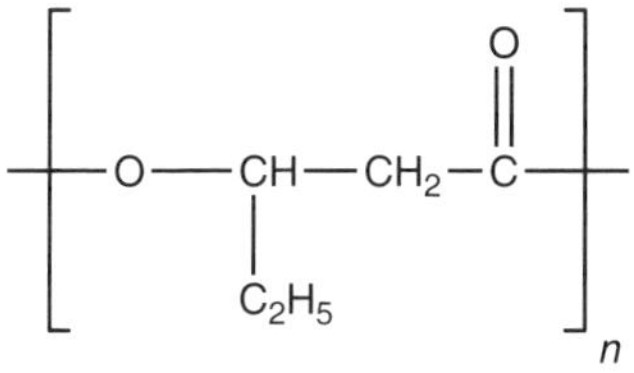 $\left[-O-CH(C_2H_5)-CH_2-C(=O)-\right]_n$
Polydioxanone (PDS)	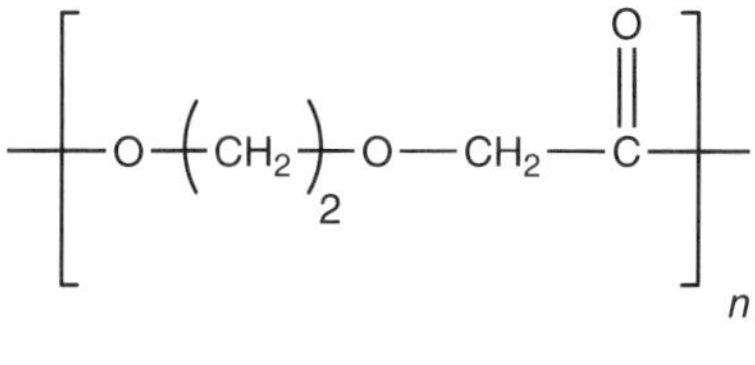 $\left[-O-(CH_2)_2-O-CH_2-C(=O)-\right]_n$

Table 4.1 (cont.)

Polymer	Monomer unit
Poly(ε-caprolactone) (PCL)	$\left[-O-(CH_2)_5-\overset{\displaystyle O}{\overset{\Vert}{C}}-\right]_n$
Poly(glycolic acid) (PGA)	$\left[-O-CH_2-\overset{\displaystyle O}{\overset{\Vert}{C}}-\right]_n$
Poly(glycolic-co-lactic acid) (PLGA)	$\left[-O-CH_2-\overset{\displaystyle O}{\overset{\Vert}{C}}-O-\underset{\displaystyle CH_3}{\underset{\vert}{CH}}-\overset{\displaystyle O}{\overset{\Vert}{C}}-\right]_n$
Polyglyconate	$\left[-CH_2-\overset{\displaystyle O}{\overset{\Vert}{C}}-O-\right]_n\left[-(CH_2)_2-O-CH_2-O-\overset{\displaystyle O}{\overset{\Vert}{C}}-O-\right]_m$
Poly(lactic acid) (PLA)	$\left[-O-\underset{\displaystyle CH_3}{\underset{\vert}{CH}}-\overset{\displaystyle O}{\overset{\Vert}{C}}-\right]_n$
Poly(β-malonic acid)	$\left[-O-\underset{\displaystyle COOH}{\underset{\vert}{CH}}-CH_2-\overset{\displaystyle O}{\overset{\Vert}{C}}-\right]_n$
Polyorthoester I (POE I)	$\left[-O-C(-O-R-)(-O-CH_2-CH_2-CH_2-)\right]_n$ (spiro C in five-membered ring containing O)

Table 4.1 (cont.)

Polymer	Monomer unit
POE II	
POE III	
POE IV	
Poly(propylene fumarate)	$HO-CH_2-CH(CH_3)-O-C(=O)-CH=CH-C(=O)-O-CH_2-CH(OH)-CH_3$
Poly(tartronic acid)	$[-O-CH(COOH)-C(=O)-]_n$
Polyvalerolactone	$[-O-(CH_2)_4-C(=O)-]_n$

susceptible to hydrolytic cleavage but, in practice, hydrophobic groups in the background preclude exclusive aqueous access to the backbone, thereby tempering the transient degradation. With these physicochemical properties in mind, polymer chemists have synthesized thousands of polyesters through polycondensation of diacids and diolos, self-polycondensation of hydroxyacids or ring-opening polymerization of cyclic diesters, lactones, glycolides and lactides. Polycondensation reactions, indicative of a small by-product such as water, combine difunctional AB monomers (hydroxy acids) or AA and BB difunctional monomers for stepwise polyester synthesis. As such, to prevent unwanted polymer cleavage during high-molecular-weight polymerization, elimination of the hydrolytic by-product is necessary. Hydrolytic cleavage of polyesters, and other hydrolytically degradable polymers, is based upon three properties: chemical composition, hydrophobicity and crystallinity. As previously discussed, the chemical composition and hydrophobicity are directly linked to the rate and degree of polymer degradation; moreover, amorphous polymers, those lacking high degrees of crystallinity, suffer from higher rates of degradation.[89]

4.3.1 Poly(ε-caprolactone)

Compared with the previous polymers discussed, polycaprolactones (PCLs) degrade at a much slower rate and are commonly used for implantable long-term biostable drug delivery systems based upon well-established biocompatibility studies over 30 years.[90] Long-term degradation studies of polylactones have reported degradation times of the order of 2 years,[91] a process occurring through hydrolytic cleavage of the ester linkages. However, kinetic degradation studies show that random hydrolytic cleavage does not operate alone; hence it is proposed that bulk hydrolysis contributes to PCL biodegradation. Bulk hydrolysis leads to autocatalytic hydrolysis of the remaining esters by the exposed carboxylic acid end groups. Synthesis of PCL from the cheap ε-caprolactone monomer (Fig. 4.6) may be achieved by at least four different mechanisms including anionic polymerization,[92] cationic polymerization,[93] coordination polymerization[94] and free-radical polymerization.[95] PCL has an intrinsic, highly favorable property to form a variety of polymer blends where this copolymerization

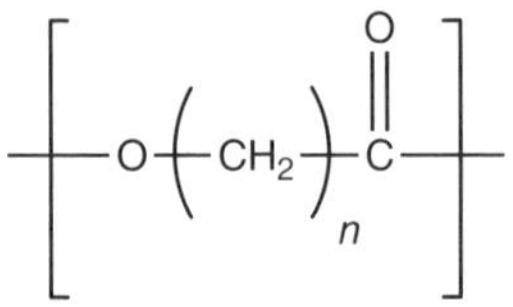

$$\left[-O-(CH_2)_n-\overset{O}{\overset{\|}{C}}- \right]$$

4.6 PPE monomer unit.

greatly reduces the degradation of the PCL. Block copolymers incorporating caprolactone include PEG–PCL,[96,97] PCL–PLA,[98] PEG–PLA–PCL,[99] PCL–chitooligosaccharide–PEG,[100], poly(3-hydroxyoctanoate)–PCL[101] and thermosensitive biodegradable polymeric micelles.[102]

Thus inspired, PCL became a key component for macromolecular drug delivery utilizing the copolymer systems aforementioned; yet, interest in lactone homopolymers for monolithic drug delivery remains. In 1985 the Research Triangle Institute was granted the patent for Capronor, a PCL-based subdermal implant for contraception, control of menstrual disorders, and endometriosis treatment through zeroth-order release of levonorgestrel over a 12–18-month period.[103] PCL block copolymers have been used to deliver doxorubicin,[100] cyclosporine A,[104,105] geldanamycin,[96] rapamycin,[97] amphotericin B,[106,107] dihydrotestosterone,[108] indomethacin[109,110] and paclitaxel.[111]

4.3.2 Poly(glycolic acid), poly(lactic acid), and poly(D,L-lactic acid-co-glycolic acid)

As early as 1970, PGA was targeted as a highly biocompatible biogradable polymer marketed as Dexon for use as surgical sutures.[112] PGA was originially synthesized by ring-opening polymerization of glycolide, a six-membered cyclic dimer of glycolic acid (GA). Modern techniques have shown successful PGA synthesis by polycondensation of diacids and diols and self-polycondensation of poly(α-hydroxy acids). Several biodegradable polyesters, many of which are PGA derivatives, have also been used in nonviral gene delivery primarily to alleviate cytotoxicity such as poly[α-(4-aminobutyl)-L-glycolic acid] (PAGA),[113,114] poly(D,L-lactic acid-co-glycolic acid) (PLGA),[115–117] PEG–PLGA–PEG[118] and poly(4-hydroxyl-1-proline esters).[119,120] PGA is a semicrystalline polymer, which limits its solubility in organic solvents, with a glass transition temperature T_g of 36 °C and melt temperature T_m 225 °C. The PGA polyester backbone has minimal methylene spacing, clearly allowing for hydrolytic cleavage; in fact, this rapid degradation into natural metabolites, coupled with the acidity of the degradation product, has limited the applications of PGA as a functional biomaterial. The biodegradation of PGA has been extensively reported in the seminal papers by Chu[121–123] wherein a two-stage erosion mechanism was proposed: firstly, the ester bonds within the amorphous polymer matrix are hydrolytically cleaved by the diffusion of bulk water followed by, secondly, hydrolytic degradation of the exposed ester bonds within the crystalline region. As with other polyesters, degradation of PGA results in an autocatalytic loop wherein the nascent carboxylic end groups accelerate further biodegradation. The ultimate *in vivo* fate of GA is widely debated. Gilding[124] has stated that glycolic acid is metabolized into water and CO_2 subsequently cleared by respiration while Hollinger[125] and Williams and Mort[126] have proposed enzymatic conversion of GA into glyoxylate followed by glycine.

PAGA is a biodegradable analogue of PGA and poly(L-lysine) (PLL) that rapidly degrades into L-oxylysine.[113,114] Systemic administration of PAGA–DNA complexes has shown promising results for the treatment of diabetes by co-expression of interleukin-4 and interleukin-10.[127–129] It was also shown that the polymer did not compromise biocompatibility as the systemically administered PAGA–DNA decreased insulitis by more than 50% and was not exacerbated by the polymer or the DNA alone.[127]

PLA, akin to PGA, has been widely accepted as a biocompatible homopolymers, in addition to PLGA blends at various ratios.[130] Similar in scope to PGA, PLA degrades into lactic acid (LA) which enters the Krebs cycle and subsequently produces water and CO_2 reaction products. Unlike the polymeric glycolide, the chiral LA monomer exists as one of three enantiomeric forms including L-lactide, D-lactide and *meso*-lactide. These stereoisomers allow for multiple forms of PLA including poly(L-lactic acid) (PLLA), poly(D-lactic acid) (PDLA), poly(D,L-lactic acid) (PDLLA) and *meso*-PLA. Polycondensation results in PLA from LA and so by definition denotes water as a reaction side product; hence, high molecular polymerization may pose problems owing to ester bond hydrolysis. An alternative polymerization scheme utilizes the cyclic lactide dimer. PLLA is synthesized by ring-opening polymerization of L-lactide, PDLA by the D-lactide, and PDLLA by the cyclic D,L-lactide diester. By differential scanning calorimetry, isotactic PLLA and PDLA are semicrystalline whereas syndiotactic PDLLA is amorphous. The effects of the stereochemistry on the physicochemical parameters of T_m and T_g are shown in Table 4.2. Although degradation occurs by the same mechanism, hydrolytic cleavage of the ester bonds, the rate is slower than that of PGA. As seen in Table 4.1, the monomer units differ by one α-methyl unit that increases the local hydrophobicity, thereby impeding hydrolytic cleavage. In practice, PLLA is most often chosen because its degradation is more readily recognized *in vivo*.

Table 4.2 Values of the glass transition temperature T_g and melting temperature T_m for three PLA species, illustrating the effects of stereochemistry on physicochemical parameters

PLA derivative	T_g (°C)	T_m (°C)
PDLA	50[131]	180[132]
PLLA	57–60,[133] 60–65[134,135]	173–178,[134] 170[135]
PDLLA	50–54,[133] 55–60[134,135]	Amorphous

PLGA alternating block copolymers are obtained from ring-opening polymerization of 6-methyl-morpholine-2,5-dione[136] and random block copolymers by copolymerization with D,L-lactic acid.[137] Numerous reports exist on characterization of PLGA multiblock copolymers[138] with variations in composition stemming from Gilding *et al.*[139] Briefly, PLGA compositions ranging from PLLA–GA 25–75% and PDLLA–GA 0–70% are amorphous;[139] however, it is interesting to note that, at the limits of the PLLA–GA composition, PLGA copolymers are more resistant to hydrolytic cleavage,[140] which is intuitively obvious as the more hydrophobic PLLA block increases but not so for the other extreme. Next, LA–GA 50–50 was shown by Miller *et al.*[141] to be the most unstable, whereas LA–GA 30–70 readily degraded owing to the rate and extent of bulk water uptake. PLGA composed of LA–GA 10–90 has long found utility as Vicryl (polyglactin 910), a biodegradable surgical suture licensed by Ethicon (Somerville, New Jersey) and, in 2002, Vicryl Plus became the first marketed suture designed to contain an antibacterial agent, Triclosan or 5-chloro-2-(2,4-dichlorophenoxy)phenol. In addition to comprising sutures, PLGA microspheres have been extensively used in drug and gene delivery;[138,142–145] however, concerns have been raised about the results following a significant drop in pH at the sites of PLGA degradation. An excellent study by Taylor *et al.*[146] showed head-to-head degradation comparisons of PGA, PLA and PCL amongst others wherein PGA exhibited toxic degradation effects after incubation for 10 days in Tris buffer whereas PLA was non-toxic in buffer up to 16 weeks but became toxic in water after 4 weeks. Gene therapy with PLGA microspheres has been met with mixed success, possibly owing in part to formulation techniques that continue to be optimized. Biodegradable PLGA formulations have resulted in variable amounts of intact DNA,[147,148] possibly because of residual levels of high acidity from degrading PLGA, thereby leading to PEG–PLGA–PEG triblock copolymers. When mixed with DNA, these copolymers gel at core temperature with zeroth-order release up to 12 days with a 5-day half-life of DNA from PEG–PLGA–PEG gels.[118]

4.3.3 Polyorthoesters

Polyorthoesters (POEs) were developed and reported by Heller *et al.* nearly 40 years ago for use as implanted biomaterials and drug delivery vehicles. POEs are typically synthesized by the addition of polyols to diketene acetals resulting in[149] POE IV or by the less common anachronistic route of diol and diethoxytetrahydrofuran transesterification used to produce the first POE generation, POE I. Degradation of POEs is through hydrolysis of the ester backbone with concomitant generation of diols and acidic levels significantly lower than PLGA. Furthermore, POEs have an added advantage because the degradation is pH sensitive. At physiological pH, POEs are stable; however, upon an interstitial drop to about pH 5, POEs begin to degrade with minimal levels of autohydrolysis, a property exploited for tumor-targeted drug delivery where the pH is commonly compromised to acidic levels.[150] This degradation profile of POEs has allowed for application of POEs to the delivery of a broader range of therapeutics including peptides or proteins, nucleic acids and traditional small molecules. The absence of a highly acidic environment favors its use to deliver nucleic acids, namely DNA wherein a low pH promotes DNA degradation, and peptides or proteins from denaturation and proteolysis. In contrast with the hydrolysis mechanism of PLGA and PAGA that degrade primarily by bulk erosion, POE hydrolysis is surface limited as a result of the hydrophobic hydrocarbon–ether ring. Researchers quickly found a zeroth-order drug release profile with POE-drug matrices because the drug release was exclusive to erosion of the surface polymer and not through Fickian diffusion.

Despite the promise of POEs as polymer-drug therapeutics in the 1970s[151–155] known as POE I (Table 4.1), POEs have had a long and arduous iterative process to the current POE IV (Table 4.1) at which the majority of pharmaceutical research is directed. Firstly, intial POE syntheses found that POE I formed by transesterification degraded into γ-hydroxybutyric acid side products, the presence of which further autocatalyzed local POE I degradation. Secondly, POE II (Table 4.1) was developed to alleviate this autocatalysis by producing neutrally charged reaction products incapable of promoting acidic degradation; however, these polymers proved almost too stable owing to their significant hydrophobicity requiring formulations with an acidic component to initiate degradation. The third generation of POEs, POE III, was plagued by extremely complex synthesis schemes in efforts to limit the backbone hydrophobicity (Table 4.1). Finally, POE IV tempered the poor degradation of POE II by incorporating GA and/or LA blocks in the polymer backbone. These multiblock copolymers allowed for tight control of degradation kinetics as a function of the acidic block composition and size. Phase II clinical trials with POE IV have been completed. A.P. Pharma (Redwood, California) has two proprietary formulations of POE IV: Biochronomer™, a POE IV and LA block copolymer for local depot drug delivery applications and Bioerodimer™, diblock copolymers of POE IV and PEG. A phase II clinical trial of Biochoronomer™ encapsulated granisetron for use as an anti-emetic agent for chemotherapy patients showed more than a 90% response with acute (within 24 h post-chemotherapy) phase patients; currently, a phase III clinical trial is ongoing. A phase II clinical trial for mepivacaine delivery with Biochronomer™ for post-operative surgical pain has been completed despite a revision of the trial protocol in 2002 owing to incidents of acute irritation. Results from this study are unknown.

4.3.4 Poly(ether esters) and Poly(ester carbonates)

The last examples of polyesters in this review are the poly(ether esters) represented by polydioxanones (PDS); and poly(ester carbonates) represented by polyglyconate. PDSs are synthesized by ring-opening polymerization of *p*-dioxanone and are biodegradable, biocompatible and semicrystalline (Table 4.1) with T_m-115 °C and $T_g \approx 10 - 0$ °C.[151] Polymer fibers composed of PDS were first tested for use as monofilament biodegradable surgical sutures and the degradation profile was later found to be affected by gamma irradiation.[156] Poly(ester carbonates) are synthesized by mixed ring-opening polymerization including lactide–glycolide–lactone monomer units; however, Schappacher *et al.*[157] constructed a diblock copolymer composed of trimethylene carbonate (TMC) and ε-caprolactone (ECL) which, at nearly equal molar ratios, produced poly(TMC-co-ECL) with $T_m = 58$ °C and $T_g = 51$ °C. In 1985, Katz *et al.*[158] reported biodegradable, poly(trimethylene carbonates) for monofilament surgical sutures currently marketed as Maxon.

4.4 Polyethylenimine and poly(ethylene glycol)-co-poly(L-lysine)-γ-histidine

4.4.1 Polyethylenimine

Biodegradable branched polyethylenimine (BPEI) has been synthesized to alleviate the putative cytotoxic effects of high-molecular-weight BPEI by coupling low-molecular-weight BPEI with difunctional PEG producing a hydrolytic-sensitive ester backbone. This novel system has shown a threefold increase in transgene expression above the base BPEI.[159] Further advances have produced biodegradable polyethylenimine (PEI) derivatives by coupling BPEI 1200 Da blocks to oligo(L-lactic acid-co-succinic acid),[160] BPEI 800 Da with small diacrylate cross-linkers to molecular weights (14–30 kDa) comparable with the BPEI 25 kDa control;[161] BPEI 1800 Da cross-linked through acid-labile imine,[162] BPEI 2000 Da cross-linked with linear nonaethylenimine (LPEI) 423 Da via amide and ester linkages,[163] LPEI 423 Da cross-linked with PEG–diacrylates[164] and LPEI–PEG–LPEI.[165]

4.4.2 Poly(ethylene glycol)-co-poly(L-lysine)-γ-histidine

A biodegradable derivative of PEG–PLL with grafted histidine residues has been synthesized for local gene therapy with transgene expression levels fourfold higher than PLL alone.[166,167] This multiblock copolymer possesses ester-linked PEG–PLL blocks with grafted *N*,*N*-dimethylhistidine for pH buffering in the late endosomal stage. The naked polymer alone, poly(ethylene glycol)-co-poly(L-lysine)-*g*-histidin, showed a half-life of nearly 5 h in isotonic phosphate-buffered saline (pH 7.4; 37 °C); however, an interesting side note is that upon the addition of plasmid DNA the subsequent complexes were stable for up to 6 days.[167] This increased stability could result from the loss of a formal charge on the primary amines, thus increasing the relative hydrophobicity and preventing hydrolytic cleavage of the ester linkages.

4.5 Synthetic block copolypeptides

Based upon the success with glycolic acid derivatives (PAGA) and copolymerization with lactic acid (PLGA), the logical extrapolation would be investigation of incorporating of multiple poly(amino acids), as the amino acid side chains offer sites for drug conjugation and cross-linking. Additionally, synthetic polypeptides have an added advantage by degrading into non-immunogenic amino acid oligomers and monomers. However, it has been shown that including three or more amino acid residues in poly(amino acids) results in an antigenic response *in vivo*;[168] consequently, researchers have relied upon one- or two-amino-acid-based systems. These properties do not necessarily have a correlation with PGA, PLA or PLGA polymers and copolymers.

4.6 Future trends

Biodegradable polymers have truly revolutionized controlled drug delivery design and biomaterial applications for implants and tissue engineering. With the help of biodegradable stents,[169,170] clinicians can site-specifically control drug release to treat coronary artery disease through delivery of traditional small molecules[171] and now gene therapy.[172,173] Implantable drug delivery that used to be limited to days is now being performed in weeks or months. While the promise is alluring, these polymer systems continue to require rigorous *in vitro* and *in vivo* biocompatibility studies to mini-mize or more ideally to eliminate immunogenic or otherwise unfavorable responses. Until such protocols are established to coordinate *in vivo* predictions with alternative sources, the 'design–synthesis–characterization–evaluation' mantra will continue to be followed.

Biodegradable block copolymers and block copolypeptides have significantly endowed novel drug delivery systems with beneficial pharmacokinetic and biocompatible properties. Synthetic chemistry and now genetically engineered copolymers provide numerous polymers capable of kinetically controlled degradation *in vitro* and more importantly *in vivo*. Traditional synthetic polymers have long been the stalwarts of biodegradable polymers for drug delivery. Now, molecular biology has given birth to a waking giant in biodegradable macromolecular drug delivery. While recombinant polymers can be designed for facile degradation by ubiquitous proteases (e.g. elastases and collagenases) resulting in oligopeptide fragments, synthetic chemists design polymers with chemical and/or hydrolytic bonds for ease of decomposition. These reaction products must not elicit a physiological response nor produce an environmental compromise such as the pH drop in PLGA systems. In the future, it may probably be a synthetic–recombinant hybrid that provides the ideal physicochemical and pharmacotherapeutic effects for a wide range of drug delivery applications. However, beyond PEGylated proteins and antibody-targeted drug delivery systems, which are not the scope of this review, substantial strides in this area are yet to made but the promise is bright.

4.7 References

1 Ravin H A, Seligman A M and Fine J, 'Polyvinyl pyrrolidone as a plasma expander; studies on its excretion, distribution and metabolism', *J Nucl Med*, 1952 **247**(24) 921–929.

2 Ammon R and Depner E, 'Elimination and retention of various polyvinylpyrrolidone types in the body', *Z Gesamte Exp Med*, 1957 **128**(6) 607–628.

3 Hulme B, Dykes P W, Appleyard I and Arkell D W, 'Retention and storage sites of radioactive polyvinylpyrrolidone', *J Nucl Med*, 1968 **9**(7) 389–393.

4 Mück K-F, Christ O and Kellner H-M, 'Das Verhalten von isotaktischen Polyacrylsäuren im Organismus. Verteilung und Ausscheidung bei Mäusen', *Makromol Chem*, 1977 **178**(10) 2785–2797.

5 Azori M, Szinai I, Veres Z, Pato J, Otvos L and Tudos F, 'Polymeric Prodrugs 3. Synthesis, elimination and whole-body distribution of 14C-labelled drug carrier', *Macromol Chem Phys*, 1986 **187**(2) 297–302.

6 Bucher J E and Slade W C, 'The anhydrides of isophthalic and terephthalic acids', *J Am Chem Soc*, 1909 **31**(12) 1319–1321.

7 Leong K W, Simonte V and Langer R, 'Synthesis of polyanhydrides: melt-polycondensation, dehydrochlorination, and dehydrative coupling', *Macromolecules* 1987 **20**(4) 705–712.

8 Lundmark S, Sjoling M and Albertsson A C, 'Polymerization of oxepan-2,7-dione in solution and synthesis of block copolymers of oxepan-2,7-dione and 2-oxepanone', *J Macromol Sci Part A: Pure Appl Chem*, 1991 **28**(1) 15–29.

9 Domb A J and Langer R, 'Polyanhydrdies 1. Preparation of high-molecular-weight polyanhydrides', *J Polym Sci Part A: Polym Chem*, 1987 **25**(12) 3373–3386.

10 Rosen H B, Chang J, Wnek G E, Linhardt R J and Langer R, 'Bioerodible polyanhydrides for controlled drug delivery', *Biomaterials*, 1983 **4**(2) 131–133.

11 Leong K W, Brott B C and Langer R, 'Bioerodible polyanhydrides as drug-carrier matrices. I. Characterization, degradation and release characteristics', *J Biomed Mater Res*, 1985 **19**(8) 941–955.

12 Leong K W, D'Amore P D, Marletta M and Langer R, 'Bioerodible polyanhydrides as drug-carrier matrices. II. Biocompatibility and chemical reactivity', *J Biomed Mater Res*, 1986 **20**(1) 51–64.

13 D'Emanuele A, Hill J, Tamada J A, Domb A J and Langer R, 'Molecular weight changes in polymer erosion', *Pharm Res*, 1992 **9**(10) 1279–1283.
14 Park M C, Weaver C E J, Donahue J E and Sampath P, 'Intracavitary chemotherapy (Gliadel) for recurrent esthesioneuroblastoma: case report and review of the literature', *J Neurooncol*, 2006 **77**(1) 47–51.
15 Shikanov A and Domb A J, 'Poly(sebacic acid-co-ricinoleic acid) biodegradable injectable in situ gelling polymer', *Biomacromolecules*, 2006 **7**(1) 288–296.
16 Shikanov A, Vaisman B, Krasko M Y, Nyska A and Domb A J, 'Poly(sebacic acid-co-ricinoleic acid) biodegradable carrier for paclitaxel: *in vitro* release and *in vivo* toxicity', *J Biomed Mater Res Part A* 2004 **69**(1) 47–54.
17 Furtado S, Abramson D, Simhkay L, Wobbekind D and Mathiowitz E, 'Subcutaneous delivery of insulin loaded poly(fumaric-co-sebacic anhydride) microspheres to type 1 diabetic rats', *Eur J Pharm Biopharm*, 2006 **63**(2) 229–236.
18 Couvreur P, Kante B, Roland M, Guiot P, Bauduin P and Speiser P, 'Polycyanoacrylate nanocapsules as potential lysosomotropic carriers: preparation, morphological and sorptive properties', *J Pharm Pharmacol*, 1979 **31**(5) 331–332.
19 Couvreur P, Kante B, Roland M and Speiser P, 'Adsorption of antineoplastic drugs to polyalkylcyanoacrylate nanoparticles and their release in calf serum', *J Pharm Sci*, 1979 **68**(12) 1521–1524.
20 Andrieu V, Fessi H, Dubrasquet M, Devissaguet J P, Puisieux F and Benita S, 'Pharmacokinetic evaluation of indomethacin nanocapsules', *Drug Des Deliv*, 1989 **4**(4) 295–302.
21 Polato L, Benedetti L M, Callegaro L and Couvreur P, '*In vitro* evaluation of nanoparticle formulations containing gangliosides', *J Drug Target*, 1994 **2**(1) 53–59.
22 Godard G, Boutorine A S, Saison-Behmoaras E and Helene C, 'Antisense effects of cholesterol-oligodeoxynucleotide conjugates associated with poly(alkylcyanoacrylate) nanoparticles', *Eur J Biochem*, 1995 **232**(2) 404–410.
23 Fresta M, Cavallaro G, Giammona G, Wehrli E and Puglisi G, 'Preparation and characterization of polyethyl-2-cyanoacrylate nanocapsules containing antiepileptic drugs', *Biomaterials*, 1996 **17**(8) 751–758.
24 Aboubakar M, Puisieux F, Couvreur P, Deyme M and Vauthier C, 'Study of the mechanism of insulin encapsulation in poly(isobutylcyanoacrylate) nanocapsules obtained by interfacial polymerization', *J Biomed Mater Res*, 1999 **47**(4) 568–576.
25 Boudad H, Legrand P, Lebas G, Cheron M, Duchene D and Ponchel G, 'Combined hydroxypropyl-beta-cyclodextrin and poly(alkylcyanoacrylate) nanoparticles intended for oral administration of saquinavir', *Int J Pharm*, 2001 **218**(1–2) 113–124.
26 Chauvierre C, Marden M C, Vauthier C, Labarre D, Couvreur P and Leclerc L, 'Heparin coated poly(alkylcyanoacrylate) nanoparticles coupled to hemoglobin: a new oxygen carrier', *Biomaterials*, 2004 **25**(15) 3081–3086.
27 Hillaireau H, Le Doan T and Couvreur P, 'Polymer-based nanoparticles for the delivery of nucleoside analogues', *J Nanosci Nanotechnol*, 2006 **6**(9–10) 2608–2617.

28 Lherm C, Muller R H, Puisieux F and Couvreur P, 'Alkylcyanoacrylate drug carriers: II. Cytotoxicity of cyanoacrylate nanoparticles with different alkyl chain length', *Int J Pharm*, 1992 **84**(1) 13–22.
29 Muller R H, Lherm C, Herbort J and Couvreur P, '*In vitro* model for the degradation of alkylcyanoacrylate nanoparticles', *Biomaterials*, 1990 **11**(8) 590–595.
30 Peracchia M T, Vauthier C, Desmaele D, Gulik A, Dedieu J C, Demoy M, d'Angelo J and Couvreur P, 'PEGylated nanoparticles from a novel methoxy-polyethylene glycol cyanoacrylate-hexadecyl cyanoacrylate amphiphilic copolymer', *Pharm Res*, 1998 **15**(4) 550–556.
31 Peracchia M T, Vauthier C, Puisieux F and Couvreur P, 'Development of sterically stabilized poly(isobutyl 2-cyanoacrylate) nanoparticles by chemical coupling of poly(ethylene glycol)', *J Biomed Mater Res*, 1997 **34**(3) 317–326.
32 Stella B, Arpicco S, Peracchia M T, Desmaele D, Hoebeke J, Renoir M, D'Angelo J, Cattel L and Couvreur P, 'Design of folic acid-conjugated nanoparticles for drug targeting', *J Pharm Sci*, 2000 **89**(11) 1452–1464.
33 Peracchia M T, Fattal E, Desmaele D, Besnard M, Noel J P, Gomis J M, Appel M, d'Angelo J and Couvreur P, 'Stealth PEGylated polycyanoacrylate nanoparticles for intravenous administration and splenic targeting', *J Control Release*, 1999 **60**(1) 121–128.
34 Crommen J H, Schacht E H and Mense E H, 'Biodegradable polymers. II. Degradation characteristics of hydrolysis-sensitive poly[(organo)phosphazenes]', *Biomaterials*, 1992 **13**(9) 601–611.
35 Singh A, Krogman N R, Sethuraman S, Nair L S, Sturgeon J L, Brown P W, Laurencin C T and Allcock H R, 'Effect of side group chemistry on the properties of biodegradable L-alanine cosubstituted polyphosphazenes', *Biomacromolecules*, 2006 **7**(3) 914–918.
36 Allcock H R and Kugel R L, 'Synthesis of high polymeric alkoxy- and aryloxy-phosphonitriles', *J Am Chem Soc*, 1965 **87**(18) 4216–4217.
37 Allcock H R, Singh A, Ambrosio A M and Laredo W R, 'Tyrosine-bearing polyphosphazenes', *Biomacromolecules*, 2003 **4**(6) 1646–1653.
38 Caliceti P, Lora S, Marsilio F and Veronese F M, 'Preparation and characterisation of polyphosphazene-based controlled release systems for naproxen', *Farmaco*, 1995 **50**(12) 867–874.
39 Veronese F M, Marsilio F, Lora S, Caliceti P, Passi P and Orsolini P, 'Polyphosphazene membranes and microspheres in periodontal diseases and implant surgery', *Biomaterials*, 1999 **20**(1) 91–98.
40 Allcock H R, Pucher S R and Scopelianos A G, 'Poly[(amino acid ester)phosphazenes] as substrates for the controlled release of small molecules', *Biomaterials*, 1994 **15**(8) 563–569.
41 De Scheerder I K, Wilczek K L, Verbeken E V, Vandorpe J, Lan P N, Schacht E, De Geest H and Piessens J, 'Biocompatibility of polymer-coated oversized metallic stents implanted in normal porcine coronary arteries', *Atherosclerosis*, 1995 **114**(1) 105–114.
42 Allcock H R, 'Inorganic–organic polymers as a route to biodegradable materials', *Macromol Symp*, 1999 **144** 33–46.
43 Neenan T X and Allcock H R, 'Synthesis of a heparinized poly(organophosph azene)', *Biomaterials*, 1982 **3**(2) 78–80.

44 Zhang J X, Qiu L Y, Jin Y and Zhu K J, 'Physicochemical characterization of polymeric micelles constructed from novel amphiphilic polyphosphazene with poly(*N*-isopropylacrylamide) and ethyl 4-aminobenzoate as side groups', *Colloids Surf B: Biointerfaces*, 2005 **43**(3–4) 123–130.
45 Allcock H R, Kwon S, Riding G H, Fitzpatrick R J and Bennett J L, 'Hydrophilic polyphosphazenes as hydrogels: radiation cross-linking and hydrogel characteristics of poly[bis(methoxyethoxyethoxy)phosphazene]', *Biomaterials*, 1988 **9**(6) 509–513.
46 Allcock H R, Neenan T X and Kossa W C, 'Coupling of cyclic and high polymeric aminoaryloxyphosphazenes to carboxylic acids: prototypes for bioactive polymers', *Macromolecules*, 1982 **15**(3) 693–696.
47 Allcock H R and Scopelianos A G, 'Synthesis of sugar-substituted cyclic and polymeric phosphazenes and their oxidation, reduction, and acetylation reactions', *Macromolecules*, 1983 **16**(5) 715–719.
48 Laurencin C T, Koh H J, Neenan T X, Allcock H R and Langer R, 'Controlled release using a new bioerodible polyphosphazene matrix system', *J Biomed Mater Res*, 1987 **21**(10) 1231–1246.
49 Veronese F M, Marsilio F, Caliceti P, De Filippis P, Giunchedi P and Lora S, 'Polyorganophosphazene microspheres for drug release: polymer synthesis, microsphere preparation, *in vitro* and *in vivo* naproxen release', *J Control Release*, 1998 **52**(3) 227–237.
50 Luten J, van Steenis J H, van Someren R, Kemmink J, Schuurmans-Nieuwenbroek N M, Koning G A, Crommelin D J, van Nostrum C F and Hennink W E, 'Water-soluble biodegradable cationic polyphosphazenes for gene delivery', *J Control Release*, 2003 **89**(3) 483–497.
51 Crommen J H, Schacht E H and Mense E H, 'Biodegradable polymers. I. Synthesis of hydrolysis-sensitive poly[(organo)phosphazenes]', *Biomaterials*, 1992 **13**(8) 511–520.
52 Aldini N N, Caliceti P, Lora S, Fini M, Giavaresi G, Rocca M, Torricelli P, Giardino R and Veronese F M, 'Calcitonin release system in the treatment of experimental osteoporosis. Histomorphometric evaluation', *J Orthop Res*, 2001 **19**(5) 955–961.
53 Ibim S M, el-Amin S F, Goad M E, Ambrosio A M, Allcock H R and Laurencin C T, '*In vitro* release of colchicine using poly(phosphazenes): the development of delivery systems for musculoskeletal use', *Pharm Dev Technol*, 1998 **3**(1) 55–62.
54 Song S C and Soo Sohn Y, 'Synthesis and hydrolytic properties of polyphosphazene/(diamine)platinum/saccharide conjugates', *J Control Release*, 1998 **55**(2–3) 161–170.
55 Song R, Joo Jun Y, Ik Kim J, Jin C and Sohn Y S, 'Synthesis, characterization and tumor selectivity of a polyphosphazene–platinum(II) conjugate', *J Control Release*, 2005 **105**(1–2) 142–150.
56 Caliceti P, Veronese F M and Lora S, 'Polyphosphazene microspheres for insulin delivery', *Int J Pharm*, 2000 **211**(1–2) 57–65.
57 Andrianov A K, Marin A and Roberts B E, 'Polyphosphazene polyelectrolytes: a link between the formation of noncovalent complexes with antigenic proteins and immunostimulating activity', *Biomacromolecules*, 2005 **6**(3) 1375–1379.

58 Seong J Y, Jun Y J, Kim B M, Park Y M and Sohn Y S, 'Synthesis and characterization of biocompatible poly(organophosphazenes) aiming for local delivery of protein drugs', *Int J Pharm*, 2006 **314**(1) 90–96.

59 Huang Y, Liu X, Wang L, Verbeken E, Li S and De Scheerder I, 'Local methylprednisolone delivery using a BiodivYsio phosphorylcholine-coated drug-delivery stent reduces inflammation and neointimal hyperplasia in a porcine coronary stent model', *Int J Cardiovasc Intervent*, 2003 **5**(3) 166–171.

60 Wang L, Salu K, Verbeken E, Bosmans J, Van de Werf F, De Scheerder I and Huang Y, 'Stent-mediated methylprednisolone delivery reduces macrophage contents and in-stent neointimal formation', *Coron Artery Dis*, 2005 **16**(4) 237–243.

61 Huang Y, Salu K, Liu X, Li S, Wang L, Verbeken E, Bosmans J and De Scheerder I, 'Methotrexate loaded SAE coated coronary stents reduce neointimal hyperplasia in a porcine coronary model', *Heart*, 2004 **90**(2) 195–199.

62 Huang Y, Salu K, Wang L, Liu X, Li S, Lorenz G, Wnendt S, Verbeken E, Bosmans J, Van de Werf F and De Scheerder I, 'Use of a tacrolimus-eluting stent to inhibit neointimal hyperplasia in a porcine coronary model', *J Invasive Cardiol*, 2005 **17**(3) 142–148.

63 Huang Y, Wang L, Li S, Liu X, Lee K, Verbeken E, van de Werf F and de Scheerder I, 'Stent-based tempamine delivery on neointimal formation in a porcine coronary model', *Acute Card Care*, 2006 **8**(4) 210–216.

64 Kawakami H, Kanezaki S, Sudo M, Kanno M, Nagaoka S and Kubota S, 'Biodegradation and biocompatibility of polyorganophosphazene', *Artif Organs*, 2002 **26**(10) 883–890.

65 Caliceti P, Nicoli Aldini N, Fini M, Rocca M, Gnudi S, Lora S, Giavaresi G, Monfardini C, Giardino R and Veronese F M, 'Bioabsorbable polyphosphazene matrices as systems for calcitonin controlled release', *Farmaco*, 1997 **52**(11) 697–702.

66 De Scheerder I K, Wilczek K L, Verbeken E V, Vandorpe J, Lan P N, Schacht E, Piessens J and De Geest H, 'Biocompatibility of biodegradable and nonbiodegradable polymer-coated stents implanted in porcine peripheral arteries', *Cardiovasc Intervent Radiol*, 1995 **18**(4) 227–232.

67 Huang Y, Liu X, Wang L, Li S, Verbeken E and De Scheerder I, 'Long-term biocompatibility evaluation of a novel polymer-coated stent in a porcine coronary stent model', *Coron Artery Dis*, 2003 **14**(5) 401–408.

68 Lapienis G and Penczek S, 'Toward nucleic-acid like backbones by ionic polymerizations-kinetics and thermodynamics of polymerization of cyclic phosphate esters. 2. Cationic polymerization of 2-methoxy-2-oxo-1,3,2-dioxaphosphorinane 1,3-propylene methyl phosphate', *Macromolecules*, 1974 **7**(2) 166–174.

69 Qiu J J, Liu CM, H u F, Guo X D and Zheng Q X, 'Synthesis of unsaturated polyphosphoester as a potential injectable tissue engineering scaffold material', *J Appl Polym Sci*, 2006 **102**(4) 3095–3101.

70 Sen Gupta A and Lopina S T, 'Synthesis and characterization of L-tyrosine based novel polyphosphates for potential biomaterial applications', *Polymer*, 2004 **45**(14) 4653–4662.

71 Chaubal M V, Wang B, Su G and Zhao Z, 'Compositional analysis of biodegradable polyphosphoester copolymers using NMR spectroscopic methods', *J Appl Polym Sci*, 2003 **90**(14) 4021–4031.
72 Wang J and Zhuo R X, 'Synthesis and characterization of phosphoester linkage-containing hydrogels', *Eur Polym J*, 1999 **35**(3) 491–497.
73 Xiao C S, Wang Y C, Du J Z, Chen X S and Wang J, 'Kinetics and mechanism of 2-ethoxy-2-oxo-1,3,2-dioxaphospholane polymerization initiated by stannous octoate', *Macromolecules*, 2006 **39**(20) 6825–6831.
74 Wang J, Zhang P C, Mao H Q and Leong K W, 'Enhanced gene expression in mouse muscle by sustained release of plasmid DNA using PPE-EA as a carrier', *Gene Ther*, 2002 **9**(18) 1254–1261.
75 Wang J, Mao H Q and Leong K W, 'A novel biodegradable gene carrier based on polyphosphoester', *J Am Chem Soc*, 2001 **123**(38) 9480–9481.
76 Huang S W, Wang J, Zhang P C, Mao H Q, Zhuo R X and Leong K W, 'Water-soluble and nonionic polyphosphoester: synthesis, degradation, biocompatibility and enhancement of gene expression in mouse muscle', *Biomacromolecules*, 2004 **5**(2) 306–311.
77 Wen J, Mao H Q, Li W, Lin K Y and Leong K W, 'Biodegradable polyphosphoester micelles for gene delivery', *J Pharm Sci*, 2004 **93**(8) 2142–2157.
78 Mao H Q and Leong K W, 'Design of polyphosphoester–DNA nanoparticles for non-viral gene delivery', *Adv Genet*, 2005 **53** 275–306.
79 Xu X, Yu H, Gao S, Ma H Q, Leong K W and Wang S, 'Polyphosphoester microspheres for sustained release of biologically active nerve growth factor', *Biomaterials*, 2002 **23**(17) 3765–3772.
80 Mao H Q, Shipanova-Kadiyaia I, Zhao Z, Dang W and Leong K W, *Encyclopedia of Controlled Drug Delivery*, New York, Wiley, 1999.
81 Harper E, Dang W, Lapidus R G and Garver R I J, 'Enhanced efficacy of a novel controlled release paclitaxel formulation (Paclimer delivery system) for local-regional therapy of lung cancer tumor nodules in mice', *Clin Cancer Res*, 1999 **5**(12) 4242–4248.
82 Li K W, Dang W, Tyler B M, Troiano G, Tihan T, Brem H and Walter K A, 'Polilactofate microspheres for Paclitaxel delivery to central nervous system malignancies', *Clin Cancer Res*, 2003 **9**(9) 3441–3447.
83 Pradilla G, Wang P P, Gabikian P, Li K, Magee C A, Walter K A and Brem H, 'Local intracerebral administration of paclitaxel with the paclimer delivery system: toxicity study in a canine model', *J Neurooncol*, 2006 **76**(2) 131–138.
84 Lapidus R G, Dang W, Rosen D M, Gady A M, Zabelinka Y, O'Meally R, DeWeese T L and Denmeade S R, 'Anti-tumor effect of combination therapy with intratumoral controlled-release paclitaxel (Paclimer microspheres) and radiation', *Prostate*, 2004 **58**(3) 291–298.
85 Armstrong D K, Fleming G F, Markman M and Bailey H H, 'A phase I trial of intraperitoneal sustained-release paclitaxel microspheres (Paclimer) in recurrent ovarian cancer: a Gynecologic Oncology Group study', *Gynecol Oncol*, 2006 **103**(2) 391–396.
86 Grigat E, Koch R and Timmermann R, 'BAK 1095 and BAK 2195: coompletely biodegradable synthetic thermoplastics', *Polym Degrad Stab*, 1998 **59**(1–3) 223–226.

87 Carothers W H, 'Studies on polymerization and ring formation. I. An introduction to the general theory of condensation polymers', *J Am Chem Soc*, 1929 **51**(8) 2548–2559.
88 Carothers W H and Arvin J A, 'Studies on polymerization and ring formation. II. Polyesters', *J Am Chem Soc*, 1929 **51**(8) 2560–2570.
89 Cutright D E, Perez B, Beasley J Dr, Larson W J and Posey W R, 'Degradation rates of polymers and copolymers of polylactic and polyglycolic acids', *Oral Surg Oral Med Oral Pathol*, 1974 **37**(1) 142–152.
90 Kronenthal R L, Oser Z and Martin E, *Polymers in Medicine and Surgery*, New York, Plenum, 1975.
91 Middleton J C and Tipton A J, 'Synthetic biodegradable polymers as orthopedic devices', *Biomaterials*, 2000 **21**(23) 2335–2346.
92 Brode G L and Koleske J V, 'Lactone polymerization and polymer properties', *J Macromol Sci Part A: Pure Appl Chem*, 1972 **6**(6) 1109–1144.
93 Horlbeck G, Siesler H W, Tittle B and G T, 'Characterization of polyether and polyester homopolymers and copolymers prepared by ring-opening polymerization with a new catalytic system', *Macromolecules*, 1977 **10**(2) 284–287.
94 Kricheldorf H R, Berl M and Scharnagl N, 'Poly(lactones). 9. Polymerization mechanism of metal alkoxide initiated polymerizations of lactide and various lactones', *Macromolecules*, 1988 **21**(2) 286–293.
95 Bailey W J, Ni Z and Wu S R, 'Synthesis of poly-epsilon-caprolactone via a free-radical mechanism – free-radical ring-opening polymerization of 2-methylene-1,3-dioxepane', *J Polym Sci Part A: Polym Chem*, 1982 **20**(11) 3021–3030.
96 Forrest M L, Zhao A, Won C Y, Malick A W and Kwon G S, 'Lipophilic prodrugs of Hsp90 inhibitor geldanamycin for nanoencapsulation in poly(ethylene glycol)-β-poly(epsilon-caprolactone) micelles', *J Control Release*, 2006 **116**(2) 139–149.
97 Forrest M L, Won C Y, Malick A W and Kwon G S, '*In vitro* release of the mTOR inhibitor rapamycin from poly(ethylene glycol)-β-poly(epsilon-caprolactone) micelles', *J Control Release*, 2006 **110**(2) 370–377.
98 Cohn D and Salomon A H, 'Designing biodegradable multiblock PCL/PLA thermoplastic elastomers', *Biomaterials*, 2005 **26**(15) 2297–2305.
99 Jo S, Kim J and Kim S W, 'Reverse thermal gelation of aliphatically modified biodegradable triblock copolymers', *Macromol Biosci*, 2006 **6**(11) 923–928.
100 Chung T W, Liu D Z, Hsieh J H, Fan X C, Yang J D and Chen J H, 'Characterizing poly(epsilon-caprolactone)-β-chitooligosaccharide-β-poly(ethylene glycol) (PCP) copolymer micelles for doxorubicin (DOX) delivery: effects of crosslinked of amine groups', *J Nanosci Nanotechnol*, 2006 **6**(9–10) 2902–2911.
101 Timbart L, Renard E, Langlois V and Guerin P, 'Novel biodegradable copolyesters containing blocks of poly(3-hydroxyoctanoate) and poly(epsilon-caprolactone): synthesis and characterization', *Macromol Biosci*, 2004 **4**(11) 1014–1020.
102 Nakayama M, Okano T, Miyazaki T, Kohori F, Sakai K and Yokoyama M, 'Molecular design of biodegradable polymeric micelles for temperature-responsive drug release', *J Control Release*, 2006 **115**(1) 46–56.
103 Research Triangle Institute, 'Capronor', *Hypotenuse*, 1985 (May–June) 2–5.

104 Aliabadi H M, Mahmud A, Sharifabadi A D and Lavasanifar A, 'Micelles of methoxy poly(ethylene oxide)-β-poly(epsilon-caprolactone) as vehicles for the solubilization and controlled delivery of cyclosporine A', *J Control Release*, 2005 **104**(2) 301–311.

105 Aliabadi H M, Brocks D R and Lavasanifar A, 'Polymeric micelles for the solubilization and delivery of cyclosporine A: pharmacokinetics and biodistribution', *Biomaterials*, 2005 **26**(35) 7251–7259.

106 Vandermeulen G, Rouxhet L, Arien A, Brewster M E and Preat V, 'Encapsulation of amphotericin B in poly(ethylene glycol)-block-poly(epsilon-caprolactone-co-trimethylenecarbonate) polymeric micelles', *Int J Pharm*, 2006 **309**(1–2) 234–240.

107 Vakil R and Kwon G S, 'Poly(ethylene glycol)-β-poly(epsilon-caprolactone) and PEG–phospholipid form stable mixed micelles in aqueous media', *Langmuir*, 2006 **22**(23) 9723–9729.

108 Allen C, Han J, Yu Y, Maysinger D and Eisenberg A, 'Polycaprolactone-b-poly(ethylene oxide) copolymer micelles as a delivery vehicle for dihydrotestosterone', *J Control Release*, 2000 **63**(3) 275–286.

109 Kim S Y, Shin I G, Lee Y M, Cho C S and Sung Y K, 'Methoxy poly(ethylene glycol) and epsilon-caprolactone amphiphilic block copolymeric micelle containing indomethacin. II. Micelle formation and drug release behaviours', *J Control Release*, 1998 **51**(1) 13–22.

110 Shin I G, Kim S Y, Lee Y M, Cho C S and Sung Y K, 'Methoxy poly(ethylene glycol)/epsilon-caprolactone amphiphilic block copolymeric micelle containing indomethacin. I. Preparation and characterization', *J Control Release*, 1998 **51**(1) 1–11.

111 Cheon Lee S, Kim C, Chan Kwon I, Chung H and Young Jeong S, 'Polymeric micelles of poly(2-ethyl-2-oxazoline)-block-poly(epsilon-caprolactone) copolymer as a carrier for paclitaxel', *J Control Release*, 2003 **89**(3) 437–446.

112 Katz A R and Turner R J, 'Evaluation of tensile and absorption properties of polyglycolic acid sutures', *Surg Gynecol Obstet*, 1970 **131**(4) 701–716.

113 Lim Y, Kim C, Kim K, Kim S W and Park J, 'Development of a safe gene delivery system using biodegradable polymer, poly[α-(4-aminobutyl)-L-glycolic acid]', *J Am Chem Soc*, 2000 **122**(27) 6524–6525.

114 Lim Y B, Han S O, Kong H U, Lee Y, Park J S, Jeong B and Kim S W, 'Biodegradable polyester, poly[α-(4-aminobutyl)-L-glycolic acid], as a non-toxic gene carrier', *Pharm Res*, 2000 **17**(7) 811–816.

115 Lim Y B, Kim S M, Suh H and Park J S, 'Biodegradable, endosome disruptive and cationic network-type polymer as a highly efficient and nontoxic gene delivery carrier', *Bioconjug Chem*, 2002 **13**(5) 952–957.

116 Panyam J, Zhou W Z, Prabha S, Sahoo S K and Labhasetwar V, 'Rapid endo-lysosomal escape of poly(DL-lactide-co-glycolide) nanoparticles: implications for drug and gene delivery', *FASEB J*, 2002 **16**(10) 1217–1226.

117 Denis-Mize K S, Dupuis M, MacKichan M L, Singh M, Doe B, O'Hagan D, Ulmer J B, Donnelly J J, McDonald D M and Ott G, 'Plasmid DNA adsorbed onto cationic microparticles mediates target gene expression and antigen presentation by dendritic cells', *Gene Ther*, 2000 **7**(24) 2105–2112.

118 Li Z, Ning W, Wang J, Choi A, Lee P Y, Tyagi P and Huang L, 'Controlled gene delivery system based on thermosensitive biodegradable hydrogel', *Pharm Res*, 2003 **20**(6) 884–888.

119 Putnam D and Langer R, 'Poly(4-hydroxy-L-proline ester): low-temperature polycondensation and plasmid DNA complexation', *Macromolecules*, 1999 **32**(11) 3658–3662.
120 Lim Y, Choi Y H and Park J, 'A self-destroying polycationic polymer: biodegradable poly(4-hydroxy-L-proline ester)', *J Am Chem Soc*, 1999 **121**(24) 5633–5639.
121 Chu C C, 'An *in vitro* study of the effect of buffer on the degradation of poly(glycolic acid) sutures', *J Biomed Mater Res*, 1981 **15**(1) 19–27.
122 Chu C C, 'The *in vitro* degradation of poly(glycolic acid) sutures – effect of pH', *J Biomed Mater Res*, 1981 **15**(6) 795–804.
123 Chu C C, 'Hydrolytic degradation of polyglycolic acid – tensile-strength and crystallinity study', *J Appl Polym Sci*, 1981 **26**(5) 1727–1734.
124 Gilding, K, 'Biodegradable polymers', in *Biocompatibility of Clinical Implant Materials*, Vol II (Ed D F Williams), Boca Raton, Florida, CRC Press, 1981, pp. 209–232.
125 Hollinger J O, 'Preliminary report on the osteogenic potential of a biodegradable copolymer of polyactide (PLA) and polyglycolide (PGA)', *J Biomed Mater Res*, 1983 **17**(1) 71–82.
126 Williams D F and Mort E, 'Enzyme-accelerated hydrolysis of polyglycolic acid', *J Bioeng* 1977 **1**(3) 231–238.
127 Koh J J, Ko K S, Lee M, Han S, Park J S and Kim S W, 'Degradable polymeric carrier for the delivery of IL-10 plasmid DNA to prevent autoimmune insulitis of NOD mice', *Gene Ther*, 2000 **7**(24) 2099–2104.
128 Lee M, Ko K S, Oh S and Kim S W, 'Prevention of autoimmune insulitis by delivery of a chimeric plasmid encoding interleukin-4 and interleukin-10', *J Control Release*, 2003 **88**(2) 333–342.
129 Ko K S, Lee M, Koh J J and Kim S W, 'Combined administration of plasmids encoding IL-4 and IL-10 prevents the development of autoimmune diabetes in nonobese diabetic mice', *Mol Ther*, 2001 **4**(4) 313–316.
130 Ignatius A A and Claes L E, '*In vitro* biocompatibility of bioresorbable polymers: poly(L, DL-lactide) and poly(L-lactide-co-glycolide)', *Biomaterials*, 1996 **17**(8) 831–839.
131 Steendam R, van Steenbergen M J, Hennink W E, Frijlink H W and Lerk C F, 'Effect of molecular weight and glass transition on relaxation and release behaviour of poly(DL-lactic acid) tablets', *J Control Release*, 2001 **70**(1–2) 71–82.
132 Ikada Y, Jamshidi K, Tsuji H and Hyon S-H, 'Stereocomplex formation between enantiomeric poly(lactides)', *Macromolecules*, 1987 **20**(4) 904–906.
133 Vert M, 'Bioresorbable polymers for temporary therapeutic applications', *Angew Makromol Chem*, 1989 **166**(February) 155–168.
134 Gunatillake P A and Adhikari R, 'Biodegradable synthetic polymers for tissue engineering', *Eur Cell Mater J*, 2003 **5** 1–16; discussion, 16.
135 Nair L S and Laurencin C T, 'Polymers as biomaterials for tissue engineering and controlled drug delivery', *Adv Biochem Eng Biotechnol*, 2006 **102**(October) 47–90.
136 Helder J, Kohn F E, Sato S, Vandenberg J W and Feijen J, 'Synthesis of poly[oxyethylidenecarbonylimino-(2-oxoethylene)] [poly(glycine-D,L-lactic acid)] by ring-opening polymerization', *Makromol Chem, Rapid Commun*, 1985 **6**(1) 9–14.

137 Helder J, Feijen J, Lee S J and Kim S W, 'Copolymers of D,L-lactic acid and glycine', *Makromol Chem, Rapid Commun*, 1986 **7**(4) 193–198.

138 Astete C E and Sabliov C M, 'Synthesis and characterization of PLGA nanoparticles', *J Biomater Sci, Polym Edn*, 2006 **17**(3) 247–289.

139 Gilding D K and Reed A M, 'Biodegradable polymers for use in surgery – polyglycolic/poly(actic acid) homo- and copolymers: 1', *Polymer*, 1979 **20**(12) 1459–1464.

140 Reed A M and Gilding D K, 'Biodegradable polymers for use in surgery – poly(glycolic)/poly(lactic acid) homo and copolymers: 2. *In vitro* degradation', *Polymer*, 1981 **22**(4) 494–498.

141 Miller R A, Brady J M and Cutright D E, 'Degradation rates of oral resorbable implants (polylactates and polyglycolates): rate modification with changes in PLA/PGA copolymer ratios', *J Biomed Mater Res*, 1977 **11**(5) 711–719.

142 Jiang W, Gupta R K, Deshpande M C and Schwendeman S P, 'Biodegradable poly(lactic-co-glycolic acid) microparticles for injectable delivery of vaccine antigens', *Adv Drug Deliv Rev*, 2005 **57**(3) 391–410.

143 Bala I, Hariharan S and Kumar M N, 'PLGA nanoparticles in drug delivery: the state of the art', *Crit Rev Ther Drug Carrier Syst*, 2004 **21**(5) 387–422.

144 Panyam J and Labhasetwar V, 'Targeting intracellular targets', *Curr Drug Deliv*, 2004 **1**(3) 235–247.

145 Panyam J and Labhasetwar V, 'Biodegradable nanoparticles for drug and gene delivery to cells and tissue', *Adv Drug Deliv Rev*, 2003 **55**(3) 329–347.

146 Taylor M S, Daniels A U, Andriano K P and Heller J, 'Six bioabsorbable polymers: *in vitro* acute toxicity of accumulated degradation products', *J Appl Biomater*, 1994 **5**(2) 151–157.

147 Hsu Y Y, Hao T and Hedley M L, 'Comparison of process parameters for microencapsulation of plasmid DNA in poly(D,L-lactic-co-glycolic) acid microspheres', *J Drug Target*, 1999 **7**(4) 313–323.

148 Walter E, Moelling K, Pavlovic J and Merkle H P, 'Microencapsulation of DNA using poly(DL-lactide-co-glycolide): stability issues and release characteristics', *J Control Release*, 1999 **61**(3) 361–374.

149 Wang C, Ge Q, Ting D, Nguyen D, Shen H R, Chen J, Eisen H N, Heller J, Langer R and Putnam D, 'Molecularly engineered poly(ortho ester) microspheres for enhanced delivery of DNA vaccines', *Nat Mater*, 2004 **3**(3) 190–196.

150 Gerweck L E and Seetharaman K, 'Cellular pH gradient in tumor versus normal tissue: potential exploitation for the treatment of cancer', *Cancer Res*, 1996 **56**(6) 1194–1198.

151 Choi N S and Heller J, 'Erodible agent releasing device comprising poly(ortho esters) and poly(ortho carbonates)', *US Pat 4,138,344*, Alza Corporation, 1979.

152 Choi N S and Heller J, 'Novel ortho ester polymers and orthocarbonate polymers', *US Pat 4,180,646*, Alza Corporation, 1979.

153 Choi N S and Heller J, 'Polycarbonates', *US Pat 4,079,038*, Alza Corporation, 1978.

154 Choi N S and Heller J, 'Drug delivery devices manufactured from poly(ortho esters) and poly(ortho carbonates)', *US Pat 4,093,709*, Alza Corporation, 1978.

155 Choi N S and Heller J, 'Structured ortho ester and ortho carbonate delivery devices', *US Pat 4,131,648*, Alza Corporation, 1978.
156 Yang K K, Wang X L and Wang Y Z, 'Poly(*p*-dioxanone) and its copolymers', *J Macromol Sci*, 2002 **42**(3) 373–398.
157 Schappacher M, Fabre T, Mingotaud A F and Soum A, 'Study of a (trimethylenecarbonate-co-epsilon-caprolactone) polymer. Part 1: preparation of a new nerve guide through controlled random copolymerization using rare earth catalysts', *Biomaterials*, 2001 **22**(21) 2849–2855.
158 Katz A R, Mukherjee D P, Kaganov A L and Gordon S, 'A new synthetic monofilament absorbable suture made from polytrimethylene carbonate', *Surg Gynecol Obstet*, 1985 **161**(3) 213–222.
159 Ahn C H, Chae S Y, Bae Y H and Kim S W, 'Biodegradable poly(ethylenimine) for plasmid DNA delivery', *J Control Release*, 2002 **80**(1–3) 273–282.
160 Petersen H, Merdan T, Kunath K, Fischer D and Kissel T, 'Poly(ethylenimine-co-L-lactamide-co-succinamide): a biodegradable polyethylenimine derivative with an advantageous pH-dependent hydrolytic degradation for gene delivery', *Bioconjug Chem*, 2002 **13**(4) 812–821.
161 Forrest M L, Koerber J T and Pack D W, 'A degradable polyethylenimine derivative with low toxicity for highly efficient gene delivery', *Bioconjug Chem*, 2003 **14**(5) 934–940.
162 Kim Y H, Park J H, Lee M, Kim Y H, Park T G and Kim S W, 'Polyethylenimine with acid-labile linkages as a biodegradable gene carrier', *J Control Release*, 2005 **103**(1) 209–219.
163 Thomas M, Ge Q, Lu J J, Chen J and Klibanov A M, 'Cross-linked small polyethylenimines: while still nontoxic, deliver DNA efficiently to mammalian cells *in vitro* and *in vivo*', *Pharm Res*, 2005 **22**(3) 373–380.
164 Park M R, Han K O, Han I K, Cho M H, Nah J W, Choi Y J and Cho C S, 'Degradable polyethylenimine-alt-poly(ethylene glycol) copolymers as novel gene carriers', *J Control Release*, 2005 **105**(3) 367–380.
165 Zhong Z, Feijen J, Lok M C, Hennink W E, Christensen L V, Yockman J W, Kim Y H and Kim S W, 'Low molecular weight linear polyethylenimine-β-poly(ethylene glycol)-β-polyethylenimine triblock copolymers: synthesis, characterization and *in vitro* gene transfer properties', *Biomacromolecules*, 2005 **6**(6) 3440–3448.
166 Bikram M, Lee M, Chang C W, Janát-Amsbury M M, Kern S E and Kim S W, 'Long-circulating DNA-complexed biodegradable multiblock copolymers for gene delivery: degradation profiles and evidence of dysopsonization', *J Control Release*, 2005 **103**(1) 221–233.
167 Bikram M, Ahn C H, Chae S Y, Lee M Y, Yockman J W and Kim S W, 'Biodegradable poly(ethylene glycol)-co-poly(L-lysine)-γ-histidine multiblock copolymers for nonviral gene delivery', *Macromolecules*, 2004 **37**(5) 1903–1916.
168 Anderson J M, Spilizewski K L and Hiltner A, 'Poly-α-amino acids as biomedical polymers', in *Biocompatibility of Tissue Analogs* (Ed D F Williams), Boca Raton, Florida, CRC Press, 1985, pp. 67–88.
169 Perin E C, 'Choosing a drug-eluting stent: a comparison between CYPHER and TAXUS', *Rev Cardiovasc Med*, 2005 **6** (Suppl 1) S13–S21.
170 Kohn J and Zeltinger J, 'Degradable, drug-eluting stents: a new frontier for the treatment of coronary artery disease', *Expert Rev Med Devices*, 2005 **2**(6) 667–671.

171 Westedt U, Wittmar M, Hellwig M, Hanefeld P, Greiner A, Schaper A K and Kissel T, 'Paclitaxel releasing films consisting of poly(vinyl alcohol)-graft-poly(lactide-co-glycolide) and their potential as biodegradable stent coatings', *J Control Release*, 2006 **111**(1–2) 235–246.
172 Sharif F, Hynes S O, McMahon J, Cooney R, Conroy S, Dockery P, Duffy G, Daly K, Crowley J, Bartlett J S and O'Brien T, 'Gene-eluting stents: comparison of adenoviral and adeno-associated viral gene delivery to the blood vessel wall *in vivo*', *Hum Gene Ther*, 2006 **17**(7) 741–750.
173 Jewell C M, Zhang J, Fredin N J, Wolff M R, Hacker T A and Lynn D M, 'Release of plasmid DNA from intravascular stents coated with ultrathin multilayered polyelectrolyte films', *Biomacromolecules*, 2006 **7**(9) 2483–2491.

5

Polymers as replacement materials for heart valves and arteries

D M ESPINO, University of Birmingham, UK

5.1 Introduction

Failure of heart valves or arteries reduces the flow of blood to the body. If vital organs do not receive sufficient blood, a person may die, unless the condition is remedied. Myxomatous degeneration of heart valves, for example, can lead to their failure, with the end result of insufficient blood flowing out from the heart, while atherosclerosis or thrombus formation (or an embolism) may, for example, block small arteries, which can lead to strokes or heart attacks.

Devices or natural tissues can be used to replace heart valves or arteries. These replacement materials are used when the natural heart valves or arteries fail to function properly, which can cause death or severe disability if left uncorrected. Such replacement materials help to restore the flow of blood that the body needs in order to function properly. Natural tissues are commonly used as replacement materials; alternatively pyrolytic carbon mechanical valves are used to replace heart valves, while metal stents can be used to hold arteries open. However, there is interest in the development of polymers as replacement materials for heart valves and for use with stents. There is also much interest in developing natural tissues by tissue engineering.

This chapter briefly introduces the tissues present in heart valves and arteries and then describes the materials and devices used to replace them. Section 5.2 provides an overview of both the heart and arteries (i.e. the cardiovascular system). Heart valve prostheses are then discussed in Section 5.3, followed by arterial replacement in Section 5.4 and tissue-engineered arteries in Section 5.5. A summary, and potential future developments, of the devices described is provided in Section 5.6. Section 5.7 suggests sources of further information, with references provided in Section 5.9.

5.2 The cardiovascular system

This section provides an introduction to the cardiovascular system; more detailed information on its anatomy, function and subsequent diseases can be found elsewhere (see, for example, Guyton and Hall (1996) and Levick (1998)). Sections 5.2.1 and 5.2.2 provide brief overviews on natural heart valves and arteries respectively.

The heart is at the centre of the cardiovascular system and contracts to pump blood around the body. It consists of four chambers that act as two separate pumping systems. These are the left atrium and left ventricle, and the right atrium and right ventricle. The left ventricle pumps blood through the aorta (an artery) and this circulates around the body through arteries; cells extract nutrients (such as O_2) from the blood and deposit waste into it (such as CO_2). The deoxygenated blood returns to the right atrium (through the venous system) and passes to the right ventricle. The right ventricle pumps the blood through the pulmonary artery towards the lungs, where the blood is oxygenated again and CO_2 released. This oxygenated blood passes to the left atrium and into the left ventricle, and the cycle is repeated.

The atria contract at the same time and, following a small delay, so do the ventricles. So, atria pump blood to the ventricles, before the ventricles pump blood to the body through arteries. The filling with blood of the left ventricle is known as diastole, whereas the stage of ventricular contraction (i.e. when the ventricles pump blood) is called systole. The right side of the heart pumps blood to the lungs and does so at mean systolic pressures of about 15–20 mmHg (or 2.0–2.7 kPa; 1 mmHg = 133 Pa). The left side of the heart works at higher mean systolic pressures (about 120 mmHg; i.e. about 16 kPa), in order to pump blood all around the body.

5.2.1 Valves

Heart valves allow blood to flow in the correct direction through the heart, to ensure that oxygenated blood is supplied to the body, and deoxygenated blood (high in CO_2) flows through to the lungs. Valves are vital to effective cardiac function.

Semilunar valves are present between the outflow duct of the ventricles, and the large arteries that carry blood to the body. They are the aortic and pulmonary valves and are present within the aorta and pulmonary artery outflow tract respectively (i.e. left and right sides, respectively, of the heart). Semilunar valves have three cusps that seal together to close the valve or move towards the vessel wall to open the valve (allowing forward flow). These valves prevent reflux of blood from the arteries into the ventricles during diastole and allow forward flow of blood through to the arteries during systole.

Atrioventricular valves, namely the mitral and tricuspid valves, are found in the left and right sides, respectively, of the heart, in between the atria and ventricles. The mitral valve has two cusps that seal to close the valve, whereas the tricuspid valve has three cusps. Atrioventricular valves have string-like chordae tendineae that connect to the ventricular wall through papillary muscles (see the discussion on mitral valve repair as an alternative to replacement given in Section 5.3). These valves prevent blood from flowing back into atria during systole and allow forward flow of blood into ventricles during diastole.

A range of possible complications exists that can damage heart valves (see, for example, Stevens and Lowe (1997)). Functionally, however, this generally consists of two complications: regurgitation and stenosis. Regurgitation occurs when the reflux of blood is not prevented by a closed valve; stenosis occurs when an open valve does not allow the forward flow of blood.

Heart valves are composed of connective tissue (collagen, elastin and glycosaminoglycans (Stevens and Lowe, (1997)), and open or close in response to pressure gradients and haemodynamics (Caro *et al.*, 1978).

5.2.2 Arteries

Arteries are composed of three layers: the intima, media and adventitia (Fig. 5.1). A layer of endothelial cells rests on the intima, which is made mostly of connective tissue (i.e. collagen, elastin and glycosaminoglycans). The media contains smooth muscle cells within a network of elastin and collagen fibres, while the adventitia consists of connective tissue. Blood flows through the lumen of blood vessels and is in contact with the endothelial layer (or endothelium). This endothelial layer is composed of endothelial cells and protects arteries (see below).

Arteries have different compositions, depending on their function. The aorta, for example, is a large artery (approximately 25 mm in diameter) with a greater proportion of connective tissue and less smooth muscle than smaller arteries such as coronary or popliteal arteries (smaller than 6 mm in diameter). The smooth muscle (in the media) in arteries allows them to vary their diameter, i.e. they vary their resistance to flow (through the nervous system, which sends impulses to these blood vessels through nerves; for further details on the nervous system see Guyton and Hall (1996)).

Atherosclerosis occurs when fatty deposits are present on blood vessel walls; this may thicken and occlude the vessel lumen (Fig 5.2(a) and Fig. 5.2(b)), forming an atheromatous plaque. Atherosclerosis disrupts the vessel endothelium and encourages thrombus formation. The endothelium naturally protects against thrombus formation or clotting of blood on its surface (platelet aggregation), which may occlude the lumen of the vessel (Yang *et al.*, 1994). Segments of the thrombus that break away are known

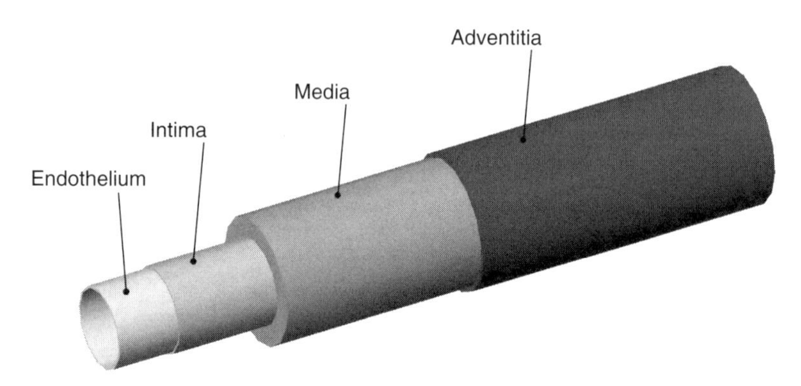

5.1 The endothelial, intimal, medial and adventitial layers are denoted; blood flows through the lumen of the artery (which is in contact with the endothelium). The endothelium consists of endothelial cells that protect the artery; these are in contact with the intima which is composed of connective tissue. The media contains a high proportion of smooth muscle cells, while the adventitia is composed mostly of connective tissue. A higher proportion of smooth muscle allows the artery more control over its diameter (and therefore its resistance to flow), while a higher proportion of connective tissue increases the elastic compliance of the artery. Large vessels such as the aorta have a higher proportion of connective tissue, while smaller arteries such as coronary or popliteal arteries have a higher proportion of smooth muscle (i.e. a thicker media).

as embolisms. These may flow through the arterial system and occlude smaller blood vessels.

Occluded blood vessels can lead to complications. Coronary arteries supply heart muscle with nutrients and, if they become blocked, the heart tissue becomes ischaemic; that is to say that the heart tissue has poor blood supply (and, therefore, poor supply of nutrients). A heart attack or ischaemic heart disease, for example, may follow. Occluded popliteal arteries may lead to ischaemia, causing complications such as gangrene, which may require leg amputations.

5.3 Replacing heart valves

This section describes valves used for heart valve replacement. The replacement of left ventricular valves are dealt with first (Section 5.3.1), followed

5.2 Arteries. (a) View through the lumen of the artery. (b) Atherosclerotic plaques occlude the lumen of arteries. Such plaques reduce the blood flow through arteries, which can cause death or disease of the tissue it supplies with blood. (c) A bypass graft (arrowed) can be placed to provide an alternative route for blood to flow around the plaque in the stenosed artery.

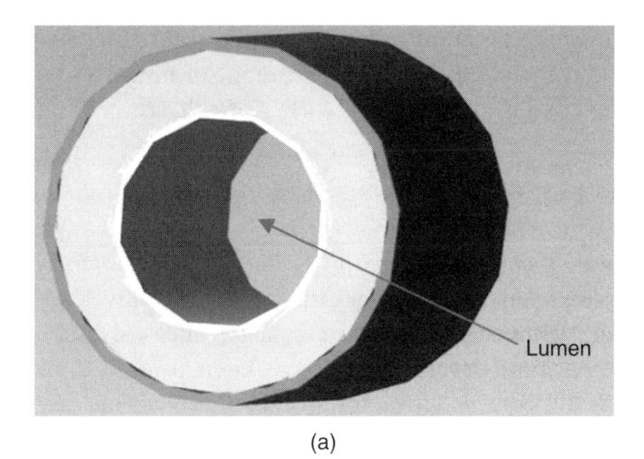

(a)

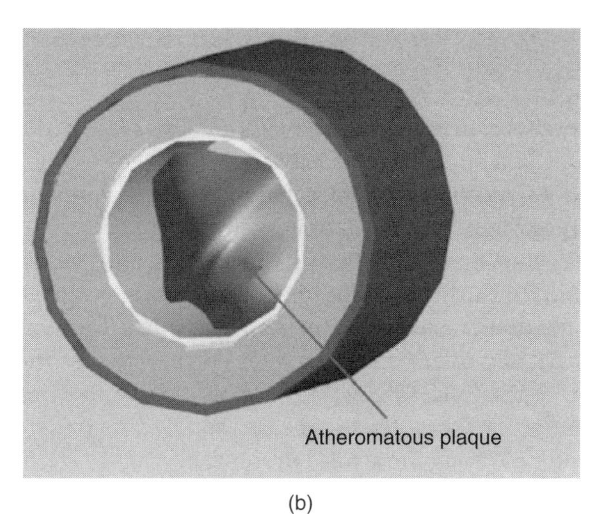

(b)

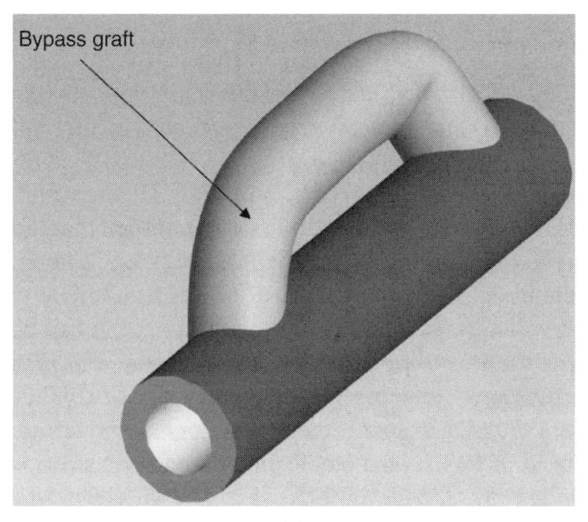

(c)

by the current state of repair of valves from the right side of the heart (Section 5.3.2). Also included is the development of mitral valve surgical repair, as an alternative to replacement with a prosthesis.

5.3.1 Replacing mitral and aortic valves

Similar replacement techniques have often been employed for replacing mitral and aortic valves, despite the fact that the aortic valve is a trileaflet valve in a conduit, while the mitral valve is a bileaflet valve covering an opening. Mechanical and tissue valves have been used with their own advantages and disadvantages. However, polymeric valves may represent a way forward for the future.

Mechanical valves

Mechanical valves were first implanted with clinical success during the 1960s; these were ball-and-cage valves (Starr *et al.*, 1967). These valves initially consisted of a silicone rubber ball contained within a Lucite (poly(methyl methacrylate)) cage. A stainless steel ring and steel wire were used to attach a Teflon sheet to the valve, the Teflon was then stitched to the heart (Starr and Edwards, 1961). Initial developments saw the development of a silicone rubber shield to prevent thrombus formation from occluding the orifice, and use of a stainless steel cage to reduce the dimensions required (Starr and Edwards, 1961). Variants of this valve were developed, e.g. with open struts (i.e. not a closed cage) and Dacron (poly(ethylene terephthalate)) cloth covering the struts (Braunwald *et al.*, 1971). The principle behind the function of these valves was essentially the same, the ball responded to pressure gradients, for closing and opening, whilst the cage held the ball in place.

Similar mechanical valves were developed that consisted of caged- and tilting-disc prostheses (Schoen *et al.*, 1982). Discs are typically made from pyrolytic carbon (i.e. produced by pyrolysis, a process of thermal decomposition, followed by carbon recrystallization (Wnek and Bowlin, 2004)), and cages from cobalt–chromium or titanium alloy (Padera and Schoen, 2004). The caged disc consists of a cage with a disc rather than a ball held in place. The disc blocks the orifice or moves away from it, depending on the pressure gradient. Tilting discs consist of a disc at an angle that leads to asymmetrical flow; in the mitral position, for example, it can be used to direct flow towards the posterior part of the ventricular wall (Fontaine *et al.*, 1996). Tilting discs have small cage-like restraints to control their motion (Bjork and Henze, 1979). Dacron or e-PTFE (expanded polytetrafluoroethylene: a single strand of PTFE which is expanded and has a ratio of about

50% air by volume; see, for example, Zussa (1995)) sewing rings on mechanical valves (including bileaflet valves; see below) are used to attach valves to the heart (see, for example, Padera and Schoen (2004)).

Mechanical failure associated with ball-and-cage valve prosthesis include sticking of the ball in between the struts (owing to swelling of the ball), and failure of the struts; caged-disc prosthesis suffered similar complications such as sticking of the discs, uneven motion of the disc within the cage or wear of the disc leading to leakage of blood (Schoen *et al.*, 1982).

Bileaflet valves, such as the St Jude Medical bileaflet valve, were developed in the 1970s (Emery *et al.*, 1979). These valves consist of a ring and two rigid leaflets (Emery *et al.*, 1979). They respond to pressure gradients, but the two-leaflet design leads to improved haemodynamics when compared with caged-valve prosthesis (see, for example, Fontaine *et al.* (1996)). It is thought that improved hydrodynamic flow through heart valves reduces problems related to blood coagulation (i.e. thrombus formation; see Section 5.2.2). Bileaflet valves are made from pyrolytic carbon, also thought to reduce platelet aggregation and thrombus formation, while being durable (Cao, 1995). However, it has been shown that platelets are still activated (i.e. they begin to aggregate and to form blood clots) by pyrolytic carbon (Goodman *et al.*, 1996) and thrombus formation can only be avoided by lifelong anticoagulation therapy, i.e. by using prescribed drugs (such as warfarin or heparin), that act pharmacologically, to prevent blood from clotting. Anticoagulation therapy has the disadvantage of increasing the risk of haemorrhages (i.e. uncontrolled bleeding that might occur after an injury), because blood clotting normally acts to stop such bleeding.

The main problems currently associated with mechanical valves include the need for long term anticoagulants (including the increased risk of haemorrhages), haemolysis (of red blood cells), endocarditis and wear of mechanical valves (Schoen *et al.*, 1982; Starr *et al.*, 2002). Haemolysis, is believed to be caused by the fast closing action of the valve leaflets, damaging the red blood cells (Kingsbury *et al.*, 1993; Garrison *et al.*, 1994; Wu *et al.*, 1994); this can be either relatively trivial or in a few cases can lead to severe anaemia (Schoen *et al.*, 1982). Developments of valves that close more physiologically, such as starting to close before systole, are being investigated (Naemura *et al.*, 1999). However, in its severe form, haemolysis is more likely to be caused by blood leakage, either through poor attachment of the valve to the heart, or through wear of the prosthesis (Padera and Schoen, 2004). Endocarditis is an infection of the valve tissue caused by the insertion of the prosthetic valve (Schoen *et al.*, 1982) with an incidence of less than 0.3% per patient year in either the mitral or the aortic position (Piper *et al.*, 2001). While it is always important to improve prosthesis resistance to wear, current mechanical valves are more durable than replacement with tissue valves (see below (Starr *et al.*, 2002)). Despite the use of anticoagulants with replacement valves, the incidence of thromboembolism (i.e. complications related to thrombus formation and embolisms; see Section 5.2.2) is about 1.5–3% per year and represents the main area of improvement required for mechanical valves (Starr *et al.*, 2002).

Tissue valves

Natural heart valves, termed bioprostheses, include the bovine pericardial tissue valve, and porcine aortic valves. They can be used to overcome some of the complications associated with mechanical heart valves.

Bioprostheses do not lead to the excessive thrombus formation seen with mechanical valves, and therefore drugs do not have to be prescribed for lifelong anticoagulation (unlike mechanical valves). While this is not a mechanical or material improvement, it improves the quality of life of patients. Another benefit of these valves is that they produce better haemodynamics than mechanical valves owing to the more natural structure and flexible leaflet material used (Fontaine *et al.*, 1996; Starr *et al.*, 2002; Padera and Schoen, 2004). However, the main problem with bioprosthetic valves is the poor long-term durability as compared with mechanical valves. It has been estimated that only between 30 and 40% of tissue valves may still be functioning after 15 years (Starr *et al.*, 2002). This can be a concern especially in the young, where degeneration occurs at a faster rate than in older patients (Starr *et al.*, 2002). To reduce degeneration, tissue valves are fixed using glutaraldehyde (Carpentier, 1977). Glutaraldehyde fixation encourages calcification (Schoen and Levy, 1999), which leads to valve failure. However, alternative methods of tissue preservation by cross-linking such as that caused by polyepoxy compounds (e.g. poly(glycidyl ether)) and dye-mediated photo-oxidation are under investigation (Schmidt and Baier, 2000).

Bovine pericardial tissue is used to produce tissue valves. The tissue is attached to a frame (metal or plastic) and is covered in synthetic material (e.g. e-PTFE or Dacron (Padera and Schoen, 2004)). Glutaraldehyde-fixed bovine pericardial valves are made to have three leaflets (i.e. to replicate aortic valve structure).

Porcine aortic valves, fixed in glutaraldehyde, are also used for valve replacement. The main difference between porcine aortic valves and bovine pericardial valves is that porcine valves have leaflets that are naturally connected to the rest of the valve (unlike pericardial valves where the leaflets have to be attached to a frame).

Tissue valves can be either stentlesss or stented. Stented valves usually have three stents that allow easier surgical placement (Schoen and Levy, 1999). However, stented valves may suffer from inferior leaflet biomechanics that may promote calcification (Fisher, 1995). This may be corrected by improved fixation processes (Fisher, 1995).

An alternative to using animal tissue valves is to use human valves (or homografts). Aortic valve homografts can be used to replace heart valves, but their availability is usually limited (e.g. see the discussion given by Breymann *et al.* (2002)). Homografts can be cryopreserved, to prevent their degradation, until they are used for implantation (Padera and Scheon, 2004). Also used for aortic valve replacement can be the patient's own pulmonary valve (i.e. an autograft). The pulmonary valve is then replaced with another valve, such as a homograft valve (see, for example, Lupinetti *et al.* (1997)). The use of homografts and autografts in children is particularly useful, because it provides an alternative either to using tissue valves that calcify quickly in children, or to the use of anticoagulants with mechanical valves (Lupinetti *et al.*, 1997). Human replacement valves in children are thought to grow as the heart grows (Elkins *et al.*, 1994).

Polymeric valves

Flexible leaflet aortic replacement valves were developed in the 1960s (Roe *et al.*, 1966). These had three silicone rubber leaflets, and Roe *et al.* (1966) suggested that including the use of a surface coating that prevented clotting might result in a clinically successful prosthesis. Other flexible synthetic valves were also developed, such as those made from Teflon (Braunwald *et al.*, 1965). However, previous polymeric valves have suffered from poor durability and thrombus formation (see, for example, Fishbein *et al.* (1975)).

There has been recent interest in developing polymeric valves made from polyurethanes. Polyurethanes have good blood compatibility (Zdrahala and Zdrahala, 1999) and can be made into physiological shapes, forming valves which are flexible (Mackay *et al.*, 1996). Synthetic poly(carbonate urethane) valves have been recently developed, for both the aortic (Daebritz *et al.*, 2004) and the mitral (Daebritz *et al.*, 2003) positions, as have poly(ether urethane) valves (Mackay *et al.*, 1996) and valves made from poly(ether urethane) frames coated with poly(ether urethane urea) (Bernacca *et al.*, 1997). *In vivo* results are promising, with tests being performed without anticoagulants in some cases (Daebritz *et al.*, 2003, 2004), and showing greater signs of durability than bioprostheses when tested in calves (Daebritz *et al.*, 2003, 2004) or sheep (Wheatley *et al.*, 2000). It has been proposed that the composition of such polyurethane valves may affect their calcification and wear (Bernacca *et al.*, 1997). Therefore, further developments of polyurethane synthesis technology may offer promise for developments of valves in future.

The development of these valves into successful clinical implants will ultimately depend on their long-term function, which can only be determined clinically. Furthermore, its long-term durability will also be an important determinant of its clinical value. The hope would be that these valves could combine the benefits of both mechanical and bioprosthetic valves, with improved durability but also leading to physiological hydrodynamics and reduced thrombus formation.

Mitral valve repair as an alternative to replacement

Replacement of mitral valves with bioprostheses or mechanical prosthesis have several limitations (Section 5.3.1). Advantages of mitral valve repair reported include long-term clinical results equivalent to those from replacement with a prosthesis, reduced or no use of anticoagulants, reduced risk of endocarditis, reduced surgical mortality risk, as well as better long-term survival rates (Perier *et al.*, 1984; Sand *et al.*, 1987; Loop *et al.*, 1991; Enriquez-Sarano *et al.*, 1995). Moreover, an increase in reoperation rates has not been observed when comparing long-term mitral valve repair results with replacement prosthetic valves (Perier *et al.*, 1984). One point that needs to be made is that no randomised trial comparing mitral valve repair and replacement has been performed (Enriquez-Sarano *et al.*, 1995). Typically, mitral valve repair is performed on healthier patients (see, for example, Sand *et al.* (1987) and Enriquez-Sarano *et al.* (1995)).

Chordae tendineae are mostly composed of collagen, elastin and glycosaminoglycans (Lis *et al.*, 1987) and hold leaflets in place during valve closure. Rupture of chordae causes mitral valve regurgitation (Espino *et al.*, 2005, 2006b). Chordal rupture can be repaired by several techniques (Espino *et al.*, 2006a) including edge to edge repair (where stitches are placed to allow the prolapsing leaflet to be supported by the non-prolapsing leaflet (Maisano *et al.*, 1999)); chordal transposition (where a chord from a separate part of the valve is placed at the area of leaflet prolapse, while the healthy leaflet from where it was removed is restitched together (Carpentier, 1983)) or chordal replacement where a synthetic material is used to replace the ruptured chord or chordae (Tomita *et al.*, 2002). Such mitral valve repairs are often accompanied by the placement of annuloplasty rings (these reduce the orifice area at the opening of the mitral valve) to reduce dilation that causes mitral valve failure (see, for example, Perier *et al.* (1984)).

Materials such as braided polyester, polybutester (a butylene terephthalate and poly(tetramethylene ether glycol) copolymer), polypropylene, PTFE or e-PTFE can be used for such repairs. For chordal transposition and edge-to-edge repair, the sutures are there to hold the leaflet tissue in place. However, during chordal replacement, the synthetic suture acts as a neochord. PTFE has been found to have the material properties closer to natural chordae than other materials such as braided polyester (Cochran and Kunzelman, 1991). However, the values of Young's modulus for all these replacement materials were much higher than those of natural chordae (about 7700 MPa for PTFE and 8100 MPa for braided polyester as compared with about 20 to 30 MPa for chordae, as determined by the same research group (Kunzelman and Cochran, 1990)). Ideally, replacement chordae would have similar properties to the chordae that they replace. Such a large difference in material properties may reduce valve leaflet mobility, thereby increasing the risk of stenosis during valve closure (Kobayashi *et al.*, 1996).

An alternative to synthetic chordae is the use of natural tissues, such as glutaraldehyde-tanned pericardial strips (Ng *et al.*, 2001). However, PTFE has been found to produce better clinical results than glutaraldehyde-tanned pericardial strips for chordal replacement (Kobayashi *et al.*, 1996). The use of glutaraldehyde and its induction of calcification may well have an adverse effect on clinical results (Section 5.3.1).

e-PTFE is a single strand of PTFE which has been expanded and has a porous microstructure with a ratio of more than 50% air by volume (Zussa, 1995). It is thought that the porous microstructure of e-PTFE allows cells to infiltrate it (Zussa *et al.*, 1997). Zussa (1995) reported that these cells had a strong adhesion to e-PTFE without calcification or thrombus formation. However, in the first reported case of e-PTFE chordal rupture (after 14 years), it was found that in some areas the sutures had been almost completely replaced by minerals, including calcium salts (Butany *et al.*, 2004). e-PTFE replacement chordae become covered in a smooth fibrous sheath that is surrounded by an endothelial cell layer (Zussa, 1995). From animal studies it was observed that the diameter of such synthetic chordae after cell infiltration was similar to that of natural chordae (Zussa, 1995). Whether e-PTFE synthetic replacement chordae covered in such tissues leads to beneficial or adverse mechanical properties or effects is unknown.

Developments of new chordal replacement materials may further improve mitral valve repair in the long term. Tissue-engineered synthetic chordae which have been reported have been made from cultured fibroblast and smooth muscle cells, with added type I collagen (Shi and Vesely, 2003, 2004). Under static loading, Young's modulus and the failure strength were about an order of magnitude below those required. Excess elongation of chordae (as caused by a low Young's modulus) clinically leads to regurgitation (Barber *et al.*, 2001). Higher stresses induced by stiffer chordae (i.e. high Young's modulus as seen for synthetic replacement chordae) may be more critical to the long-term success of the repair (Reimink *et al.*, 1995), or to tearing of the leaflet after being stitched in place. It is possible that strategies used for developments in blood vessels using tissue engineering may hold clues for chordal tissue engineering (see Section 5.5). Tissue-engineered chordae could, potentially, be produced to have viscoelastic material properties that match those of natural chordae (see, for example, Lim and Boughner (1975) and Lim *et al.* (1977)).

To summarise, mitral valve repair (including chordal replacement) has many benefits over replacement with a prosthesis. Several chordal replacement materials can be used, with e-PTFE often being the replacement material of choice (see, for example, Zussa *et al.* (1997)). However, replacement synthetic chordae with properties closer to real chordae may well provide benefits for mitral valve replacement. Replacement materials in future may include tissue-engineered chordae tendineae.

5.3.2 Replacing pulmonary and tricuspid valves

The gold standards for right ventricular outflow tract reconstruction (i.e. the pulmonary valve conduit) are currently aortic and pulmonary homografts. However, homografts are not always available, especially in small sizes (Allen *et al.*, 2002; Breymann *et al.*, 2002) (see Section 5.3.1). Furthermore, homografts undergo faster degeneration and calcification in young patients (Hawkins *et al.*, 1992). Alternatives such as porcine xenografts (i.e. cross-species) in Dacron conduits have not met with great success, as problems such as calcification have been encountered (Tweddell *et al.*, 2000). However, porcine xenografts may be an alternative for valve conduits less than 15 mm in diameter (Lange *et al.*, 2001). Alternatives such as the use of bovine pericardial tissue valves (Section 5.3.1) with a PTFE conduit (rather than a Dacron conduit) have led to good midterm results (Allen *et al.*, 2002), while good early results have been obtained with bovine-valved venous conduits (i.e. bovine jugular vein, with its trileaflet valve in place) fixed in glutaraldehyde, available in smaller sizes (Breymann *et al.*, 2002).

Another perspective is provided by the development of acellular valves (Goldstein *et al.*, 2000; Steinhoff *et al.*, 2000; Elkins *et al.*, 2001; Simon *et al.*, 2003). In such valves, cells from the original valve structure are removed (these may be porcine valves). However, the valve structure (i.e. extracellular matrix components such as collagen, elastin and proteoglycans) remains. The idea is that host cells infiltrate the scaffold and allow it to regenerate, function and grow naturally within the body. This provides an ideal scenario for young patients undergoing growth, given the limitations with homografts (Section 5.3.1). Good *in vitro* and *in vivo* results (Steinhoff *et al.*, 2000; Elkins *et al.*, 2001) and some initial clinical trials show promise (Goldstein *et al.*, 2000). However, such acellular valves led to poor clinical results for paediatric patients (Simon *et al.*, 2003). Clearly, the use of acellular valves may hold great promise for valve replacement, with further understanding of how such structures react and function after implantation being necessary.

Tricuspid valves

Tricuspid valves are typically repaired whenever possible (see, for example, Rizzoli *et al.* (1998), Carrier *et al.* (2003), Bernal *et al.* (2004) and Bernal *et al.* (2005)). However, replacement with a prosthesis is performed when necessary. Replacement valves are the same as those used for left ventricle valve replacement (Section 5.3.1) (Rizzoli *et al.*, 1998; Carrier *et al.*, 2003). Whether it is best to use mechanical or bioprosthetic valves for such replacement procedures remains unclear (Rizzoli *et al.*, 1998; Carrier *et al.*, 2003). The arguments for mechanical or bioprosthetic valves are similar as those presented in Section 5.3.1, with mechanical valves having better durability but requiring lifelong anticoagulation. However, bioprosthesis are more durable in the right side of the heart than in the left side, but high rates of bioprosthetic degeneration are common after about 7 years post-implantation (Rizzoli *et al.*, 1998).

5.4 Replacing arteries

Large arteries have been found to be successfully replaced with synthetic materials, such as e-PTFE or Dacron. However, replacement of smaller arteries (less than about 6 mm) with such synthetic materials has been less successful (Conte *et al.*, 1998). This section, therefore, discusses the repair and replacement of small-diameter arteries. Natural tissues (Section 5.4.1) as bypass grafts, and stents (Section 5.4.2) to maintain the vessel structure, have been used to improve blood flow in small occluded vessels. Stents and better anticoagulation therapies have improved restenosis rates but have not eradicated it. Other strategies are therefore being adopted, such as tissue engineering of blood vessels (Section 5.5).

5.4.1 Natural tissues

Replacement of small-diameter arteries has so far proven most successful using segments from other parts of the vascular system, as bypass grafts (Fig. 5.2(c)). The internal mammary artery has been used to replenish flow in coronary and popliteal arteries (Okies *et al.*, 1984) and is considered as the best graft candidate (Cox *et al.*, 1991). However, it is not always possible to use the internal mammary artery, because of limited availability of the vessel, or because it has been used previously. The other common alternative is the use of the saphenous vein for bypass grafting (Cox *et al.*, 1991; Sayers *et al.*, 1998).

Saphenous veins (Fig. 5.3) are not always healthy to begin with (Cox *et al.*, 1991). Furthermore, while veins are compliant over the venous pressure range, they are not designed to support higher pressures of the arterial

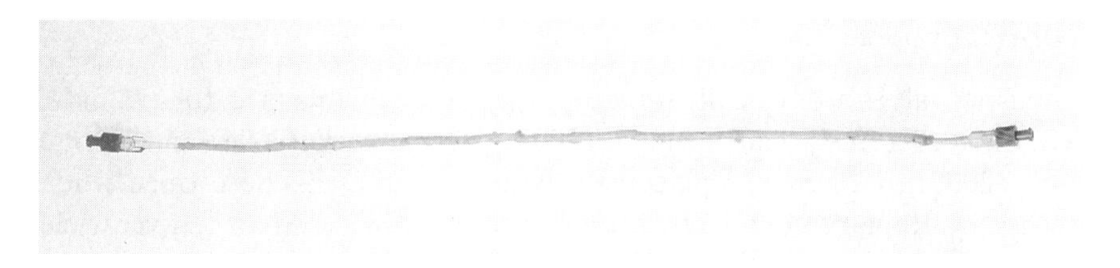

5.3 Saphenous vein. Section of vein that can be used for arterial bypass grafting. (Picture reprinted with permission from CryoLife, Inc., Kennesaw, Georgia.)

system. This can lead to a mismatch in compliance compared with neighbouring arteries (Cox *et al.*, 1991).

After grafting of saphenous veins, occlusion may occur (Cox *et al.*, 1991). The development of intimal hyperplasia may start as early as a few weeks post-operatively. Intimal hyperplasia is believed to be caused by excessive smooth muscle growth and proliferation (into the intima), as well as growth of the extracellular matrix, occluding the lumen. This remains the main problem associated with graft occlusion after 5 years. The thickening occurs over time, occluding the flow into the artery from the vein graft (Bassiouny *et al.*, 1992). In the longer term, atherosclerosis becomes the main cause for concern and progresses quickly. Furthermore, patients that require multiple operations to small arterial vessels can require reoperations, limiting the available tissue.

Therefore, given the limited availability of natural tissues, and in the case of the saphenous vein the complications that can occur, there is a clear need for surgical alternatives.

5.4.2 Stents

During balloon angioplasty an inflatable device is inserted into a stenosed artery and inflated so as to increase the diameter of the occluded lumen (for a more detailed explanation of this, see Padera and Schoen (2004)). While it can be successful in some cases, restenosis does occur. Stents are often used with balloon angioplasty, in order to prevent restenosis. Stents are typically made from a wire mesh (see below) and hold the artery open, preventing its collapse, i.e. the stent keeps the artery open at the diameter required for adequate blood flow.

Materials

Stents are usually composed of metal wires forming the outer boundaries of an open cylinder. The most widely used stents are made from stainless steel (Bertrand *et al.*, 1998; Topol and Serruys, 1998; Padera and Schoen,

2004) and are relatively inert when in place. Nitinol stents (a nickel–titanium alloy) are also popular; Nitinol is said to be superelastic and has thermal shape memory (Ryhanen *et al.*, 1997). So, it can be inserted in one state and heated so as to regain the required shape *in vivo*. Processing during manufacture can allow the shape after heating to be programmed.

One potential problem with Nitinol is the release of toxic nickel into surrounding tissues. However, passivation of the surface of the Nitinol stent (e.g. with nitric acid) increases the amount of titanium oxide on the surface. This is thought to improve corrosion resistance and to reduce the amount of nickel released (O'Brien *et al.*, 2002).

Self-expanding stents can be used as an alternative to balloon expandable stents (Topol and Serruys, 1998). Some stainless steel stents, for example, expand until tissue resistance prevents the stent from further expansion, while Nitinol stents can be designed to expand to a programmed size. Topol and Serruys (1998) also reported several types of custom-made stent that are available commercially, such as bifurcating stents, and stents with holes (to improve flow through side branches).

Stents have been very successful clinically and may well be used in over 50% of angioplasty (Section 5.4.2) procedures (Topol and Serruys, 1998). However, arteries held open by stents sometimes become occluded (i.e. restenosis may still occur). Such occlusion may be caused, in the short term (i.e. days after surgery), by the formation of a thrombus (Section 5.2.2) in the lumen of the artery (Section 5.2.2 (see Fig. 5.2(a) and Fig. 5.2(b)). Intimal hyperplasia (see Section 5.4.1) may occur in the longer term (i.e. months after surgery (Topol and Serruys, 1998)). The placement of stents may damage the arterial endothelial layer (by abrasion; for more detail see Padera and Schoen (2004)), which may cause some of the problems associated with stents. This is because (as explained in Section 5.2.2), the endothelial layer prevents thrombus formation on the artery surface and may prevent smooth muscle cell proliferation (Yang *et al.*, 1994) that leads to intimal hyperplasia (see Section 5.4.1).

To prevent the formation of thrombus on stents, drugs are used (Topol and Serruys, 1998). These drugs are usually used in the short term (as thrombus occlusion occurs in the short term after stent implantation; see above); stents do not usually require the same long-term anticoagulation therapy necessary with mechanical heart valves (Topol and Serruys, 1998). However, the ideal stent would not require prescribed drugs to function effectively (i.e. they would not cause thrombus formation).

Introduction to coatings

Initially stents were designed to be bioinert (by using materials such as stainless steel). However, coatings may be necessary to avoid restenosis after stent implantation. Polymer coatings, including natural polymers such as heparin (a polysaccharide), have been used on stents. In this instance, heparin is used to coat the material, and not as a pharmacological agent (as with mechanical valves (Section 5.3.1)). Degradation of polymer coatings, however, raises concerns of possible toxicity. However, a similar approach has been used as a drug delivery system, where substances of choice are released (e.g. to reduce thrombosis or prevent excessive smooth muscle cell proliferation).

Polymer coatings

Several non-degradable coatings have been tested in animal studies for covering stents (Bertrand *et al.*, 1998), including polyurethane (De Scheerder *et al.*, 1994) and silicon carbide (Ozbek *et al.*, 1997). Fewer, however, have reached human trials; one such coating is silicon carbide, which reduces fibrinogen activation (this may be important in the development of restenosis). However, restenosis was not eliminated, and Ozbek *et al.* (1997) suggested that further investigation into the use of anticoagulation with this stent was needed. Other haemocompatible substances such as diamond-like carbon coating have been suggested for stainless steel (Santin *et al.*, 2004), while a gold coating led to poor clinical results (Kastrati *et al.*, 2000).

Stents coated with resorbable polymers are also under investigation. Polymers such as polycaprolactone and polyorthoester, and copolymers such as polyglycolic–polylactic acid, poly(hydroxybutyrate valerate) and poly(ethylene oxide)–poly(butylene terephthalate) have been compared *in vivo* as resorbable stent coatings (van der Giessen *et al.*, 1996). However, during examination after they were implanted on metallic stents *in vivo* (in pigs, over a 4-week period), these polymer coatings led to signs of both chronic and acute inflammation, as well as proliferation of cells (which may cause intimal hyperplasi; see Section 5.4.1). Thrombus deposits were also detected, and in some cases acute thrombotic occlusion led to death, within 2 days of being implanted. As part of this study, three non-biodegradable polymers were also tested (polyurethane, silicone and poly(ethylene terephthalate)) with similar results to the resorbable polymers tested.

Natural coatings

Stents have been coated with phosphorylcholine, in order to mimic the natural membrane that surrounds cells. The natural cell membrane is made from phospholipids, composed of two fatty acid groups and one phosphorylated alcohol group bound to glycerol (for more details see Raven and Johnson (1996)). Initial clinical reports show good clinical results at 6 months follow-up, but these results did not show an improvement over uncoated stents (Bakhai *et al.*, 2005). Phosphorylcholine applied to the stents has the potential of preventing the stent from inducing the formation of a thrombus on its surface. This is because platelet adhesion (see Section 5.2.2) is reduced (as is protein absorption), which reduces the formation of thrombus (Grenadier *et al.*, 2002). Such a phosphorylcholine synthetic coating has been found to be non-inflamatory and biocompatible (Whelan *et al.*, 2000). It has been proposed that phosphorylcholine could be used, as a coating, for drug delivery (Whelan *et al.*, 2000) because of its good biocompatibility, and because other candidates are other polymers that have led to poor biocompatibility (see above), especially as regards inflammation (van der Giessen *et al.*, 1996).

The use of a vein graft cuff within a stent has also been used clinically, with good results after a 4-year follow-up period (Stefanidis *et al.*, 2000). However, whether the vein cuff would suffer similar injury to that observed by normal vein grafts (Section 5.4.1) remains to be seen.

The ideal stent may well be lined with endothelial cells (see Section 5.2.2), to replicate their protective nature. Reports of stents coated with endothelial cells have been available since the 1980s (Dichek *et al.*, 1989); however, retaining endothelial cells on their scaffold has been a limitation. More recent efforts have therefore consisted of encouraging endothelial cell growth and proliferation on the scaffold surface, with *in vivo* results showing that thrombus formation was inhibited and intimal hyperplasia was reduced (Van Belle *et al.*, 1997).

Coatings to inhibit thrombus formation have been used on stents, with heparin being of particular promise. Heparin is a mucopolysaccharide, made of sulphated glycosaminoglycans. Heparin binds to antithrombin III, which normally inhibits thrombus formation (by inactivating thrombin) and, when heparin is bound to it, the rate of this inhibition is increased (for more details see Rang *et al.* (1999)). *In vitro* studies have shown that, while heparin reduces endothelial cell growth, smooth muscle cell growth is also reduced (important in reducing intimal hyperplasia, see Section 5.4.1 (Chupa *et al.*, 2000; Letourneur *et al.*, 2002)).

Initial clinical trials using heparin are promising (Serruys *et al.*, 1996, 1998; Vrolix *et al.*, 2000). Attachment of heparin to stents has been through either ionic (Bertrand *et al.*, 1998) or covalent bonding (Topol and Serruys, 1998), or through end point attachment on to a polyamine–dextran sulphate layer on a stent surface (Serruys *et al.*, 1996). The end-point attachment method has the benefit that it does not depend on initial concentration and release of heparin for its durability (Bertrand *et al.*, 1998; Topol and Serruys, 1998). Instead, heparin is bound to the stent, with its active site free to bind to antithrombin III (Bertrand *et al.*, 1998), which then inhibits the formation of thrombus (see above). The process of inhibition of thrombus formation can then be repeated.

Another method proposed is to release heparin (or other substances) at a site separate from the stent, in a controlled manner. For example, resorbable hydrophobic (poly-D,L lactide-co-glycolide) microspheres containing heparin were suspended in a hydrophilic alginate film (a hydrogel). The degradation of the microspheres led to the controlled release of heparin. *In vivo*, this method inhibited smooth muscle cell proliferation (i.e. intimal hyperplasia) and allowed the suture line to heal (Edelman *et al.*, 2000).

Drug releasing stents

Another strategy is that of drug-releasing stents. These drugs are attached to the stent by a polymer coating, which may lead to their release by degradation (i.e. resorbable polymer) or without degradation (i.e. by diffusion through a non-degradable polymer). The most promising polymers at present for drug delivery (Sousa *et al.*, 2003b, 2003c) appear to be the non-biodegradable poly(*n*-butyl methacrylate) and poly(ethylene vinyl acetate) copolymer (Suzuki *et al.*, 2001), and the degradable poly(lactide-co-ε-caprolactone) copolymer (Drachman *et al.*, 2000).

Initial clinical trials of drug-releasing stents have produced good clinical results and hold promise for the future (Morice *et al.*, 2002; Park *et al.*, 2003; Sousa *et al.*, 2003a). However, concerns over potential inflammatory response induced by the polymer, polymer degradation and possible local toxic effects by the released drug have been raised, with the possible outcome that restenosis is not prevented but delayed (Fattori and Piva, 2003). A similar process was observed with radioactive stents, used to reduce excessive cell growth (Hehrlain *et al.*, 1995, 1996), where late thrombus formation and restenosis occurred clinically after good initial results (Salame *et al.*, 2001). Long-term clinical results will be required to determine the effectiveness of drug release in preventing restenosis.

Use of polymers for stents

Resorbable polymer stents have not been as successful as metallic stents during animal testing (Bertrand *et al.*, 1998). Such stents may be desirable because they may be used as a temporary structure that allows the vessel to heal and subsequently to function as normal, by which point the stent can biodegrade. However, much research is still needed for their development into stents that are as effective as currently available metal stents. Currently, polymers within stents hold most promise as coatings used to control drug delivery or release from or near stents (aiming to reduce restenosis and thrombus formation).

5.5 Tissue-engineered arteries

Limitations of stents, natural tissues and synthetic materials for small-diameter arterial replacement has led to the development of tissue-engineered arteries. Several approaches are being investigated, presented here under the titles of synthetic constructs (5.5.1) and natural constructs (5.5.2). Synthetic constructs cover synthetic materials lined with endothelial cells, and biodegradable materials. Natural constructs cover the development of blood vessels using reconstituted extracellular matrices, naturally created extracellular matrices or cell removal to use already available extracellular matrix scaffolds.

5.5.1 Synthetic constructs

Synthetic arterial replacement materials for small-diameter blood vessels have typically produced poor results (Conte, 1998) compared with saphenous vein grafts, or other natural materials (see, for example, Sandusky *et al.* (1995)), owning to their occlusion by platelet aggregation and thrombus formation. However, lining of an arterial scaffold, with endothelial cells may prevent such occlusion (Section 5.2.2). Therefore, lining of synthetic scaffolds such as e-PTFE with endothelial cells may reduce its tendency to occlude when used for small-diameter blood vessel replacement.

As with stents (Section 5.4.2), maintaining endothelial cells bound to the replacement blood vessel has proved challenging (see, for example, Rosenman *et al.* (1985) and Greisler *et al.* (1990)). However, attaching these cells to e-PTFE has been achieved and long-term studies have shown the value of such vascular grafts, with improved patency rates over a 9-year study during femoropopliteal (i.e. lower-limb) artery replacement (Deutsch *et al.*, 1999). One disadvantage of this method, however, is the time needed for seeding of endothelial cells. This type of replacement artery was, hence, not available for acute vascular replacement surgery during that clinical study. Another concern is the possibility of immune response to the synthetic material. Lining of PTFE with a vein cuff has also been reported from long-term clinical experience (Sayers *et al.*, 1998). This was found to produce better results than using bare PTFE.

Non-degradable synthetic materials behave differently from natural arteries. Biodegradable polymers, however, may allow the remodelling of the replacement artery within its environment, so that it could gain properties like those of its surrounding vessel. A poly(glycolic acid) scaffold has been used to develop such a construct (Niklason *et al.*, 1999). Smooth muscle and endothelial cells were seeded on to the scaffold. These constructs were shown to resist pressures of about 2150 mmHg *in vitro*. These constructs are therefore promising, but their value can only be determined by long-term clinical use and are not currently available.

5.5.2 Natural constructs

An alternative approach to synthetic scaffolds is the development of a purely tissue-engineered structure, i.e. without synthetic materials. One of the first attempts to develop such a construct was by Weinberg and Bell (1986). This consisted of using reconstituted collagen matrices and smooth muscle cells. Endothelial cell lining was also present. However, the collagen matrix was too weak and these constructs failed owning to low strength. Methods to increase this strength have included by the use of a Dacron sleeve (Weinberg and Bell, 1986), by glycation of the collagen matrix (Girton *et al.*, 1999) or by dynamic loading (Seliktar *et al.*, 2000). Suitable mechanical properties were only achieved by the use of a Dacron sleeve. However, this does not avoid the use of synthetic materials.

A separate approach to using a reconstituted extracellular matrix is using a naturally created matrix in culture. One such approach used layers of smooth muscle and fibroblast cells rolled up in culture over a mandrel to generate a blood vessel construct (L'Heureux *et al.*, 1998). Luminal flow was applied to the construct in a bioreactor during development. The cells produced their own extracellular matrix (i.e. as opposed to a reconstituted matrix). Finally, endothelial cells were seeded on the lumen. This method led to high mechanical strength (with burst pressures of about 2500 mmHg), and morphology similar to that of native blood vessels. Of concern was the fact that the strength of the construct was provided by the adventitial layer rather than the medial layer (Nerem and Seliktar, 2001). The advantage of this construct (apart from its mechanical integrity) is that it was developed using human cells. However, the process took about 3 months; therefore, this method is not suitable for acute arterial replacement surgery. Long-term clinical trials are also needed to determine its value. However, initial *in vivo* testing led to occlusion in three of six dogs within a week. Because human cells were being transplanted into a dog, excess immune response was anticipated, and endothelial cells were not included. However, Deutsch *et al.* (1999) expected that the use of endothelial cells would have prevented such occlusion.

Acellular vascular grafts can be used to produce replacement arteries (Schmidt and Bayer, 2000; Nerem and Seliktar, 2001). Extraction via detergent or enzyme-detergent methods have been used to remove cells from the tissues, leaving the extracellular matrix intact (see, for example, Courtman *et al.* (1994)). The small-intestine submucosa has been used to develop such an acellular vascular replacement vessel (Sandusky *et al.*, 1995). Initial testing in dogs showed promising results when compared with e-PTFE grafts. Methods involving natural tissues (such as the small-intestine submucosa), which are made into arterial replacement conduits, rely on endothelial cell covering *in vivo*, in order to prevent occlusion of the blood vessel.

5.6 Summary and future trends

At present, heart valves (when not repaired) are typically replaced by mechanical or bioprosthetic valves. While bioprosthetic valves allow more natural haemodynamics and do not need long-term anticoagulation, mechanical valves are more durable. Bileaflet mechanical valves and porcine or bovine pericardial bioprostheses are the most commonly used replacement valves. Natural valves such as homografts are used as well, although their availability can be limited.

Large arteries can be successfully replaced using synthetic materials such as e-PTFE or Dacron. Smaller arteries (less than 6 mm in diameter) occlude when such materials are used. Arterial or vein bypass grafts may be used to replenish blood flow but their availability is sometimes limited. Balloon angioplasty can be used to expand the occluded vessel, and a stent may be placed to prevent the vessel from occluding again. At present, metal stents are typically used. Development in stent technology at present includes either stents coated with substances to prevent restenosis, or stents that elute drugs aiming to prevent restenosis.

Developments in tissue engineering, to produce replacement blood vessels and heart valves, offer great potential. Development of acellular replacement tissues (composed mostly of extracellular matrix) have led to replacement arteries and heart valves that can potentially allow host cell infiltration. A tissue-engineered artery with an extracellular matrix made by cells in culture also led to a replacement artery with suitable properties for implantation. It is likely that further advances with these technologies and optimisation of their production will occur; very useful techniques will be available that may form prominent cardiovascular replacement materials.

Developments in polymers for use with stents in drug delivery systems, and to produce heart valves may allow further developments in replacement devices. While, at present, polymer stents have not met with success, improvements in such technology may allow their use in the future.

For all new devices used to repair or replace arteries or heart valves, the ultimate test is how well they perform clinically, and how they compare with other devices available. Inevitably, this takes time. It should be noted, however, that, for cardiovascular surgery, developments in surgical methods and clinical treatment may also be important in such developments. The development of better anticoagulation therapy, for example, may improve clinical results, as might developments in surgical methods (e.g. percutaneous surgical techniques for heart valve repair (Block, 2003)). The use of genetic therapies, with implanted materials, has also been advocated (Topol and Serruys, 1998).

5.7 Sources of further information and advice

Good explanations in cardiovascular physiology can be found in general physiology textbooks, such as that by Guyton and Hall (1996) or in cardiovascular physiology textbooks such as that by Levick (1998), while biology textbooks such as that by Raven and Johnson (1996) include several illustrative figures that aid understanding. Anatomy and histology of heart valves are described quite nicely, with figures and diagrams having been given by Stevens and Lowe (1997). A good account of the physical considerations of the cardiovascular circulation has been provided by Caro *et al.* (1978).

Several articles are available on the topic of biomaterials, connective tissue composition and their biomechanics, such as those by Hukins (1982), Hukins and Aspden (1985), Fratzl *et al.* (1997), Hukins *et al.* (1999) and Goh *et al.* (2004).

Stent coatings used so far, and future directions, have been nicely covered by Gunn and Cumberland (1999). These factors and related strategies have also been dealt with by Topol and Serruys (1998). Bertrand *et al.* (1998), on the other hand, covered the topic of advances in stent technology. The subject of drug-eluting stents has been discussed by Fattori and Piva (2003) and Sousa *et al.* (2003b, 2003c).

Some interesting articles on tissue engineering of blood vessels are available as provided by Conte (1998) or with more detail by Nerem and Seliktar (2001). The use of acellular tissues used for tissue replacement has been covered by Schmidt and Bayer (2000).

Good commentaries on the development of replacement heart valves by Starr *et al.* (2002) and Schoen *et al.* (1982) are available. The latter does not include much about bileaflet mechanical valves. Tissue valves and their calcification, on the other hand, have been well covered by Schoen and Levy (1999). Hyde *et al.* (1999) described the development of research into the topic of polymer heart valves, although most recent advances in this field must be taken into account (see, for example, Daebritz *et al.* (2003, 2004)).

5.8 Acknowledgements

The author thanks both Professor David W L Hukins and Dr Duncan E T Shepherd for discussion and comments on this chapter.

5.9 References

Allen B S, El-Zein C, Cuneo B, Cava J P, Barth M J and Ilbawi M N (2002), 'Pericardial tissue valves and Gore-Tex conduits as an alternative for right ventricular outflow tract replacement in children', *Ann Thorac Surg*, **74** 771–777.

Bakhai A, Booth J, Delahunty N, Nugara F, Clayton T, McNeill J, Davies S W, Cumberland D C and Stables R H (2005), 'The SV stent study: a prospective, multicentre, angiographic evaluation of the BiodivYsio phosphorylcholine coated small vessel stent in small coronary vessels', *Int J Cardiol*, **102** 95–102.

Barber J E, Ratliff N B, Cosgrove D M, Griffin B P and Vesely I (2001b), 'Myxomatous mitral valve chordae. I: mechanical properties', *J Heart Valve Dis*, **10** 320–324.

Bassiouny H S, White S, Glagov S, Choi E, Giddens D P and Zarins C K (1992), 'Anastomotic intimal hyperplasia: mechanical injury or flow induced', *J Vasc Surg*, **15** 708–717.

Bernacca G M, Mackay T G, Wilkinson R and Wheatley D J (1997), 'Polyurethane heart valves: fatigue failure, calcification, and polyurethane structure', *J Biomed Mater Res*, **34** 371–379.

Bernal J M, Gutierrez-Morlote J, Llorca J, San Jose J M, Morales D and Revuelta J M (2004), 'Tricuspid valve repair: an old disease, a modern experience', *Ann Thorac Surg*, **78** 2069–2075.

Bernal J M, Morales D, Revuelta C, Llorca J, Gutierrez-Morlote J and Revuelta J M (2005), 'Reoperations after tricuspid valve repair', *J Thorac Cardiovasc Surg*, **130** 498–503.

Bertrand O F, Sipehia R, Mongrain R, Rodes J, Tardif J C, Bilodeau L, Cote G and Bourassa M G (1998), 'Biocompatible aspects of new stent technology', *J Am Coll Cardiol*, **32** 562–571.

Bjork V and Henze A (1979), 'Ten years experience with the Bjork–Shiley tilting disc valve', *J Thorac Cardiovasc Surg*, **78** 331–342.

Block P C (2003), 'Percutaneous mitral valve repair for mitral regurgitation', *J Interv Cardiol*, **16** 93–96.

Braunwald N S, Tatooles C, Turina M and Detmer D (1971), 'New developments in the design of fabric-coated prosthetic heart valves', *J Thorac Cardiovasc Surg*, **62** 673–682.

Breymann T, Thies W R, Boethig D, Goerg R, Blanz U and Koerfer R (2002), 'Bovine valved xenografts for RVOT reconstruction: results after 71 implantations', *Eur J Cardiothorac Surg*, **21** 703–710.

Butany J, Collins M J and David T E (2004), 'Ruptured synthetic expanded polytetrafluoroethylene chordae tendineae', *Cardiovasc Pathol*, **13** 182–84.

Cao H (1995), 'Mechanical performance of pyrolytic carbon in prosthetic heart valve applications', *J Heart Valve Dis*, **5** S32–S49.

Caro C G, Pedley T J, Schroter R C and Seed W A (1978), *The Mechanics of the Circulation*, Oxford, Oxford University Press.

Carpentier A (1977), 'From vascular xenograft to valvular bioprosthesis (1965–77)', *J Assoc Adv Med Instrum*, **11** 98–101.

Carpentier A (1983), 'Cardiac valve surgery – the "French correction" ', *J Thorac Cardiovasc Surg*, **86** 323–337.

Carrier M, Hebert Y, Pellerin M, Bouchard D, Perrault L P, Cartier R, Basmajian A, Page P and Poirier N C (2003), 'Tricuspid valve replacement: an analysis of 25 years of experience at a single centre', *Ann Thorac Surg*, **75** 47–50.

Chupa J M, Foster A M, Sumner S R, Madihally S V and Matthew H W T (2000), 'Vascular cell responses to polysaccharide materials: *in vitro* and *in vivo* evaluations', *Biomaterials*, **21** 2315–2322.

Cochran R P and Kunzelman K S (1991), 'Comparison of viscoelastic properties of suture versus porcine mitral valve chordae tendineae', *J Card Surg*, **6** 508–513.

Conte M S (1998), 'The ideal small arterial substitute: a search for the Holy Grail?', *FASEB J*, **12** 43–45.

Courtman D W, Pereira C A, Kashef V, McComb D, Lee J M and Wilson G J (1994), 'Development of a pericardial acellular matrix biomaterial: biochemical and mechanical effects of cell extraction', *J Biomed Mater Res*, **28** 655–666.

Cox J L, Chiasson D A and Gotlieb A I (1991), 'Stranger in a strange land: the pathogenesis of saphenous vein graft stenosis with emphasis on structural and functional differences between veins and arteries', *Prog Cardiovasc Dis*, **34** 45–68.

Daebritz S H, Fausten B, Hermanns B, Schroeder J, Groetzner J, Autschbach R, Messmer B J and Sachweh J S (2004), 'Introduction of a flexible polymeric heart valve prosthesis with special design for the aortic position', *Eur J Cardiothorac Surg*, **25** 946–952.

Daebritz S H, Sachweh J S, Hermanns B, Fausten B, Franke A, Groetzner J, Klosterhalfen B and Messmer B J (2003), 'Introduction of a flexible polymeric heart valve prosthesis with special design for mitral position', *Circulation*, **108**(Suppl. II) II134–II139.

De Scheerder I K, Wilczek K L, Verbeken E V, Vandorpe J, Lan P N, Schacht E, De Geest H and Piessens J (1994), 'Biocompatbility of polymer coated tantalum stents', *Atherosclerosis*, **114** 105–114.

Deutsch M, Meinhart J, Fischlein T, Preiss P and Zilla P (1999), 'Clinical autologous *in vitro* endothelialization of infrainguinal ePTFE grafts in 100 patients: a 9-year experience', *Surgery*, **126** 847–855.

Dichek D A, Neville R F, Zwiebel J A, Freeman S M, Leon M B and Anderson W F (1989), 'Seeding of intravascular stents with genetically engineered endothelial cells', *Circulation*, **80** 1347–1353.

Drachman D E, Edelman E R, Seifert P, Groothuis A R, Bornstein D A, Kamath K R, Palasis M, Yang D, Nott S H and Rogers C (2000), 'Neointimal thickening after stent delivery of paclitaxel: change in composition and arrest of growth over six months', *J Am Coll Cardiol*, **36** 2325–2332.

Edelman E R, Nathan A, Katada M, Gates J and Karnovsky M J (2000), 'Perivascular graft heparin delivery using biodegradable polymer wraps', *Biomaterials*, **21** 2279–2286.

Elkins R C, Dawson P E, Goldstein S, Walsh S P and Black K S (2001), 'Decellularized human valve allografts', *Ann Thorac Surg*, **71** S428–S432.

Elkins R C, Knott-Craig C J, Ward K E, McCue C and Lane M M (1994), 'Pulmonary autograft in children: realized growth potential', *Ann Thorac Surg*, **57** 1387–1394.

Emery R W, Mettler E and Nicoloff D M (1979), 'A new cardiac prosthesis. The St Jude medical cardiac valve: *in vivo* results', *Circulation*, **60**(Suppl. I) I48–I54.

Enriquez-Sarano M, Schaff H V, Orszulak T A, Tajik A J, Bailey K R and Frye R L (1995), 'Valve repair improves the outcome of surgery for mitral regurgitation: a multivariate analysis', *Circulation*, **91** 1022–1028.

Espino D M, Hukins D W L, Shepherd D E T, Watson M A and Buchan K (2006a), 'Determination of the pressure required to cause mitral valve failure', *Med Eng Phys*, **28** 36–41.

Espino D M, Hukins D W L, Shepherd D E T and Buchan K (2006b), 'Mitral valve repair: an *in vitro* comparison of the effect of surgical repair on the pressure required to cause mitral valve regurgitation', *J Heart Valve Dis*, **15** 375–381.

Espino D M, Shepherd D E T, Hukins D W L and Buchan K (2005), 'The role of chordae tendineae in mitral valve competence', *J Heart Valve Dis*, **14** 603–609.

Fattori R and Piva T (2003), 'Drug-eluting stents in vascular intervention', *Lancet*, **361** 247–249.

Fishbein M C, Roberts W C, Golden A and Hufnagel C A (1975), 'Cardiac pathology after aortic valve replacement using Hufnagel trileaflet prostheses: a study of 20 necropsy patients', *Am Heart J*, **89** 443–448.

Fisher J (1995), 'Porcine bioprosthetic valves prepared with permanent pre-dilation of the aortic root', *J Heart Valve Dis*, **4** S81–S84.

Fontaine A A, He S, Stadter R, Ellis J T, Levine R A and Yoganathan A P (1996), '*In vitro* assessment of prosthetic valve function in mitral valve replacement with chordal preservation techniques', *J Heart Valve Dis*, **5** 186–198.

Fratzl P, Misof K, Zizak I, Rapp G, Amenitsch H and Bernstorff S (1998), 'Fibrillar structure and mechanical properties of collagen', *J Struct Biol*, **122** 119–122.

Garrison L A, Lamson T C, Deutsch S, Geselowitz D B, Gaumond R P and Tarbell J M (1994), 'An *in-vitro* investigation of prosthetic heart valve cavitation in blood', *J Heart Valve Dis*, **3** S8–S24.

Girton T S, Oegema T R and Tranquillo R T (1999), 'Exploiting glycation to stiffen and strengthen tissue equivalents for tissue engineering', *J Biomed Mater Res*, **46** 87–92.

Goh K L, Aspden R M and Hukins D W L (2004), 'Review: finite element analysis of stress transfer in short-fibre composite materials', *Compos Sci Technol*, **64** 1091–1100.

Goldstein S, Clarke D R, Walsh S P, Black K S and O'Brien M F (2000), 'Transpecies heart valve transplant: advanced studies of a bioengineered xeno-autograft', *Ann Thorac Surg*, **70** 1962–1969.

Goodman S L, Tweden K S and Albrecth R M (1996), 'Platelet interaction with pyrolytic carbon heart-valve leaflets', *J Biomed Mater Res*, **32** 249–258.

Greisler H P, Johnson S, Joyce K, Henderson S, Patel N M, Alkhamis T, Beissinger R and Kim D U (1990), 'The effects of shear stress on endothelial cell retention and function on expanded polytetrafluoroethylene', *Arch Surg*, **125** 1622–1625.

Grenadier E, Roguin A, Hertz I, Peled B, Boulos M, Nikolsky E, Amikam S, Kerner A, Cohen S and Beyar R (2002), 'Stenting very small coronary narrowings (<2 mm) using the biocompatible phosphorylcholine-coated coronary stent', *Catheter Cardiovasc Interv*, **55** 303–308.

Gunn J and Cumberland D (1999), 'Stent coatings and local drug delivery', *Eur Heart J*, **20** 1693–1700.

Guyton A C and Hall J E (1996), *Textbook of Medical Physiology*, Philadelphia, Pennsylvania, W B Saunders.

Hawkins J A, Bailey W W, Dillon T and Schwartz D C (1992), 'Midterm results with cryopreserved allograft valved conduits from the right ventricle to the pulmonary arteries', *J Thorac Cardiovasc Surg*, **104** 910–916.

Hehrlein C, Gollan C, Dönges K, Metz J, Riessen R, Fehsenfeld P, von Hodenberg E and Kübler W (1995), 'Low-dose radioactive endovascular stents prevent smooth muscle cell proliferation and neointimal hyperplasia in rabbits', *Circulation*, **92** 1570–1575.

Hehrlein C, Stintz M, Kinscherf R, Schlösser K, Huttel E, Friedrich L, Fehsenfeld P and Kübler W (1996), 'Pure β-particle emitting stents inhibit neointima formation in rabbits', *Circulation*, **93** 641–645.

Hukins D W L (1982), 'Biomechanical properties of collagen', in *Collagen in Health and Disease* (Eds J B Weiss and M I V Jayson), Edinburgh, Churchill–Livingstone.

Hukins D W L and Aspden R M (1985), 'Composition and properties of connective tissues', *Trends Biochem Sci*, **10** 260–264.

Hukins D W L, Leahy J C and Mathias K J (1999), 'Biomaterials: defining the mechanical properties of natural tissues and selection of replacement materials', *J Mater Chem*, **9** 629–636.

Hyde J A J, Chinn J A and Phillips R E (1999), 'Polymer heart valves', *J Heart Valve Dis*, **8** 331–339.

Kastrati A, Schomig A, Dirschinger J, Mehilli J, von Welser N, Pache J, Schuhlen H, Schilling T, Schmitt C and Neumann F J (2000), 'Increased risk of restenosis after placement of gold-coated stents', *Circulation*, **101** 2478–2483.

Kingsbury C, Kafesjian R, Guo G, Adlparvar P, Unger J, Quijano R C, Graf T, Fisher H, Reul H and Rau G (1993), 'Cavitation threshold with respect to d*P*/d*t*: evaluation in 29 mm bileaflet, pyrolitic carbon heart valves', *Int J Artif Organs*, **16** 515–520.

Kobayashi Y, Nagata S, Ohmori F, Eishi K and Miyatake K (1996), 'Mitral valve dysfunction resulting from thickening and stiffening of artificial mitral valve chordae', *Circulation*, **94**(Suppl. II) II129–II132.

Kunzelman K S and Cochran R P (1990), 'Mechanical properties of basal and marginal mitral valve chordae tendineae', *ASAIO Trans*, **36** M405–M408.

L'Heureux N, Paquet S, Labbe R, Germain L and Auger F A (1998), 'A completely biological tissue-engineered human blood vessel', *FASEB J*, **12** 47–56.

Lange R, Weipert J, Homann M, Mendler N, Paek S U, Holper K and Meisner H (2001), 'Performance of allografts and xenografts for right ventricular outflow tract reconstruction', *Ann Thorac Surg*, **71** S365–S367.

Letourneur D, Machy D, Pelle A, Marcon-Bachari E, D'Angelo G, Vogel M, Chaubet F and Michel J B (2002), 'Heparin and non-heparin like dextrans differentially modulate endothelial cell proliferation: *in vitro* evaluation with soluble and crosslinked polysaccharide matrices', *J Biomed Mater Res*, **60** 94–100.

Levick J R (1998), *An Introduction to Cardiovascular Physiology*, Oxford, Butterworth–Heinemann.

Lim K O and Boughner D R (1975), 'Mechanical properties of human mitral valve chordae tendineae: variation with size and strain rate', *Can J Physiol Pharmacol*, **53** 330–339.

Lim K O, Boughner D R and Smith C A (1977), 'Dynamic elasticity of human mitral valve chordae tendineae', *Can J Physiol Pharmacol*, **55** 413–418.

Lis Y, Burleigh M C, Parker D J, Child A H, Hogg J and Davies M J (1987), 'Biochemical characterization of individual normal, floppy and rheumatic human mitral valves', *Biochem J*, **244** 597–603.

Loop F D, Cosgrove D M and Stewart W J (1991), 'Mitral valve repair for mitral insufficiency', *Eur Heart J*, **12**(Suppl. B) 30–33.

Lupinetti F M, Warner J, Jones T K and Herndon S P (1997), 'Comparison of human tissues and mechanical prostheses for aortic valve replacement in children', *Circulation*, **96** 321–325.
Mackay T G, Wheatley D J, Bernacca G M, Fisher A C and Hindle C S (1996), 'New polyurethane heart valve prosthesis: design, manufacture and evaluation', *Biomaterials*, **17** 1857–1863.
Maisano F, Redaelli A, Pennati G, Fumero R, Torracca L and Alfieri O (1999), 'The hemodynamic effects of double-orifice valve repair for mitral regurgitation: a 3-D computational model', *Eur J Cardiothorac Surg*, **15** 419–425.
Morice M C, Serruys P W, Sousa J E, Fajadet J, Hayashi E B, Perin M, Colombo A, Schuler G, Barragan P, Guagliumi G, Molnar F and Falotico R (2002), 'A randomized comparison of a sirolimus-eluting stent with a standard stent for coronary revascularization', *N Engl J Med*, **346** 1773–1780.
Naemura K, Umezu M and Dohi T (1999), 'Preliminary study on the new self-closing mechanical mitral valve', *Artif Organs*, **23** 869–875.
Nerem R M and Seliktar D (2001), 'Vascular tissue engineering', *Annu Rev Biomed Eng*, **3** 225–243.
Ng C K, Nesser J, Punzengruber C, Pachinger O, Auer J, Franke H and Hartl P (2001), 'Valvuloplasty with glutaraldehyde-treated autologous pericardium in patients with complex mitral valve pathology', *Ann Thorac Surg*, **71** 78–85.
Niklason L E, Gao J, Abbott W M, Hirschi K K, Houser S, Marini R and Langer R (1999), 'Functional arteries grown *in vitro*', *Science*, **284** 489–493.
O'Brien B O, Carroll W M and Kelly M J (2002), 'Passivation of nitinol wire for vascular implants – a demonstration of the benefits', *Biomaterials*, **23** 1739–1748.
Okies J E, Page U S, Bigelow J C, Krause A H and Salomon N W (1984), 'The left internal mammary artery: the graft of choice', *Circulation*, **70**(Suppl. I) I213–I221.
Ozbek C, Heisel A, Groβ B, Bay W and Schieffer H (1997), 'Coronary implantation of silicone carbide coated Palmaz–Schatz stents in patients with high risk of stent thrombosis without oral anticoagulation', *Cathet Cardiovasc Diagn*, **41** 71–78.
Padera R F and Schoen F J (2004), 'Cardiovascular medical devices', in *Biomaterials Science* (Eds BD Ratner, A S Hoffman, F J Schoen and J E Lemons), London, Elsevier, pp. 470–494.
Park S J, Shim W H, Ho D S, Raizner A E, Park S W, Hong M K, Lee C W, Choi D, Jang Y, Larn R, Weissman N J and Mintz G S (2003), 'A paclitaxel-eluting stent for the prevention of coronary restenosis', *N Engl J Med*, **348** 1537–1545.
Perier P, Deloche A, Chauvaud S, Fabiani J N, Rossant P, Bessou J P, Relland J, Bourezak H, Gomez F, Blondeau P, D'Allaines C and Carpentier A (1984), 'Comparative evaluation of mitral valve repair and replacement with Starr, Bjork, and porcine mitral valve prosthesis', *Circulation*, **70**(Suppl. I) I187–I192.
Piper C, Korfer R and Horstkotte D (2001), 'Valve disease: prosthetic valve endocarditis', *Heart*, **85** 590–593.
Rang H P, Dale M M and Ritter J M (1999), *Pharmacology*, Edinburgh, Churchill–Livingstone.
Raven P and Johnson G (1996), *Biology*, London, Wm C Brown.
Reimink M S, Kunzelman K S, Verrier E D and Cochran R P (1995), 'The effect of anterior chordal replacement on mitral valve function and stresses – a finite element study', *ASAIO J*, **41** M754–M762.

Rizzoli G, De Perini L, Bottio T, Minutolo G, Thiene G and Casarotto D (1998), 'Prosthetic replacement of the tricuspid valve: biological or mechanical?', *Ann Thorac Surg*, **66** S62–S67.

Roe B B, Kelly P B, Myers J L and Moore D W (1966), 'Tricuspid leaflet aortic valve prosthesis', *Circulation*, **33**(Suppl. I) I124–I130.

Rosenman J E, Kempczinski R F, Pearce W H and Silberstein E B (1985), 'Kinetics of endothelial cell seeding', *J Vasc Surg*, **2** 778–784.

Ryhanen J, Niemi E, Serlo W, Niemela E, Sandvik P, Pernu H and Salo T (1997), 'Biocompatibility of nickel–titanium shape memory metal and its corrosion behaviour in human cell culture', *J Biomed Mater Res*, **35** 451–457.

Salame M Y, Verheye S, Crocker I R, Chronos N A F, Robinson K A and King S B (2001), 'Intracoronary radiation therapy', *Eur Heart J*, **22** 629–647.

Sand M E, Naftel D C, Blackstone E H, Kirklin J W and Karp R B (1987), 'A comparison of repair and replacement for mitral valve incompetence', *J Thorac Cardiovasc Surg*, **94** 208–219.

Sandusky G E, Lantz G C and Badylak S F (1995), 'Healing comparison of small intestine submucosa and ePTFE grafts in the canine carotid artery', *J Surg Res*, **58** 415–420.

Santin M, Mikhalovska L, Lloyd A W, Mikhalovsky S, Sigfrid L, Denyer S P, Field S and Teer D (2004), '*In vitro* response assessment of biomaterials for cardiovascular stent manufacture', *J Mater Sci*, **15** 473–477.

Sayers R D, Raptis S, Berce M and Miller J H (1998), 'Long-term results of femorotibial bypass with vein or polytetrafluoroethylene', *Br J Surg*, **85** 934–938.

Schmidt C E and Bayer J M (2000), 'Acellular vascular tissues: natural biomaterials for tissue repair and tissue engineering', *Biomaterials*, **21** 2215–2231.

Schoen F J and Levy R J (1999), 'Tissue heart valves: current challenges and future research perspectives', *J Biomed Mater Res*, **47** 439–465.

Schoen F J, Titus J L and Lawrie G M (1982), 'Bioengineering aspects of heart valve replacement', *Ann Biomed Eng*, **10** 97–128.

Seliktar D, Black R A, Vito R P and Nerem R M (2000), 'Dynamic mechanical conditioning of collagen–gel blood vessel constructs induces remodelling *in vitro*', *Ann Biomed Eng*, **28** 351–362.

Serruys P W, Emanuelsson H, van der Giessen W, Lunn A C, Kiemeney F, Macaya C, Rutsch W, Heyndrickx G, Suryapranata H, Legrand V, Goy J J, Materne P, Bonnier H, Morice M C, Fajadet J, Belardi J, Colombo A, Garcia E, Ruygrok P, de Jaegere P and Morel M A (1996), 'Heparin coated Palmaz–Schatz stents in human coronary arteries: early outcome of the Benestent II pilot study', *Circulation*, **93** 412–422.

Serruys P W, van Hout B, Bonnier H, Legrand V, Garcia E, Macaya C, Sousa E, van der Giessen W, Colombo A, Seabra-Gomes R, Kiemeneij F, Ruygrok P, Ormiston J, Emanuelsson H, Fajadet J, Haude M, Klugmann S and Morel M A (1998), 'Randomised comparison of implantation of heparin-coated stents with balloon angioplasty in selected patients with coronary disease (Benestent II)', *Lancet*, **352** 673–681.

Shi Y and Vesely I (2003), 'Fabrication of tissue engineered mitral valve chordae using directed collagen gel shrinkage', *Tissue Eng*, **9** 1233–1242.

Shi Y and Vesely I (2004), 'Characterization of statically loaded tissue-engineered mitral valve chordae tendineae', *J Biomed Mater Res Part A*, **69** 26–39.

Simon P, Kasimiar M T, Seebacher G, Weigel G, Ullrich R, Salzer-Muhar U, Rieder E and Wolner E (2003), 'Early failure of the tissue engineered porcine heart valve SYNERGRAFT in pediatric patients', *Eur J Cardiothorac Surg*, **23** 1002–1006.
Sousa J E, Costa M A, Sousa A G M R, Abizaid A C, Seixas A C, Abizaid A S, Feres F, Mattos L A, Falotico R, Jaeger J, Popma J J and Serruys P W (2003a), 'Two-year angiographic and intravascular ultrasound follow-up after implantation of sirolimus-eluting stents in human coronary arteries', *Circulation*, **107** 381–383.
Sousa J E, Serruys P W and Costa M A (2003b), 'New frontiers in cardiology: drug-eluting stents: part I', *Circulation*, **107** 2274–2279.
Sousa J E, Serruys P W and Costa M A (2003c), 'New frontiers in cardiology: drug-eluting stents: part II', *Circulation*, **107** 2383–2389.
Starr A and Edwards M L (1961), 'Mitral replacement: the shielded ball valve prosthesis', *J Thorac Cardiovasc Surg*, **42** 673–682.
Starr A, Fessler C L, Grunkemeier G and He G W (2002), 'Heart valve replacement surgery: past, present and future', *Clin Exp Pharmacol Physiol*, **29** 735–738.
Starr A, Herr R H and Wood J A (1967), 'Mitral replacement: review of six years' experience', *J Thorac Cardiovasc Surg*, **54** 333–358.
Stefanidis C, Toutouzas K, Tsiamis E, Vlachopoulos C, Kallikazaros I, Stratos C, Vavuranakis M and Toutouzas P (2000), 'Stents covered by autologous venous grafts: Feasibility and immediate and long-term results', *Am Heart J*, **139** 437–445.
Steinhoff G, Stock U, Karim N, Mertsching H, Timke A, Meliss R R, Pethig K, Haverich A and Bader A (2000), 'Tissue engineering of pulmonary heart valves on allogenic acellular matrix conduits', *Circulation*, **102**(Suppl. III) III50–III55.
Stevens A and Lowe J (1997), *Human Histology*, London, Mosby.
Suzuki T, Kopia G, Hayashi S, Bailey L R, Llanos G, Wilensky R, Klugherz B D, Papandreou G, Narayan P, Leon M B, Yeung A C, Tio F, Tsao P S, Falotico R and Carter A J (2001), 'Stent-based delivery of sirolimus reduces neointimal formation in a porcine coronary model', *Circulation*, **104** 1188–1193.
Tomita Y, Yasui H, Tominaga R, Morita S, Masuda M, Kurisu K and Nishimura Y (2002), 'Extensive use of polytetrafluoroethylene artificial grafts for prolapse of bilateral mitral leaflets', *Eur J Cardiothorac Surg*, **21** 27–31.
Topol E J and Serruys P W (1998), 'Frontiers in interventional cardiology', *Circulation*, **98** 1802–1820.
Tweddell J S, Pelech A N, Frommelt P C, Mussatto K A, Wyman J D, Fedderly R T, Berger S, Frommelt M A, Lewis D A, Friedberg D Z, Thomas J P, Sachdeva R and Litwin S B (2000), 'Factors affecting longevity of homograft valves used in right ventricular outflow tract reconstruction for congenital heart disease', *Circulation*, **102**(Suppl. III) III130–III135.
Van Belle E, Tio F O, Chen D, Maillard L, Chen D, Kearney M and Isner J M (1997), 'Passivation of metallic stents after arterial gene transfer of $phVEGF_{165}$ inhibits thrombus formation and intimal thickening', *J Am Coll Cardiol*, **29** 1371–1379.
van der Giessen W J, Lincoff A M, Schwartz R S, van Beusekom H M M, Serruys P W, Holmes D R, Ellis S G and Topol E J (1996), 'Marked inflammatory sequelae to implantation of biodegradable and nonbiodegradable polymers in porcine coronary arteries', *Circulation*, **94** 1690–1697.
Vrolix M C M, Legrand V M, Reiber J H C, Grollier G, Schalij M J, Brunel P, Martinez-Elbal L, Gomez-Recio M, Bar F W H M, Bertrand M E, Colombo A

and Brachman J (2000), 'Heparin-coated wiktor stents in human coronary arteries (MENTOR trial)', *Am J Cardiol*, **86** 385–389.

Weinberg C B and Bell E (1986), 'A blood vessel model constructed from collagen and cultured vascular cells', *Science*, **231** 397–400.

Wheatley D J, Raco L, Bernacca G M, Sim I, Belcher P R and Boyd J S (2000), 'Polyurethane: material for the next generation of heart valve prostheses?', *Eur J Cardiothorac Surg*, **17** 440–448.

Whelan D M, van der Giessen W J, Krabbendam S C, van Vliet E A, Verdouw P D, Serruys P W and van Beusekom H M M (2000), 'Biocompatibility of phosphorylcholine coated stents in normal porcine coronary arteries', *Heart*, **83** 338–345.

Wnek G E and Bowlin G L (2004), *Encyclopedia of Biomaterials and Biomedical Engineering*, New York, Marcel Dekker.

Wu Z J, Wang Y and Hwang N H (1994), 'Occluder closing behaviour: a key factor in mechanical heart valve cavitation', *J Heart Valve Dis*, **3**(Suppl. I) S25–S34.

Yang Z, Arnet U, Bauer E, von Segesser L, Siebenmann R, Turina M and Luscher T F (1994), 'Thrombin-induced endothelium dependent inhibition and direct activation of platelet-vessel wall interaction', *Circulation*, **89** 2266–2272.

Zdrahala R J and Zdrahala I J (1999), 'Biomedical applications of polyurethanes: a review of past promises, present realities, and a vibrant future', *J Biomater Appl*, **14**(1) 67–90.

Zussa C (1995), 'Artificial chordae', *J Heart Valve Dis*, **4**(Suppl. II) S249–S256.

Zussa C, Polesel E, Rocco F and Valfre C (1997), 'Artificial chordae in the treatment of anterior mitral leaflet pathology', *Cardiovasc Surg*, **5** 125–128.

6
Ultrahigh-molecular-weight polyethylene (UHMWPE) in joint replacement

F-W SHEN, University of California Los Angeles, USA

6.1 Introduction

Ultrahigh-molecular-weight polyethylene (UHMWPE) has been the material of choice for the polymeric component in total joint replacements primarily because of its excellent combination of wear resistance, structural strength and biocompatibility and remains the gold standard thus far. Nevertheless, wear of UHMWPE prostheses produces billions of submicron particles annually,[1] which may cause a foreign-body response, leading to extensive bone resorption and gross loosening of the implants.[2–5] UHMWPE wear is of particular concern for young or active patients who may face one or more revisions with accumulative bone loss in their lifetime. Thus, improving the wear resistance of UHMWPE and, thereby, reducing the volume of wear particles released to the periarticular tissues should reduce the adverse biological responses and substantially extend the clinical lifespan of total joint replacements.

This chapter covers the structure and morphology of UHMWPE, processing (fabrication and sterilization) and properties, and methods of cross-linking to improve the wear resistance of UHMWPE. Clinical studies on new cross-linked UHMWPE are discussed.

6.2 The structure of UHMWPE

UHMWPE is a linear semicrystalline polymer produced by the polymerization of ethylene, $CH_2{=}CH_2$, with the unit cell of its crystal structure being orthorhombic. As defined by ISO 11542 specification, UHMWPE has an average molecular weight of at least 10^6 g/mol, which is much greater than that of conventional high-density polyethylene (HDPE), while the American Society for Testing and Materials standard (ASTM D4020) specifies UHMWPE as having a molecular weight greater than 3.1×10^6 g/mol.[6] As a result of its extremely high molecular weight, UHMWPE exhibits excellent mechanical properties such as impact strength and toughness, and better abrasive wear resistance than other polymers.[7–9]

The UHMWPE powder or flake resulting directly from synthesis is a highly crystalline (60–75%,[10] depending on the resin type) material that is referred to as 'nascent' crystallized or crystallized at birth (i.e. simultaneous polymerization, precipitation and crystallization). The high crystallinity and melting temperature exhibited by the nascent UHMWPE powder were attributed to the presence of an extended-chain crystal morphology.[10–12] However, once melted and recrystallized, the long polyethylene chains inhibit the arrangement of molecules into crystal domains, and the crystallinity is reduced to 50–55%, implying that folded-chain crystal lamellae are formed. The crystalline lamellar thickness of fabricated UHMWPE is about 10–50 nm.[9,13] The morphology of low-crystalline UHMWPE is likely to be composed of many small and imperfect crystals connected by taut tie molecules. Taut tie molecules are parts of polyethylene chains that connect two crystals and result from the separate crystallization of parts of long polyethylene chains. Taut tie molecules were preferentially broken by irradiation, and the reorganization of broken molecules resulted in an increase in the degree of crystallinity.[14]

The physical and mechanical properties of UHMWPE are specific to the type of resin (differing in molecular weight) and the consolidation process (extrusion versus compression molding).[9,15–20] For example, when the molecular weight of UHMWPE increases from 3×10^6 to 6×10^6 g/mol, abrasion resistance improves by approximately 30%, while impact strength decreases from 140 to 80 kJ/m^2.[21] Typically, UHMWPE has a density of 0.932–0.945 g/cm^3, an elastic modulus of 0.8–1.6 GPa, a tensile yield stress of 21–28 MPa, elongation at break of 350–525% and an ultimate tensile stress of 39–48 MPa.[22] Material standards of UHMWPE powder and the fabricated forms for surgical implants are specified in the ASTM F648-04 standard. The standard provides physical and chemical requirements for fabricated forms of UHMWPE but does not imply the *in vivo* performance criteria.

Several studies that led to the understanding of UHMWPE structure and morphology have been published.[23–29] Further information on the history of UHMWPE as a bearing material has been extensively reviewed by Kurtz *et al.*,[9] Li and Burstein[30] and Li.[31]

6.3 Fabrication of implants using UHMWPE

Because of its high melt viscosity (owing to the extremely high molecular weight), UHMWPE powder is difficult to process using conventional processing techniques such as injection molding, screw extrusion or blow molding. Instead, the most common fabrication methods for UHMWPE are ram extrusion, compression molding and direct compression molding. Pressure, temperature and time are process parameters that need to be controlled. Excessive heat or time can cause degradation of the material (e.g. molecular weight and mechanical properties), whereas insufficient heat, pressure or time can result in fusion defects in the fabricated UHMWPE, which can lead to inadequate mechanical strength and poor resistance to oxidation and wear.

Ram extrusion uses a reciprocating ram to compact and transfer UHMWPE powder through a heated die.[7,21] In this process, UHMWPE powder is fed into the extruder throat through a hopper and then compressed into the die with a hydraulic ram. When the ram is retracted, fresh powder is fed into the empty chamber and the process is repeated. The compacted powder then moves through the heated die, where it is melted and fused. Since ram extrusion is a continuous process, the UHMWPE powder is consolidated into a continuous cylindrical bar with a diameter ranging from 1 to 6 in. Bar stocks are then annealed to release the residual stress induced by the forming process prior to implant fabrication (i.e. to increase the dimensional stability of implant).

Compression molding of sheets consists in filling the unheated mold with UHMWPE powder to 2.2–2.5 times the desired sheet thickness and then carefully levelling the powder with a straight edge.[21] The UHMWPE powder is then cold pressed to remove air and to compact the material. The compacted powder is heated and fused at a controlled pressure and temperature. After the powder is completely fused, the pressure is increased to prevent voids inside the block and sink marks on the surface while the mold is slowly cooled to below the melting point of UHMWPE.[21] Molded blocks are then annealed to release the residual stress induced by the forming process prior to implant fabrication.

For direct compression molding, the UHMWPE powder is placed into a mold that is in the shape of an implant and then compressed. The compacted powder is heated at a controlled pressure to consolidate the material and to form the device. Implants fabricated with direct compression molding have no external machining lines and exhibit a highly glossy surface finish.[31] Although the process is slow, direct compression molding a smaller part may have greater control for the pressure and temperature than bulk compression molding does, thereby improving the material properties of implant.

6.4 Implant sterilization

6.4.1 Gamma irradiation sterilization

Because of its chemical simplicity and wide commercial applications, the effects of high-energy irradiation on polyethylene have been extensively studied.[32–37] Ionizing radiation on polyethylene cleaves carbon–carbon and carbon–hydrogen bonds, and generates free radicals. Free radicals on adjacent polyethylene chains can recombine and form cross-links that lead to the formation of a three-dimensional network. It was suggested that radiation-induced cross-linking occurs preferentially at the fold surfaces of folded-chain lamellae or in the amorphous region of bulk polyethylene.[34–36] The absence of cross-links inside the crystal lattice had been attributed to the fact that carbon atoms on adjacent polyethylene chains are too far apart (4.1 Å) to allow a carbon–carbon bond (1.54 Å) between adjacent chains, and the crystal lattice is too rigid at room temperature to form interchain carbon–carbon bonds.[35] Free radicals also can recombine to re-form the original molecular chain (particularly in the crystalline region), decay into unsaturations, react with oxygen (if present) to form oxidized species or remain in the crystalline region (the so-called 'residual free radicals'). While the dominant effect of ionizing radiation on polyethylene is cross-linking, main chain scission also occurs. Main chain scission breaks up molecules and results in a decrease in molecular weight that can affect the mechanical properties of polyethylene.

Since the 1960s, gamma irradiation has been the sterilization method for bearing components owing to its effectiveness, reliability and simplicity. The dose range for sterilization is typically from 2.5 to 4 Mrad. The majority of UHMWPE components implanted in the past three decades were sterilized by gamma irradiation in ambient air. However, oxygen that was present in the UHMWPE when it was irradiated (i.e. primarily in the surface layer), could react with the free radicals that were generated by the radiation and initiate the oxidation process. Because oxidation and cross-linking are competing processes during gamma radiation sterilization in air, oxidation within the surface region reduces the the level of cross-linking (i.e. reducing the gel content Fig. 6.1[38]). The oxidation process can continue during shelf storage[39–43] and *in vivo*,[44] resulting in molecular chain scission that degraded the molecular weight, increased the density, stiffness and brittleness and reduced the fracture strength and elongation to failure.[43–51] These changes can reduce the wear resistance of UHMWPE[39,52–55] and cause the early failure of the implants. Consequently, alternative sterilization methods such as gamma radiation in a reduced oxygen environment (i.e. in inert gas or partial vacuum), gas plasma sterilization or ethylene oxide sterilization (nonradiation methods) were used by several orthopedic manufacturers.[54]

Gamma sterilization in a reduced oxygen environment minimizes the immediate oxidation in the surface region of UHMWPE implant and promotes cross-linking (Fig. 6.1[38]). Cross-linking has been shown to improve the wear resistance of UHMWPE acetabular cups markedly in laboratory wear simulators and in clinical studies (Fig. 6.2[54] and Fig. 6.3[56]).[57–70] In order to retain the potential benefits of gamma-induced cross-linking, while

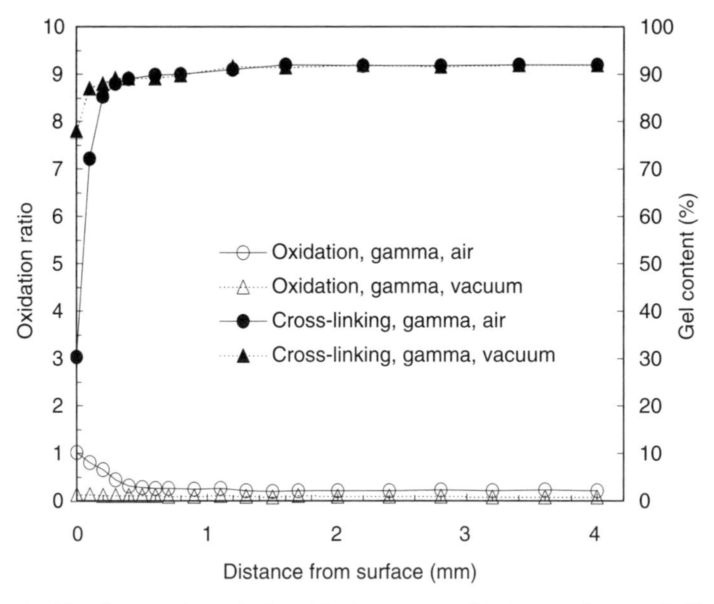

6.1 The interactive relationship between oxidation and cross-linking in the UHMWPE that was gamma irradiated (3.3 Mrad) while packaged in either air or vacuum. The measurements were made within 2 days after irradiation. One specimen for each material was analyzed. (Reproduced with permission from Shen and McKellop[38].)

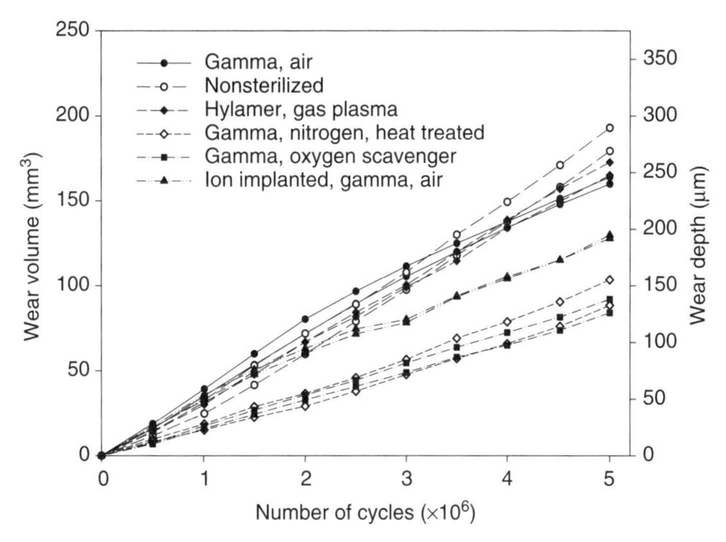

6.2 Volumetric wear of two cups of each material tested without artificial aging. The scale on the right indicates the approximate maximum depth of wear, i.e. at the center of the contact zone. (Reproduced with permission from McKellop *et al.*[54])

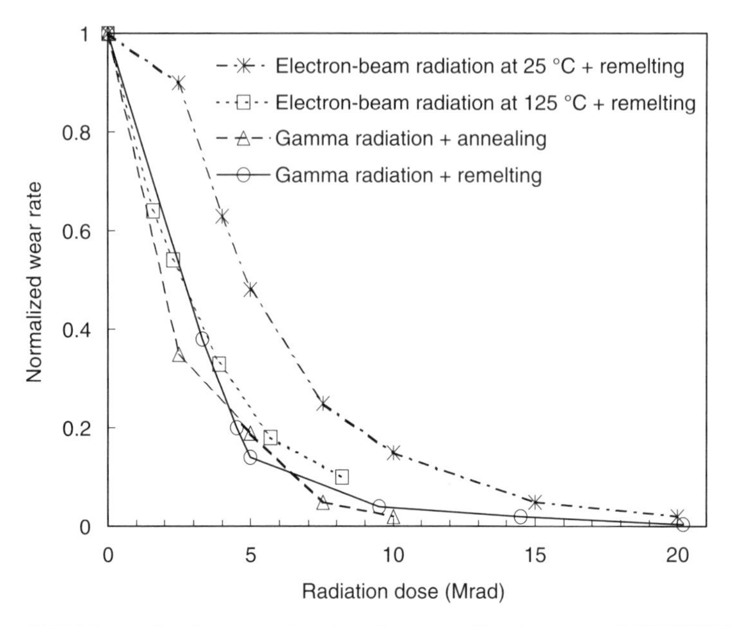

6.3 Schematic diagram showing the reduction in wear of UHMWPE with increased radiation dose (increased level of cross-linking). The curves for gamma radiation plus annealing[63] and gamma radiation plus remelting[60] were produced on hip joint wear simulators. The curves for electron beam radiation[64] were produced on a bidirectional pin-on-disk wear tester. (Reproduced with permission from McKellop.[56])

reducing the immediate and long-term oxidative degradation, in the mid-1990s, several orthopedic manufacturers began to gamma-sterilize UHMWPE components in a low-oxygen atmosphere. This could be accomplished by sealing the finished components in a partial vacuum,[71] in an inert gas such as nitrogen[72] or argon, or with a chemical scavenger to absorb the oxygen.[73] Packaging in a low-oxygen environment after fabrication minimized the diffusion of oxygen into the UHMWPE and prevented it from oxidation during the course of irradiation sterilization and shelf storage prior to implantation. However, regardless of the atmosphere in which the specimens were irradiated, once the package was open to air, the residual free radicals that remained in UHMWPE components after irradiation can combine with any oxygen that subsequently diffused in from the surface, initiating a progressive oxidation process[38,41] and thereby reducing the level of cross-linking and mechanical properties. Although it is generally recognized that oxygen diffusion will be much lower *in vivo* than during storage in air, owing to the lower concentration of oxygen in the body fluids, Currier *et al.*[39] and Kurtz *et al.*[44] have reported that the *in vivo* oxidation of gamma-sterilized UHMWPE do occur after implantation. Thus, *in vivo* oxidation can occur in the UHMWPE components gamma sterilized in a low-oxygen atmosphere. Further studies of retrieved UHMWPE components that have been treated in this way are needed.

The amount of residual free radicals present in irradiated UHMWPE may be reduced by annealing, i.e. by heating below the melt transition temperature for an extended period.[72,74,75] However, since crystalline regions remain in the polyethylene during annealing, many of the free radicals are not neutralized. Jahan and coworkers[76,77] reported that substantial amount of free radicals remained afer annealing. This renders the potential susceptible to oxidative degradation to some extent and a reduction in the wear resistance in the irradiated and annealed UHMWPE components.[54] In contrast, residual free radicals can be virtually eliminated if the polyethylene is heated above the melt transition temperature (about 150 °C) for a few hours.[60,61,64] However, since heating to this temperature could cause unacceptable distortion of a finished component, remelting to eliminate free radicals is typically applied to pre-cross-linked bulk material, before it is machined into a final component. This approach can provide a cross-linked UHMWPE component with high resistance to oxidation and wear (see discussion below).

Further information on the effects of radiation on UHMWPE, including melting behavior, tensile properties, fatigue strength and fracture toughness, free radicals and oxidation have been published.[6,45,49,51,78–100]

6.4.2 Ethylene oxide sterilization

Ethylene oxide (EtO) sterilization is a surface sterilization process that deactivates bacteria, spores and viruses.[101,102] The efficacy of an EtO sterilization cycle is dependent on stringent control of process parameters, including temperature, humidity, pressure and gas duration time.[101,102] Because of its toxicity, highly hazardous and flammable nature, and toxic residues, implant manufacturers who sterilize UHMWPE components with ethylene gas have the responsibility to comply with the federal regulations.[101]

EtO sterilization does not generate free radicals in UHMWPE.[103] Therefore, this sterilization process will not cause oxidization or form cross-linking in UHMWPE components, and it does not substantially affect the physical, chemical and mechanical properties of UHMWPE.[87,91] Sterilizing UHMWPE components with EtO can avoid the immediate and long-term oxidative degradation of the components[41,43,91,102–104] but does not improve the inherent wear resistance of UHMWPE (because of lack of cross-linking). In a hip simulator study (without thermal aging), it was shown that EtO sterilized cups exhibited about 30–50% higher wear rate than did the gamma-irradiated cups (Fig. 6.2).[54,63,105,106] In a short-term clinical follow-up, Digas *et al.*[107] reported that, after implantation for 2 years, EtO-sterilized

UHMWPE cups had almost twice the proximal and three-dimensional penetration rates, compared with the UHMWPE gamma sterilized in a low-oxygen atmosphere. In contrast, in follow-up intervals of 2 and 14 years, EtO-sterilized cups showed comparable wear rate with the cups gamma sterilized in air.[108] Clinically, the wear rate of EtO-sterilized cups might be lower than that of cups gamma sterilized in air, particularly if the cups gamma sterilized in air are shelf aged for a long period prior to implantation. Although the UHMWPE cups gamma sterilized in a low-oxygen atmosphere had the advantage of 30–50% lower wear rate than the EtO-sterilized cups, the clinical wear rate of the former cups might eventually be higher than that of the latter cups if a substantial amount of oxidation were to occur in the cups gamma sterilized in a low-oxygen atmosphere.[54] On the other hand, if the EtO-sterilized cups fails during the early stage owing to wear-induced osteolysis, the long-term benefit of greater resistance to oxidation will diminish.

6.4.3 Gas plasma sterilization

Gas plasma sterilization is a low-pressure low-temperature plasma-based process. Plasma is an ionized or partially ionized gas and is created by microwave electromagnetic field. The sterilization method uses a two-phase vapor process in which a peroxide or peracetic acid vapor is alternately introduced with a plasma-based gas mixture, rendering the implants sterile.[109] Because the process does not leave toxic residues on the implants, the implants may be used as soon as they are removed from the sterilizer with no aeration. Gas plasma sterilization also eliminates the safety and environmental issues associated with EtO sterilization.

Gas plasma sterilization is a surface sterilization process and does not produce free radicals in UHMWPE.[103] Thus, similar to EtO sterilization, gas plasma sterilization does not cause oxidative degradation and has minimal effect on the mechanical properties.[41,102,109] UHMWPE components sterilized with EtO or gas plasma will probably exhibit similar clinical outcomes. Because UHMWPE is not cross-linked by gas plasma, there is no improvement in the inherent wear resistance of the material, which is supported with a hip simulator study.[54] Clinically, Hopper *et al.*[110] reported that the UHMWPE liners that had been sterilized with gamma radiation in air exhibited a significantly lower wear rate than did the liners sterilized with gas plasma.

6.5 Cross-linking to improve implant wear properties

Polyethylene cups that were intentionally cross-linked at levels much higher than occurs with radiation sterilization (2.5–4 Mrad) were used in three clinical studies. Grobbelaar *et al.*[68,69] cross-linked finished polyethylene cups with 10 Mrad of gamma radiation. By irradiating the cups in the presence of acetylene gas, cross-linking in the surface layer (about 300 μm) was substantially increased above what would normally occur at 10 Mrad. No post-irradiation thermal treatment was carried out to reduce residual free radicals. In a 14–20 year follow-up based on radiographs, Grobbelaar *et al.*[69] reported a 'lack of measurable wear' in 56 out of 64 cases and only two revisions due to osteolytic loosening.

Oonishi *et al.*[67,111] cross-linked finished polyethylene cups with 100 Mrad of gamma radiation in an ambient atmosphere. As with the Grobbelaar *et al.* method, no post-irradiation thermal treatment was performed to reduce residual free radicals. In an early clinical follow-up, Oonishi *et al.*[67] reported steady-state wear rates of 0.247 mm/year and 0.098 mm/year for non-cross-linked polyethylene cups bearing against cobalt–chromium and alumina heads, respectively, and 0.076 mm/year and 0.072 mm/year for 100 Mrad cross-linked polyethylene cups bearing against cobalt–chromium and alumina heads, respectively. Recently, in the mean follow-up of 17.3 years, it was reported that, against cobalt–chromium femoral heads, the steady-state wear rates averaged 0.29 mm/year and 0.06 mm/year for the noncross-linked and 100 Mrad cross-linked polyethylene cups, respectively.[111]

Wroblewski *et al.*[112] chemically cross-linked polyethylene cups with silane. In a 10-year follow-up, Wroblewski *et al.* reported that, after an initial 'bedding-in' period (2 years), the average steady-state wear rate of cross-linked polyethylene against alumina ceramic head was only 0.02 mm/year. While this wear rate was well below the clinical range for cups gamma sterilized in air, it was not clear how much of the advantage was due to the head material rather than to cross-linking. Nevertheless, the results of the three clinical studies were encouraging in that, despite any reduction in material strength caused by elevated cross-linking and the lack of thermal treatment to reduce residual free radicals in the gamma-cross-linked polyethylenes, none of the investigators reported fracture or other mechanical failures from the cross-linked polyethylene cups.

6.5.1 Intentional cross-linked, thermally stabilized ultrahigh-molecular-weight polyethylenes

Current fabrication methods of intentional cross-linked, thermally stabilized UHMWPEs are illustrated in Fig. 6.4. Extruded bars or molded blocks of UHMWPE are first cross-linked by gamma or electron-beam irradiation. The cross-linked UHMWPE is then subject to thermal treatment (annealing or remelting) to reduce residual free radicals generated by irradiation and improve its resistance to oxidation. Final components are machined from the central portion of thermally treated cross-linked UHMWPE,

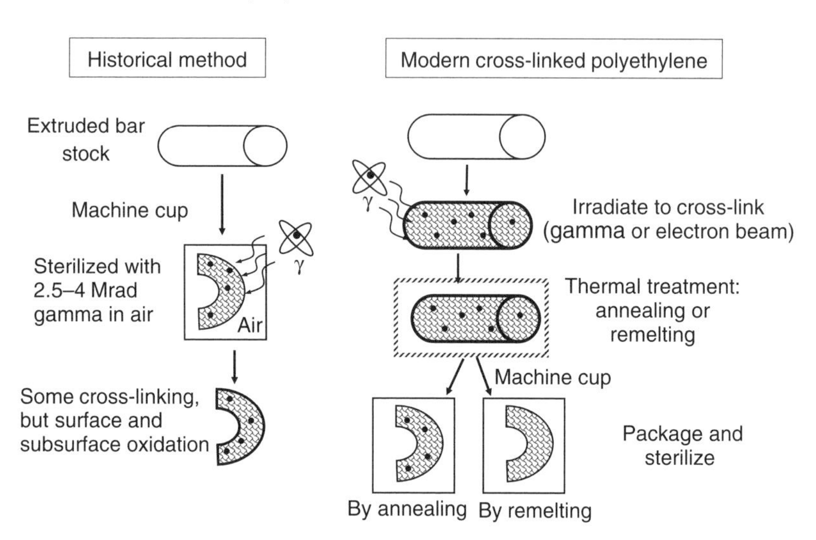

6.4 Schematic diagram showing the fabrication processes for historical (gamma sterilized in air) and new cross-linked UHMWPEs. The small full circles denotes free radicals generated by irradiation.

thereby removing the most oxidized surface layer. Implants are packaged and sterilized. Implants are preferably sterilized with nonradiation methods (EtO or gas plasma) in order not to reintroduce free radicals. The key difference between conventional polyethylene and modern cross-linked polyethylene is that, in the historical fabrication process, UHMWPE components are first machined out of raw materials, packaged and sterilized with gamma radiation in air (gamma sterilized in a low-oxygen environment for the later process) (Fig. 6.4), leading to surface oxidation and residual free radicals in UHMWPE implants. As is well known, residual free radicals lead to long-term oxidative degradation and eventually degrade the mechanical and wear properties of UHMWPE implants. Thus, compared with conventional UHMWPE, the modern cross-linked UHMWPE can provide a higher level of cross-linking to reduce the wear rate of UHMWPE while substantially improving its oxidation resistance (except for Crossfire™ polyethylene, discussed below).

A number of laboratory wear simulations have demonstrated that the wear rate of UHMWPE cups decreases markedly with an increasing level of cross-linking.[60,63,64] As shown in Fig. 6.3,[56] the greatest wear reduction per megarad occurred as the dose increased from zero to about 5 Mrad, with progressively less improvement at higher doses and no additional benefit after 10–15 Mrad. Although the baseline wear rate differed between various wear simulators owing to systematic differences in the load, sliding distance per cycles and other factors, the dose–wear curve was essentially consistent for different laboratories and with different cross-linking techniques.[56]

While the dose–wear relationship is the basis for the recent development of various intentionally cross-linked UHMW polyethylenes, orthopedic manufacturers have arrived at different opinions on the optimum dose and processing parameters for optimizing the clinical performance of a cross-linked UHMWPE implant. The fabrication and characteristics of the new, intentionally cross-linked, thermally stabilized UHMWPEs are summarized in Table 6.1.[112–115]

Marathon™ gamma-cross-linked and remelted polyethylene

In the Marathon process, extruded bars of UHMWPE are cross-linked with 5 Mrad of gamma radiation. The cross-linked bars are then heated to 155 °C (above melting temperature) for 24 h, followed by annealing at 120 °C for 24 h and then slow cooling to room temperature. Because the residual free radicals generated by irradiation are primarily trapped in the crystalline region, heating above the melting temperature enables them to combine each other, forming additional cross-links and minimizing the potential for long-term oxidation.[60,61] The acetabular cup is then machined from the central portion of the cross-linked and remelted bar, thereby removing the oxidized surface layer, and is sterilized using gas plasma to avoid reintroducing free radicals or increasing the level of cross-linking. Under clean test conditions, the Marathon™ polyethylene has shown about 85% reduction in wear compared with non-cross-linked polyethylene, while against severely roughened femoral balls, Marathon™ still shows substantially better wear resistance than non-cross-linked polyethylene.[61]

XLPE™ gamma-cross-linked and remelted polyethylene

XLPE™ is fabricated in a similar manner to Marathon™, except that the cross-linking dose is 10 Mrad and the final component is sterilized with EtO.

Longevity™ electron-beam-cross-linked and remelted polyethylene

In the Longevity process, compression-molded sheets of UHMWPE are cross-linked at room temperature with a 10 MeV electron beam to a total of 10 Mrad. The cross-linked UHMWPE is then heated at 150 °C for about 2 h to extinguish the residual free radicals. Final components are machined from the cross-linked and remelted material and sterilized with gas plasma.[116]

Durasul™ electron-beam-cross-linked and remelted polyethylene

In the Durasul process, UHMWPE is machined into short segments or pucks that are preheated to about 125 °C and cross-linked from both sides

Table 6.1 Comparison between new cross-linked, thermally stabilized polyethylenes. The processing parameters shown in this table were compiled from various publications and information provided by the manufacturers and are subject to ongoing modification. For Crossfire™ and Aeonian™, the total cross-linking dose will depend on how much irradiation is used for terminal sterilization. The allowable range is 2.5–4 Mrad. (Modified with permission from McKellop[56])

Name and manufacturer	Radiation type and dose	Thermal stabilization	Final sterilization	Total cross-linking dose and type
Marathon™, DePuy, Inc.	Gamma radiation to 5 Mrad at room temperature	Remelted at 155 °C for 24 h	Gas plasma	5 Mrad, gamma
XLPE™, Smith & Nephew–Richards, Inc.	Gamma radiation to 10 Mrad at room temperature	Remelted at 150 °C for 2 h	Eto	5 Mrad, gamma
Longevity™, Zimmer, Inc.	Electron-beam radiation to 10 Mrad at warm room temperature	Remelted at 150 °C for about 6 h	Gas plasma	10 Mrad, electron beam
Durasul™, Zimmer, Inc.	Electron-beam radiation to 9.5 Mrad at 125 °C	Remelted at 150 °C for about 2 h	Eto	9.5 Mrad, electron beam
Crossfire™, Stryker Osteonics Howmedica, Inc.	Gamma radiation to 7.5 Mrad at room temperature	Annealed at about 120 °C for a proprietary duration	Gamma at 2.5–3.5 Mrad while packaged in nitrogen	10–11 Mrad, gamma
SXL™,[113] Stryker Osteonics Howmedica, Inc.	Gamma radiation to 3 Mrad at room temperature (first cycle)	Annealed at about 130 °C for 8 h. The cycle of gamma radiation (3 Mrad) and annealing is repeated twice more to a total dose of 9 Mrad	Gas plasma	9 Mrad, gamma
Aeonian™, Kyocera, Inc.	Gamma radiation to 3.5 Mrad at room temperature	Annealed at 110 °C for 10 h	Gamma at 2.5–4 Mrads while packaged in nitrogen	6–7.5 Mrad, gamma
ArComXL™,[114] Biomet, Inc.	Gamma radiation to 5 Mrad at room temperature	Annealed at 130 °C for a proprietary duration while applying solid-state hydrostatic extrusion. After mechanical deformation, annealed at 130 °C for stress relief	Gas plasma	5 Mrad, gamma

with a 10 MeV electron beam to a total of 9.5 Mrad. The cross-linked UHMWPE is then heated above the melting temperature to extinguish free radicals. Components are machined from the cross-linked and remelted material and sterilized with EtO.[62] Comparative tests indicated that electron-beam cross-linking at warm temperature provided less reduction in elongation to break and toughness than that at room temperature.[62]

Although there is no difference in the type of radiolytic event induced with electron-beam or gamma radiation, the spatial profiles of these events (i.e. the penetration of radiation) are substantially different for the two radiation methods. In general, gamma irradiation can penetrate the entire thickness of raw UHMWPE material (e.g. a rod of 3 in diameter or compression-molded block), while the penetration of electron-beam radiation is dependent on the beam energy and the density of the absorbing material. Thus, to assure the dose uniformity (i.e. uniform cross-linking) with electron-beam radiation, attention to the control of process parameters is required. A study on the spatial distribution of electron-beam penetration in UHMWPE indicated that the extent of beam penetration increased with increasing irradiation temperature and that the optimum thicknesses with maximum uniformity in the dose–depth profile for double-sided irradiation were 85 mm and 90 mm for irradiation temperatures of 25 °C and 125 °C, respectively.[117]

Crossfire™ gamma-cross-linked and annealed polyethylene

Different from the Marathon process, in which the cross-linked polyethylene is heated above the melting temperature to extinguish residual free radicals, in the Crossfire process, extruded bars of UHMWPE are cross-linked with 7.5 Mrad of gamma radiation and then the cross-linked bars are annealed below the melting temperature for a proprietary duration. Cups are machined out of the cross-linked and annealed bars, packaged in a nitrogen atmosphere and sterilized by exposure to an additional 2.5–3.5 Mrad of gamma radiation. After the final gamma sterilization, no thermal treatment is applied to extinguish residual free radicals.

Developers of the Crossfire process prefer annealing to remelting of irradiated UHMWPE on the basis that annealing induces less change in material morphology and properties.[118] However, unless the cross-linked UHMWPE is heated above its melting temperature, residual free radicals that are trapped in the crystalline regions would remain in the polyethylene, i.e. annealing (heating below the melting temperature) is not as effective as remelting (heating above the melt temperature) in extinguishing the residual free radicals. For example, in one study,[119] it was reported that the Crossfire UHMWPE contained 58% more residual free radicals than control UHMWPE (gamma sterilized in either air or nitrogen). Therefore, after artificial aging at 80 °C in air for 3 weeks, Crossfire UHMWPE exhibited substantial oxidative degradation in its strength and wear resistance.[119] In contrast, artificial aging had negligible effect on the wear and mechanical properties of cross-linked and remelted polyethylenes.[61] In a separate study of real-time aging (up to 128 weeks),[121] the Crossfire UHMWPE exhibited higher oxidation than the conventional UHMWPE (gamma sterilized in a low-oxygen atmosphere), while the irradiated and melted UHMWPE showed no detectable oxidation. In a limited series of retrieved, highly cross-linked UHMWPE acetabular cups, it was found that three of the nine retrieved Crossfire components showed markedly elevated oxidation and crystallinity after *in vivo* service of less than 3 years, whereas none of the Durasul or Longevity components showed detectable oxidation after *in vivo* durations up to 3 years.[121] Thus, *in vivo* oxidation of the Crossfire UHMWPE may become a clinical issue in the long term.

Sequentially cross-linked and annealed polyethylene

In this process, compression-molded blocks of UHMWPE are first cross-linked by irradiating with gamma rays to 3 Mrad and then annealed at 130 °C for 8 hours.[113,122] The cross-linked and annealed UHMWPE is then processed twice more with the above procedures to give a cumulative dose of 9 Mrad (SXL™).[113,122] Components are then machined from the cross-linked and annealed UHMWPE and sterilized with gas plasma. In hip and knee wear simulator studies, the SXL™ UHMWPE showed reductions of 97% and 79%, respectively, over the control UHMWPE that was gamma sterilized in nitrogen to 3 Mrad.[113,123,124]

The key differences between SXL™ and Crossfire™ UHMWPEs are that the SXL™ process irradiates (3 Mrad) and anneals the UHMWPE for three times to a cumulative dose of 9 Mrad and sterilizes the final components with gas plasma, while the Crossfire™ process irradiates the UHMWPE to 7.5 Mrad, anneals for 8 h at 130 °C and sterilizes the final components with gamma radiation in nitrogen (a total dose of 10–11.5 Mrad, depending on the sterilization dose). The manufacturer claimed that the SXL™ UHMWPE had lower free-radical concentration than its counterpart, which had been irradiated to 9 Mrad (non-sequential) and annealed at 130 °C for 8 h, such that the oxidation resistance of SXL™ UHMWPE was equivalent to that of virgin UHMWPE.[122]

Aeonian™ gamma-cross-linked and annealed polyethylene

Except for lower cross-linking dose and annealing temperature, the rationale and processing of Aeonian are similar to those for Crossfire UHMWPE.

ArComXL™ gamma-irradiated and annealed, highly cross-linked polyethylene

In the ArComXL™ process, the isostatically molded rods are cross-linked with 5 Mrad of gamma radiation. The cross-linked UHMWPE is heated to 130 °C and the heated rod is then ram extruded through a circular die, with a diametral compression ratio of 1.5.[114] This processing step reduces free-radical concentration and induces plastic deformation and orientation of the molecules in UHMWPE. In the final step, the deformed rod is annealed at 130 °C to relieve residual stresses such that, after the stress relief step, the extruded rod retains 90–95% of its initial diameter.[114] UHMWPE components are machined from the treated rod and sterilized with gas plasma.

Since the ArComXL™ UHMWPE is annealed below the melting point while applying mechanical deformation, the material shows greater similarity to annealed, highly cross-linked UHMWPE, including a higher yield stress, ultimate strength and resistance to plastic deformation than to remelted materials, presumably owing to a higher crystallinity in the annealed materials. The ArComXL™ UHMWPE contained residual free radicals, but the concentration was 90% less than the control UHMWPE that was sterilized with gamma radiation in an argon environment. After accelerated aging at 70 °C for 4 weeks in a pressure vessel containing oxygen at 5 atm, the ArComXL™ UHMWPE showed little evidence of oxidation.[114]

Several studies on the tensile properties of new cross-linked UHMWPEs are summarized in Table 6.2.[114,122,125] Other properties such as crystallinity, degree of cross-linking, concentration of residual free radicals, resistance to oxidation, and fatigue strength were also reported in these studies. Further information on the fatigue strength and fracture toughness, and other properties of cross-linked UHMWPE have been published.[126–145]

Other modifications that preserve the physical and mechanical properties and avoid oxidation include surface-gradient cross-linking with low-energy electron-beam radiation[146] and the addition of vitamin E to the irradiated UHMWPE.[147–153] Since annealing and vitamin E are applied to improve the oxidation resistance of irradiated UHMWPE, these two techniques preserve the crystallinity of irradiated materials. The idea of surface-gradient cross-linking with low-energy electron-beam radiation is to provide a UHMWPE component with a bearing surface having a wear resistance comparable with that with full-thickness cross-linking, while retaining the original strength and toughness of non-cross-linked polyethylene in the bulk of the implant.[146] Low-energy electron-beam radiation is utilized to produce cross-linking that is limited to the surface area and gradually decreases with increasing depth below the surface (Fig. 6.5),[146] thereby

Table 6.2 Mechanical properties of cross-linked UHMWPEs. (Modified with permission from Collier *et al.*[125])

Cross-linked material	Yield point (MPa)	*p* value*	Ultimate tensile strength (MPa)	*p* value*	Elongation (%)	*p* value*
ArCom®, Biomet, Inc.	24 ± 0.8	<0.01	59 ± 4.7	0.3826	240 ± 38	<0.01
Marathon™, DePuy/ Johnson & Johnson, Inc.	21 ± 0.5	<0.01	56 ± 7.0	0.1892	300 ± 14	<0.01
Reflection™ XLPE (5 Mrad), Smith & Nephew–Richards Inc.	20 ± 1.3	<0.01	56 ± 7.1	0.1895	300 ± 20	<0.01
Crossfire™, Stryker Howmedica Osteonics, Inc.	22 ± 1.0	0.8177	53 ± 5.3	<0.01	230 ± 17	<0.01
Durasul™, Zimmer, Inc.	19 ± 1.6	<0.01	34 ± 3.4	<0.01	330 ± 19	<0.01
Longevity™, Zimmer, Inc.	21 ± 1.1	0.0271	43 ± 5.3	<0.01	250 ± 25	<0.01
SXL™,[122] Stryker Howmedica Osteonics, Inc.	23.5 ± 0.3	Not applicable	56.7 ± 2.1	Not applicable	267 ± 7	Not applicable
ArComXL™,[114] Biomet, Inc.	24.2 ± 0.4†	Not applicable	64.7 ± 4.5†	Not applicable	207 ± 11†	Not applicable
HSS reference UHMWPE	21.7 ± 1.0	—	58 ± 4.7	—	380 ± 10	—

* Probability values are for the *t* test between the cross-linked materials and the Hospital for Special Surgery (HSS) reference UHMWPE.

† Specimens were taken along the long axis of the rod.

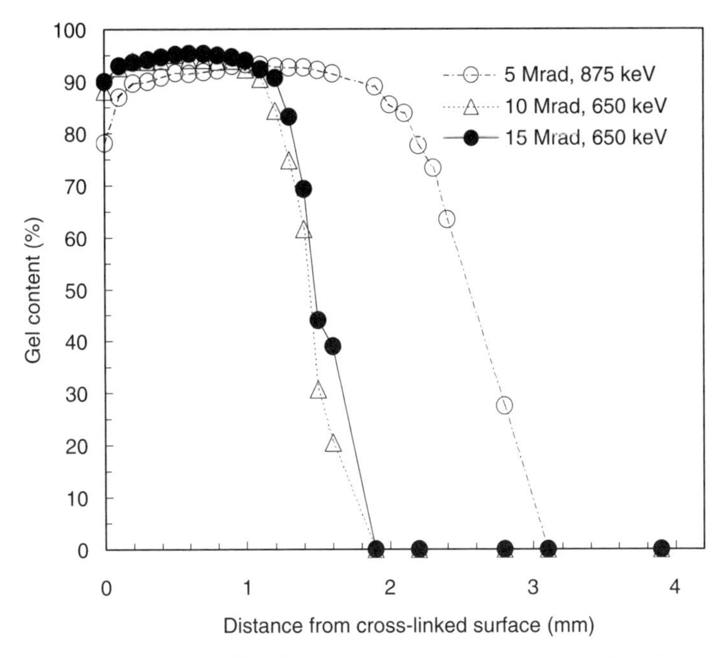

6.5 Gel content profiles (level of cross-linking) produced by low-energy electron-beam irradiation in disks 8 mm thick. One disk for each cross-linking dose was analyzed. (Reproduced with permission from Shen and McKellop.[146])

avoiding a sudden change in properties that might constitute a weak interface and lead to delamination. After radiation cross-linking, residual free radicals are markedly reduced by annealing at 100 °C for 6 days. The desired amount and depth profile of cross-linking can be obtained by adjusting the beam energy and radiation dose such that, through the lifeime of *in vivo* service, the cross-linked surface area will not be worn away. Although the wear rates at a given dose of low-energy (650 keV) electron-beam radiation tended to be higher than for cups cross-linked to the same total dose using gamma radiation or high-energy (10 MeV) electron-beam radiation, this may have been caused by the fact that the 650 keV electron beam generated fewer cross-links per megarad. If correct, then there also should be less reduction in the physical properties of the UHMWPE of the cross-linked layer, such that the electron-beam dose could be increased above 15 Mrad to provide even greater wear resistance, while preserving adequate mechanical properties of the cross-linked surface layer, and the original mechanical properties in the non-cross-linked bulk of the implant.[146]

Another technique to preserve the physical and mechanical properties of UHMWPE and to avoid oxidation is to incorporate an antioxidant (α-tocopherol or vitamin E) in the irradiated UHMWPE. There are two processes to incorporate vitamin E in the irradiated UHMWPE. In one process, vitamin E is blended with the UHMWPE powder before consolidation.[149,151,152] This process produces a uniform distribution of vitamin E in UHMWPE. After consolidating the mixture, the vitamin-E-containing raw material is subject to radiation cross-linking to improve its wear resistance. Since vitamin E acts as a scavenger for free radicals during irradiation, the level of cross-linking produced in the vitamin-E-containing UHMWPE is lower than that in the control material (with no vitamin E) that was irradiated to the same total dose.[152] The lower level of cross-linking in the irradiated vitamin-E-containing UHMWPE is supported with a hip simulator wear study in that the wear rates of the irradiated vitamin-E-containing UHMWPEs are higher than that of the control material irradiated to same total dose.[149] In another process, UHMWPE is first cross-linked by irradiation, and the irradiated material is then soaked in vitamin-E-containing solution for the diffusion of vitamin E into the interior.[147,148,150] The amount of vitamin E incorporated into irradiated UHMWPE is determined by the soaking time and temperature. Because vitamin E is doped after radiation cross-linking, the vitamin-E-doped irradiated UHMWPE shows oxidation and wear resistance comparable with those of contemporary highly cross-linked and melted UHMWPEs and a fatigue resistance higher than those of contemporary cross-linked UHMWPEs.[147] Although vitamin E is generally recognized as safe and approved for use in food contact applications, the addition of vitamin E in irradiated UHMWPE requires that the Food and Drug Administration or other international organizations approve it for implant applications.[154]

The substantial improvement of wear resistance with the cross-linked UHMWPE (between 5 and 10 Mrad (Fig. 6.3)) would provide a substantial clinical benefit. One clinical review has indicated that significant osteolysis is rare in patients whose polyethylene acetabular cups are wearing linearly less than 0.1 mm/year.[155] In contrast, if the linear wear rate exceeds 0.3 mm/year, osteolysis becomes more common. Thus, if the wear rates in the clinical use of these new cross-linked polyethylenes is as low as in the laboratory tests, the rate of accumulation of polyethylene wear particles should be well below the level that is necessary to initiate osteolysis.

However, increasing the level of cross-linking alone can reduce the strength and toughness of the UHMWPE below that necessary to avoid fracture *in vivo*.[59,156] In determining an amount of cross-linking that will retain safe values of strength and toughness, it should be recalled that the majority of polyethylene cups that were implanted during the past three decades were cross-linked to a moderate level with 2.5–4 Mrad of gamma radiation used for sterilization. Despite this, fracture *in vivo* has been rare, and the components that have fractured were typically found to be highly

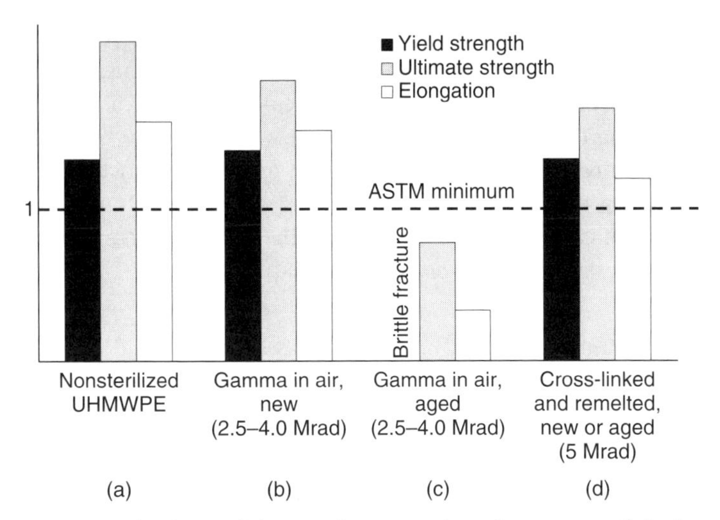

6.6 Typical values of the tensile properties of non-cross-linked and cross-linked UHMWPEs, compiled from previously published studies: (a) conventional nonirradiated (non-cross-linked) polyethylene;[60] (b) polyethylene that has been sterilized by gamma irradiation in air (as was used industrially for the past two decades) prior to aging; (c) polyethylene gamma sterilized in air after aging for 5 years or more *in vivo*;[43] (d) the cross-linked and remelted polyethylene of the present study. Although cross-linking at 5 Mrad reduces the initial tensile properties relative to non-cross-linked material, these were still above the minima used by the ASTM International to define UHMWPE. Because of the removal of the free radicals by remelting, there was little or no additional reduction in mechanical properties after extensive artificial aging (14 days at 70 °C under oxygen at 5 atm).[158] Thus, implant components fabricated from gamma-cross-linked and remelted polyethylene should not experience the progressive degradation of their mechanical properties during clinical use that has been typical of past components that had been irradiated in air.[43] (Reproduced with permission from McKellop *et al.*[61])

oxidized.[157] This historical track record implies that the strength and toughness of an UHMWPE component that has a moderate amount of intentional cross-linking and has been rendered immune to post-irradiation oxidative degradation by the application of a suitable thermal treatment to eliminate residual free radicals should be more than sufficient even for high-stress clinical applications such as knee prostheses. As shown in Fig. 6.6,[61] because of the elimination of residual free radicals, the mechanical properties of acetabular cups fabricated from cross-linked and remelted UHMWPE are significantly more stable with time than has been typical of the components gamma sterilized in air which have been clinically used in the past. Thus, it is expected that an UHMWPE acetabular cup that is moderately cross-linked and adequately stabilized against oxidative degradation will be less likely to fracture than the cups gamma sterilized in air and oxidized, which have been the clinical standard for the past three decades.[112] The optimal cross-linking dose will provide a UHMWPE with sufficient wear resistance to avoid osteolysis in even the most active patients, while retaining the strength and toughness well above that required for a lifetime of clinical use. Close monitoring the clinical performance of each of the new cross-linked polyethylenes is required.

6.5.2 Clinical studies of new cross-linked ultrahigh-molecular-weight polyethylenes

To date, there have been several clinical follow-ups available among modern cross-linked UHMWPEs. Using computer-assisted radiographic measurement techniques, Hopper *et al.*[159] reported that, based on early (2–3 years) wear data, Marathon polyethylene liners, cross-linked with 5.0 Mrad of gamma irradiation, were wearing at a mean rate of 0.08 mm/year. This rate is about half that of non-cross-linked polyethylene but represents a more modest wear reduction than *in vitro* simulator studies have predicted. Heisel *et al.*[160] reported that Marathon cross-linked UHMWPE (mean duration of follow-up, 33 months) showed 81% lower wear than conventional UHMWPE gamma sterilized in air. When accounting for differences in patient activity, the adjusted wear reduction for Marathon cross-linked UHMWPE was 72%, suggesting that the *in vivo* wear reduction with Marathon is consistent with the predictions of hip simulator studies.[160] Another clinical study reported by Sychterz *et al.*[161] indicated that Marathon cross-linked polyethylene (0.12 mm/year) had a lower true wear rate than non-irradiated Enduron polyethylene liners (0.22 mm/year) at 3.2 years, and a greater proportion of Marathon liners had true wear rates below 0.1 mm/year (62% versus 22%).

In a randomized evaulation of penetration rate in cemented and uncemented sockets using radiostereometric analysis, Digas *et al.*[162] reported that, at 2 years follow-up, Longevity, highly cross-linked polyethylene showed lower proximal penetration (62%) and lower total penetration (31%) than the control UHMWPE gamma sterilized in nitrogen. Bradford *et al.*[163] reported that a hip with a Longevity cup was revised after 2 years owing to midstem osteolysis. The cup rim was grooved because of neck–socket impingement. Although Bradford *et al.* implied that the lysis was associated with the cross-linked polyethylene cup, they also reported, but did not discuss, the fact that the grit-blasted stem was loose in the cement mantle. It is highly likely that the lysis was caused by cement and/or metal debris generated by stem–cement micromotion, rather than by the polyethylene debris from the cup.

In a 2-year follow-up study, Digas *et al.*[164] reported that Durasul, highly cross-linked polyethylene showed 50% reduction of proximal wear compared with the control UHMWPE gamma sterilized in nitrogen (when patients were studied standing). Dorr *et al.*[165] reported that, at 5-year follow-up, the annual linear wear rate of Durasul cross-linked polyethylene was 45% of that seen with the conventional polyethylene liner (i.e. 55% reduction), while the qualitative wear pattern of the highly cross-linked polyethylene liner was the same as that of the conventional polyethylene liner.

Martell *et al.*[166] reported that Crossfire, highly cross-linked polyethylene liners, had lower two- and three-dimensional linear wear rates (42% and 50%, respectively) than conventional polyethylene liners gamma sterilized in nitrogen. In a 5-year follow-up study, D'Antonio *et al.*[167] reported that the calculated annual wear was 0.036 mm/year for the Crossfire components and 0.131 mm/year for the controls (gamma sterilized in nitrogen), a reduction of 72%. Radiographic review at most recent follow-up showed a reduction in erosive osteolytic lesions of the proximal femur for the Crossfire components compared with controls, also suggesting a reduction in debris release for the Crossfire components.[167] In a case study reported by Della Valle *et al.*,[168] it was shown that titanium deposited on ceramic head after recurrent dislocation damaged (severe scratching) Crossfire, highly cross-linked polyethylene liner. Another clinical follow-up reported by Rohrl *et al.*[169] indicated that, from 2 to 24 months, the mean proximal head penetration (wear) was 156 μm for standard polyethylene (gamma sterilized in air), 138 μm for stabilized polyethylene (Duration, gamma sterilized in nitrogen and thermally stabilized) and 23 μm for Crossfire, highly cross-linked polyethylene. The low *in vivo* wear rate for highly cross-linked cups was not at the expense of higher migration or less favorable clinical outcome and looks promising.[169]

6.6 Future trends

Short-term clinical follow-up indicated that the new cross-linked UHMWPEs show a substantial improvement in wear resistance over that of conventional UHMWPE. This is encouraging because, with the use of new cross-linked UHMWPEs, the osteolysis induced by UHMWPE wear particles essentially might be eliminated, substantially extending the lifespan of implants. Future developments of new cross-linked UHMWPE include optimization between the cross-linking dose (wear resistance) and mechanical properties for specific implant applications, adjusting thermal treatment parameters to eliminate residual free radicals while preserving the material crystallinity, and any other methods that can remove residual free radicals in irradiation-cross-linked UHMWPE but maintain the mechanical properties of cross-linked UHMWPE, i.e. without further reducing the mechanical properties during the process of eliminating residual free radicals. In addition, implant design (e.g. liner thickness and locking mechanism) can also play an important role in the *in vivo* performance of new cross-linked UHMWPEs, and optimization between design parameters and material properties should be taken into account. In the future, close monitoring of the clinical performance of the new cross-linked UHMWPE is required.

6.7 Sources of further information and advice

www.uhmwpe.org
www.uhmwpe.unito.it
www.jnjgateway.com/marathon
www.smithnephew.com
www.howost.com
www.zimmer.com
www.biomet.com

6.8 References

1 McKellop H A, Campbell P, Park S H, Schmalzried T P, Grigoris P, Amstutz H C and Sarmiento A, 'The origin of submicron polyethylene wear debris in total hip arthroplasty', *Clin Orthop Relat Res*, 1995 **311** 3–20.
2 Amstutz H C, Campbell P, Kossovsky N and Clarke I, 'Mechanisms and clinical significance of wear debris induced osteolysis', *Clin Orthop Relat Res*, 1992 **276** 7–18.
3 Harris W H, 'The problem is osteolysis', *Clin Orthop Relat Res*, 1995 **311** 46–53.
4 Schmalzried T P, Jasty M and Harris W H, 'Periprosthetic bone loss in total hip arthroplasty. Polyethylene wear debris and the concept of the effective joint space', *J Bone Jt Surg Am*, 1992 **74** 849–863.
5 Willert H G, Bertram H and Buchhorn G H, 'Osteolysis in alloarthroplasty of the hip. The role of ultra-high molecular weight polyethylene wear particles', *Clin Orthop Relat Res*, 1990 **258** 95–107.
6 Rimnac C and Kurtz S, 'Ionizing radiation and orthopaedic protheses', *Nucl Instrum Methods Phys Res B*, 2005 **236** 30–37.
7 Kelly J M, 'Ultrahigh molecular weight polyethylene', *J Macromol Sci, Part C: Polym Rev*, 2002 **42** 355–371.
8 Edidin A A and Kurtz S M, 'Influence of mechanical behavior on the wear of 4 clinically relevant polymeric biomaterials in a hip simulator', *J Arthroplasty*, 2000 **15** 321–331.
9 Kurtz S M, Muratoglu O K, Evans M and Edidin A A, 'Advances in the processing, sterilization and crosslinking of ultra-high molecular weight polyethylene for total joint arthroplasty', *Biomaterials*, 1999 **20** 1659–1688.
10 Wang X and Salovey R, 'Melting of ultra high molecular weight polyethylene', *J Appl Polym Sci*, 1987 **34** 593–599.

11 Smith P, Chanzy H D and Rotzinger B P, 'Drawing of virgin ultrahigh molecular weight polyethylene: an alternative route to high strength/high modulus materials. Part 2 Influence of polymerization temperature', *J Mater Sci*, 1987 **22** 523–531.
12 Zachariades A E and Logan J A, 'The melt anisotropy of UHMWPE', *J Polym Sci, Polym Phys Edn*, 1983 **21** 821–830.
13 Bellare A, Schnablegger H and Cohen R E, 'A small-angle x-ray scattering study of high-density polyethylene and ultrahigh molecular weight polyethylene', *Macromolecules*, 1995 **28** 7585–7588.
14 Bhateja S K, Andrews E H and Young R J, 'Radiation-induced crystallinity changes in linear polyethylene', *J Polym Sci, Polym Phys Edn*, 1983 **21** 523–536.
15 Bellare A and Cohen R E, 'Morphology of rod stock and compression-moulded sheets of ultra-high-molecular-weight polyethylene used in orthopaedic implants', *Biomaterials,* 1996 **17** 2325–2333.
16 Greer K and King R, 'The mechanical and physical properties of four different crosslinked UHMWPE materials', in *Transactions of the 27th Annual Meeting of the Society for Biomaterials*, Saint Paul, Minnesota, USA, 2001, Mt Laurel, New Jersey, Society for Biomaterials, 2001, p. 85.
17 Lykins M D and Evans M A, 'A comparision of extruded and molded UHMWPE', in *Transactions of the 21st Annual Meeting of the Society for Biomaterials*, San Francisco, California, USA, 1995, Mt Laurel, New Jersey, Society for Biomaterials, 1995, p. 385.
18 Poggie R A, Takeuchi M T and Averill R, 'Effects of resin type, consolidation method and sterilization of UHMWPE', in *Transactions of the 23rd Annual Meeting of the Society for Biomaterials*, New Orleans, Louisiana, USA, 1997, Mt Laurel, New Jersey, Society for Biomaterials, 1997, p. 216.
19 Barbour P S M, Stone M H and Fisher J, 'A study of the wear resistance of three types of clinically applied UHMWPE for total replacement hip prostheses', *Biomaterials*, 1999 **20** 2101–2106.
20 Currier B H, Currier J H, Collier J P and Mayor M B, 'Effect of fabrication method and resin type on performance of tibial bearings', *J Biomed Mater Res*, 2000 **53** 143–151.
21 Stein H L, 'Ultrahigh molecular weight polyethylene', in *Engineered Materials Handbook*, Vol. 2: *Engineering Plastics*, Materials Park, Ohio, ASM International, 1998, pp. 167–171.
22 Kurtz S, *The UHMWPE Handbook, Ultrahigh Molecular Weight Polyethylene in Total Joint Replacement*, New York, Elsevier Academic Press, 2004.
23 Pienkowski D, Jacob R, Hoglin D, Saum K, Kaufer H and Nicholls P J, 'Low-voltage scanning electron microscopic imaging of ultrahigh-molecular weight polyethylene', *J Biomed Mater Res*, 1995 **29** 1167–1174.
24 Pienkowski D, Hoglin D P, Jacob R J, Saum K A, Nicholls P J and Kaufer H, 'Shape and size of virgin ultrahigh molecular weight GUR 4150 HP polyethylene powder', *J Biomed Mater Res*, 1996 **33** 65–71.
25 Jacob R J, Pienkowski D, Hoglin D, Saum K A, Kaufer H and Nicholls P J, 'Molecular anatomy of freeze-fractured ultra-high-molecular-weight polyethylene as determined by low-voltage scanning electron microscopy', *J Biomed Mater Res*, 1997 **37** 489–496.

26 Lee K-Y and Pienkowski D, 'Compressive creep characteristics of extruded ultra-high-molecular-weight polyethylene', *J Biomed Mater Res*, 1998 **39** 261–265.
27 Cook J T E, Klein P G, Ward I M, Brain A A, Farrar D F and Rose J, 'The morphology of nascent and molded UHMWPE. Insights from solid-state NMR, nitric acid etching, GPC and DSC', *Polymer*, 2000 **41** 8615–8623.
28 Phillips R A, 'Morphology and melting behavior of nascent UHMWPE', *J Polym Sci Part B: Polym Phys*, 1998 **36** 495–517.
29 Farrar D F and Brain A A, 'The microstructure of ultra-high molecular weight polyethylene used in total joint replacements', *Biomaterials*, 1997 **18** 1677–1685.
30 Li S and Burstein A H, 'Ultra-high molecular weight polyethylene. The material and its use in total joint implants', *J Bone Jt Surg Am*, 1994 **76** 1080–1090.
31 Li S, 'Polyethylene', in *The Adult Hip* (Eds J Callaghan, A Rosenberg and H Rubash), Philadelphia, Lippincott–Raven, 1998, pp. 105–122.
32 Charlesby A, *Atomic Radiations and Polymers*, London, Pergamon, 1960.
33 Salovey R, 'Irradiation of cyrstalline polyethylene', *J Polym Sci*, 1962 **61** 463–473.
34 Salovey R and Yager W A, 'Electron spin resonance of irradiated solution crystallized polyethylene', *J Polym Sci*, 1964 **2** 219–224.
35 Patel G N and Keller A, 'Crystallinity and the effect of ionizing radiation in polyethylene', *J Polym Sci, Polym Phys Edn*, 1975 **13** 303–321, 323–331, 333–338.
36 Ungar G, 'Radiation effects in polyethylene and *n*-alkanes', *J Mater Sci*, 1981 **16** 2635–2656.
37 Premnath V, Harris W H, Jasty M and Merrill E W, 'Gamma sterilization of UHMWPE articular implants: an analysis of the oxidation problem', *Biomaterials*, 1996 **17** 1741–1753.
38 Shen F-W and McKellop H A, 'Interaction of oxidation and crosslinking in gamma-irradiated ultrahigh molecular-weight polyethylene', *J Biomed Mater Res*, 2002 **61** 430–439.
39 Currier B H, Currier J H, Collier J P, Mayor M B and Scott R D, 'Shelf life and in vivo duration. Impacts on performance of tibial bearings', *Clin Orthop Relat Res*, 1997 **342** 111–122.
40 Jacob R J, Pienkowski D, Lee K Y, Hamilton D M, Schroeder D and Higgins J, 'Time- and depth-dependent changes in crosslinking and oxidation of shelf-aged polyethylene acetabular liners', *J Biomed Mater Res*, 2001 **56** 168–176.
41 Willie B M, Ashrafi S, Alajbegovic S, Burnett T and Bloebaum R D, 'Quantifying the effect of resin type and sterilization method on the degradation of ultrahigh molecular weight polyethylene after 4 years of real-time shelf aging', *J Biomed Mater Res Part A*, 2004 **69** 477–489.
42 Pienkowski D, Patel A, Lee K Y, Hamilton D M, Jacob R J, Higgins J and Schroeder D W, 'Solubility changes in shelf-aged ultra-high molecular weight polyethylene acetabular liners', *J Long Term Eff Med Implants*, 1999 **9** 273–288.
43 Sutula L C, Lollier D E, Saum K A, Currier B H, Currier J H, Sanford W M, Mayor M B, Wooding R E, Sperling D K, Williams I R, Kaspizak D J and Surprenant V A, 'Impact of gamma sterilization on clinical performance of polyethylene in the hip', *Clin Orthop Relat Res*, 1995 **319** 28–40.

44 Kurtz S M, Rimnac C M, Hozack W J, Turner J, Marcolongo M, Goldberg V M, Kraay M J and Edidin A A, '*In vivo* degradation of polyethylene liners after gamma sterilization in air', *J Bone Jt Surg Am*, 2005 **87** 815–823.
45 Roe R J, Grood E S, Shastri R, Gosselin C A and Noyes F R, 'Effect of radiation sterilization and ageing on ultrahigh molecular weight polyethylene', *J Biomed Mater Res*, 1981 **15** 209–230.
46 Eyerer P and Ke Y C, 'Property changes of UHMW polyethylene hip cup endoprostheses during implantation', *J Biomed Mater Res*, 1984 **18** 1137–1151.
47 Eyerer P, Kurth M, McKellop H and Mittlmeier T, 'Characterization of UHMWPE hip cups run on joint simulators', *J Biomed Mater Res*, 1987 **21** 275–291.
48 Kurth M, Eyerer P, Ascherl R, Dittel K and Holz U, 'An evaluation of retrieved UHMWPE hip joint cups', *J Biomed Mater Appl*, 1988 **3** 33–51.
49 Collier J P, Sperling D K, Currier J H, Sutula L C, Saum K A and Mayor M B, 'Impact of gamma sterilization on clinical performance of polyethylene in the knee', *J Arthroplasty*, 1996 **11** 377–389.
50 Rimnac C M, Klein R W, Betts F and Wright T, 'Post-irradiation aging of ultra-high molecular weight polyethylene', *J Bone Jt Surg Am*, 1994 **76** 1052–1056.
51 Deng M and Shalaby S W, 'Long-term irradiation effects on ultrahigh molecular weight polyethylene', *J Biomed Mater Res*, 2001 **54** 428–435.
52 Shen C and Dumbleton J H, 'The friction and wear behavior of irradiated very high molecular weight polyethylene', *Wear*, 1974 **30** 349–364.
53 Fisher J, Chan K L, Hailey J L, Shaw D and Stone M, 'Preliminary study of the effect of aging following irradiation on the wear of ultrahigh-molecular-weight polyethylene', *J Arthroplasty*, 1995 **10** 689–692.
54 McKellop H, Shen F W, Lu B, Campbell P and Salovey R, 'Effect of sterilization method and other modifications on the wear resistance of acetabular cups made of ultra-high molecular weight polyethylene. A hip-simulator study', *J Bone Jt Surg Am*, 2000 **82** 1708–1725.
55 Besong A A, Hailey J L, Ingham E, Stone M, Wroblewski B M and Fisher J, 'A study of the combined effects of shelf ageing following irradiation in air and counterface roughness on the wear of UHMWPE', *Biomed Mater Eng*, 1997 **7** 59–65.
56 McKellop H, 'Bearing surfaces in total hip replacements. State of the art and future development', in *Instructional Course Lectures* Vol. 50 (Ed F H Sim), Rosemont, Illinois, American Academy of Orthopaedic Surgeons, 2001, pp. 165–179.
57 Chiesa R, Tanzi M C, Alfonsi S, Paracchini L, Moscatelli M and Cigada A, 'Enhanced wear performance of highly crosslinked UHMWPE for artificial joints', *J Biomed Mater Res*, 2000 **50** 381–387.
58 Shen F-W, McKellop H A and Salovey R, 'Irradiation of chemically crosslinked ultrahigh molecular weight polyethylene', *J Polym Sci Part B: Polym Phys*, 1996 **34** 1063–1077.
59 Rose R M, Cimino W R, Ellis E and Crugnola A N, 'Exploratory investigations on the structure dependence of the wear resistance of polyethylene', *Wear*, 1982 **77** 89–104.

60 McKellop H, Shen F W, Lu B, Campbell P and Salovey R, 'Development of an extremely wear resistant UHMW polyethylene for total hip replacements', *J Orthop Res*, 1999 **17** 157–167.
61 McKellop H, Shen F-W, DiMaio W and Lancaster J, 'Wear of gamma-crosslinked polyethylene acetabular cups against roughened femoral balls', *Clin Orthop Relat Res*, 1999 **369** 73–82.
62 Muratoglu O K, Bragdon C R, O'Connor D O, Jasty M and Harris W H, 'A novel method of cross-linking ultra-high-molecular-weight polyethylene to improve wear, reduce oxidation, and retain mechanical properties. Recipient of the 1999 HAP Paul Award', *J Arthroplasty*, 2001 **16** 149–160.
63 Wang A, Essner A, Polineni V K, Stark C and Dumbleton J H, 'Lubrication and wear of ultra-high molecular weight polyethylene in total joint replacements', *Tribol Int*, 1998 **31** 17–33.
64 Muratoglu O K, Bragdon C R, O'Connor D O, Jasty M, Harris W H, Gul R and McGarry F, 'Unified wear model for highly crosslinked ultra-high molecular weight polyethylenes (UHMWPE)', *Biomaterials*, 1999 **20** 1463–1470.
65 D'Lima D D, Hermida J C, Chen P C and Colwell C W Jr, 'Polyethylene cross-linking by two different methods reduces acetabular liner wear in a hip joint wear simulator', *J Orthop Res*, 2003 **21** 761–766.
66 Oonishi H, Clarke I C, Yamamoto K, Masaoka T, Fujisawa A and Masuda S, 'Assessment of wear in extensively irradiated UHMWPE cups in simulator studies', *J Biomed Mater Res Part A*, 2004 **68** 52–60.
67 Oonishi H, Takayama Y and Tsuji E, 'Improvement of polyethylene by irradiation in artificial joints', *Radiat Phys Chem*, 1992 **39** 495–504.
68 Grobbelaar C J, Plessis T A D and Marais F, 'The radiation improvement of polyethylene prostheses', *J Bone Jt Surg Br*, 1978 **60** 370–374.
69 Grobbelaar C J, Weber F A, Spirakis A, Du Plessis T A, Cappaert G and Cakic J N, 'Clinical experience with gamma irradiation-crosslinked polyethylene – a 14 to 20 year follow-up report', *S Afr Bone Jt Surg*, 1999 **9** 140–147.
70 Wroblewski B M, Siney P D, Dowson D and Collins S N, 'Prospective clinical and joint simulator studies of a new total hip arthroplasty using alumina ceramic heads and cross-linked polyethylene cups', *J Bone Jt Surg Br*, 1996 **78** 280–285.
71 Greer K W, Schmidt M B and Hamilton J V, 'The hip simulator wear of gamma-vacuum, gamma-air, and ethylene oxide sterilized UHMWPE following a severe oxidative challenge,' in *Transactions of the 44th Annual Meeting of the Orthopaedic Research Society*, New Orleans, Louisiana, USA, 1998, Rosemont, Illinois, Orthopaedic Research Society, 1998, p. 52.
72 Sun D C, Wang A, Stark C and Dumbleton J H, 'The concept of stabilization in UHMWPE', in *Transactions of the 5th World Biomaterials Congress*, Toronto, Canada, 1996, Mt Laurel, New Jersey, Society for Biomaterials, 1996, p. 195.
73 Bapst J M, Valentine R H and Vasquez R, 'Wear simulation testing of direct compression molded UHMWPE irradiated in oxygenless packaging', in *Transactions of the 23rd Annual Meeting of the Society for Biomaterials*, New Orleans, Louisiana, USA, 1997, Mt Laurel, New Jersey, Society for Biomaterials, 1997, p. 72.
74 Streicher R M, 'Influence of ionizing irradiation in air and nitrogen for sterilization of surgical grade polyethylene for implants', *Radiat Phys Chem*, 1988 **31** 693–698.

75 Streicher R M, 'Investigation of sterilization and modification of high molecular weight polyethylenes by ionizing irradiation', *Beta–Gamma*, 1989 **1** 34–43.
76 Naheed N, Jahan M S and Ridley M, 'Measurements of free radicals over a period of 4.5 years in gamma-irradiated ultrahigh molecular weight polyethylene', *Nucl Instrum Methods Phys Res B*, 2003 **208** 204–209.
77 Jahan M S, King M C, Haggard W O, Sevo K L and Parr J E, 'A study of long-lived free radicals in gamma-irradiated medical grade polyethylene', *Radiat Phys Chem*, 2001 **62** 141–144.
78 Nusbaum H J and Rose R M, 'The effects of radiation sterilization on the properties of ultrahigh molecular weight polyethylene', *J Biomed Mater Res*, 1979 **13** 557–576.
79 Bhateja S K andrews E H and Yarbrough S M, 'Radiation induced crystallinity in linear polyethyelenes: long term effects', *Polym J*, 1989 **21** 739–750.
80 Bhateja S K, Duerst R W, Martens J A and Andrews E H, 'Radiation-induced enhancement of crystallinity in polymers', *J Macromol Sci, Part C: Rev Chem Phys*, 1995 **35** 581–659.
81 Narkis M, Raiter I, Shkolnik S, Siegmann A and Eyerer P, 'Structure and tensile behavior of irradiation- and peroxide-crosslinked polyethylenes', *J Macromol Sci, Part B: Phys*, 1987 **26** 37–58.
82 Shinde A and Salovey R, 'Irradiation of ultra high molecular weight polyethylene', *J Polym Sci, Polym Phys Edn*, 1985 **23** 1681–1689.
83 Jahan M S, Wang C, Schwartz G and Davidson J A, 'Combined chemical and mechanical effects on free radicals in UHMWPE joints during implantation', *J Biomed Mater Res*, 1991 **25** 1005–1017.
84 O'Neill P, Birkinshaw C, Leahy J J and Barklie R, 'The role of long lived free radicals in the ageing of irradiated UHMWPE', *Polym Degrad Stab*, 1999 **63** 31–39.
85 Streicher R M, 'Ionizing irradiation for sterilization and modification of high molecular weight polyethylenes', *Plast Rubber Process Appl*, 1988 **10** 221–229.
86 Zhao Y, Luo Y and Jiang B, 'Effect of irradiatio on crystallinity and mechanical properties of ultrahigh molecular weight polyethylene', *J Appl Polym Sci*, 1993 **50** 1797–1801.
87 Ries M D, Weaver K, Rose R M, Gunther J, Sauer W and Beals N, 'Fatigue strength of polyethylene after sterilization by gamma irradiation or ethylene oxide', *Clin Orthop Relat Res*, 1996 **333** 87–95.
88 Deng M and Shalaby S W, 'Effects of gamma irradiation, gas environments, and postirradiation aging on ultrahigh molecular weight polyethylene', *J Appl Polym Sci*, 1995 **58** 2111–2119.
89 Minkova L, 'DSC of gamma-irradiated UHMWPE and high density polyethylene of normal molecular weight', *Colloid Polym Sci*, 1988 **266** 6–10.
90 Goldman M, Gronsky R, Ranganathan R and Pruitt L, 'The effects of gamma radiation sterilization and aging on the structure and morphology of medical grade UHMWPE', *Polymer*, 1996 **37** 2909–2913.
91 Goldman M, Lee M, Gronsky R and Pruitt L, 'Oxidation of ultrahigh molecular weight polyethylene characterized by Fourier transform infrared spectroscopy', *J Biomed Mater Res*, 1997 **37** 43–50.
92 Goldman M and Pruitt L, 'Comparison of the effects of gamma radiation and low temperature hydrogen peroxide gas plasma sterilization on the molecular

structure, fatigue resistance, and wear behavior of UHMWPE', *J Biomed Mater Res*, 1998 **40** 378–384.
93 Yu Y J, Shen F, Lu B, Salovey R and McKellop H, 'Oxidation of UHMWPE acetabular cups after sterilization and wear testing in a hip joint simulator', in *Transactions of the 43rd Annual Meeting of the Orthopaedic Research Society*, San Francisco, California, USA, 1997, Rosemont, Illinois, Orthopaedic Research Society, 1997, p. 778.
94 Daly B M and Yin J, 'Subsurface oxidation of polyethylene', *J Biomed Mater Res*, 1998 **42** 523–529.
95 Costa L, Luda M P, Trossarelli L, Brach del Prever E M, Crova M and Gallinaro P, 'Oxidation in orthopaedic UHMWPE sterilized by gamma-radiation and ethylene oxide', *Biomaterials*, 1998 **19** 659–668.
96 Kurtz S M, Pruitt L A, Jewett C W, Foulds J R and Edidin A A, 'Radiation and chemical crosslinking promote strain hardening behavior and molecular alignment in ultra high molecular weight polyethylene during multi-axial loading conditions', *Biomaterials*, 1999 **20** 1449–1462.
97 Pascaud R S, Evans W T, McCullagh P J and FitzPatrick D P, 'Influence of gamma-irradiation sterilization and temperature on the fracture toughness of ultra-high-molecular-weight polyethylene', *Biomaterials*, 1997 **18** 727–735.
98 Buchanan F J, Sim B and Downes S, 'Influence of packaging conditions on the properties of gamma-irradiated UHMWPE following accelerated ageing and shelf ageing', *Biomaterials*, 1999 **20** 823–837.
99 Blanchet T A and Burroughs B R, 'Numerical oxidation model for gamma radiation-sterilized UHMWPE consideration of dose–depth profile', *J Biomed Mater Res*, 2001 **58** 684–693.
100 Medel F J, Garcia-Alvarez F, Gomez-Barrena E and Puertolas J A, 'Microstructure changes of extruded UHMWPE after gamma irradiation and shelf-aging', *Polym Degrad Stab*, 2005 **88** 435–443.
101 Ries M D, Weaver K and Beals N, 'Safety and efficacy of ethylene oxide sterilized polyethylene in total knee arthroplasty', *Clin Orthop Relat Res*, 1996 **331** 159–163.
102 Bargmann L S, Bargmann B C, Collier J P, Currier B H and Mayor M B, 'Current sterilization and packaging methods for polyethylene', *Clin Orthop Relat Res*, 1999 **369** 49–58.
103 Collier J P, Sutula L C, Currier B H, Currier J H, Wooding R E, Williams I R, Farber K B and Mayor M B, 'Overview of polyethylene as a bearing material: comparison of sterilization methods', *Clin Orthop Relat Res*, 1996 **333** 76–86.
104 Williams I R, Mayor M B and Collier J P, 'The impact of sterilization method on wear in knee arthroplasty', *Clin Orthop Relat Res*, 1998 **356** 170–180.
105 McKellop H A, Shen F W, Campbell P and Ota T, 'Effect of molecular weight, calcium stearate, and sterilization methods on the wear of ultra high molecular weight polyethylene acetabular cups in a hip joint simulator', *J Orthop Res*, 1999 **17** 329–339.
106 Affatato S, Bordini B, Fagnano C, Taddei P, Tinti A and Toni A, 'Effects of the sterilisation method on the wear of UHMWPE acetabular cups tested in a hip joint simulator', *Biomaterials*, 2002 **23** 1439–1446.
107 Digas G, Thanner J, Nivbrant B, Rohrl S, Strom H and Karrholm J, 'Increase in early polyethylene wear after sterilization with ethylene oxide: radiostereometric analyses of 201 total hips', *Acta Orthop Scand*, 2003 **74** 531–541.

108 Orishimo K F, Hopper R H Jr and Engh C A, 'Long-term *in vivo* wear performance of porous-coated acetabular components sterilized with gamma irradiation in air or ethylene oxide', *J Arthroplasty*, 2003 **18** 546–552.
109 McNulty D E, Liao Y S and Haas B D, 'The influence of sterilization method on wear performance of low contact stress total knee system', *Orthopedics*, 2002 **25**(Suppl) S243–S246.
110 Hopper R H Jr, Young A M, Orishimo K F and Engh C A Jr, 'Effect of terminal sterilization with gas plasma or gamma radiation on wear of polyethylene liners', *J Bone Jt Surg Am*, 2003 **85** 464–468.
111 Oonishi H, Saito M and Kadoya Y, 'Wear of high-dose gamma irradiated polyethylene in total joint replacement – long term radiological evaluation', in *Transactions of the 44th Annual Meeting of the Orthopaedic Research Society*, New Orleans, Louisiana, USA, 1998, Rosemont, Illinois, Orthopaedic Research Society, 1998, 97.
112 Wroblewski B M, Siney P D and Fleming P A, 'Low-friction arthroplasty of the hip using alumina ceramic and cross-linked polyethylene. A ten-year follow-up report', *J Bone Jt Surg Br*, 1999 **81** 54–55.
113 Essner A, Schmidig G, Herrera L, Yau S S, Wang A, Dumbleton J and Manley M, 'Hip wear performance of a next generation crosslinked and annealed polyethylene', in *Transactions of the 51st Annual Meeting of the Orthopaedic Research Society*, Washington, DC, USA, 2005, Rosemont, Illinois, Orthopaedic Research Society, 2005, p. 830.
114 Kurtz S, Mazzucco D, Rimnac C and Schroeder D, 'Anisotropy and oxidative resistance of highly crosslinked UHMWPE after deformation processing by solid-state extrusion', *Biomaterials*, 2006 **27** 24–34.
115 Campbell P, Shen F W and McKellop H, 'Biologic and tribologic considerations of alternative bearing surfaces', *Clin Orthop Relat Res*, 2004 **418** 98–111.
116 Laurent M, Yao J Q, Bhambri S K, Gesll R A, Gilbertson L N, Swarts D F and Crowninshield R D, 'High cycle wear of highly crosslinked UHMWPE acetabular liners evaluated in a hip simulator', in *Transactions of the 46th Annual Meeting of the Orthopaedic Research Society*, Orlando, Florida, USA, 2000, Rosemont, Illinois, Orthopaedic Research Society, 2000, p. 567.
117 Muratoglu O K, Delaney J, O'Connor D O and Harris W H, 'The use of trans-vinylene formation in qualifying the spatial distribution of electron beam penetration in polyethylene. Single-sided, double-sided and shielded irradiation', *Biomaterials*, 2003 **24** 2021–2029.
118 Wang A and Yau S S, 'Melt-quenching vs below-melt annealing consequence on mechanical properties of radiation crosslinked UHMWPE', in *Transactions of the 49th Annual Meeting of the Orthopaedic Research Society*, New Orleans, Louisiana, USA, 2003, Rosemont, Illinois, Orthopaedic Research Society, 2003, p. 1425.
119 Muratoglu O K, Merrill E W, Bragdon C R, O'Connor D, Hoeffel D, Burroughs B, Jasty M and Harris W H, 'Effect of radiation, heat and aging on in vitro wear resistance of polyethylene', *Clin Orthop Relat Res*, 2003 **417** 253–262.
120 Wannomae K K, Christensen S D, Freiberg A A, Bhattacharyya S, Harris W H and Muratoglu O K, 'The effect of real-time aging on the oxidation and wear of highly cross-linked UHMWPE acetabular liners', *Biomaterials*, 2006 **27** 1980–1987.

121 Bhattacharyya S, Doherty A M, Wannomae K, Oral E, Freiberg A A, Harris W H and Muratoglu O, 'Severe *in vivo* oxidation in a limited series of retrieved highly-crosslinked UHMWPE acetabular components with residual free radicals', in *Transactions of the 50th Annual Meeting of the Orthopaedic Research Society*, San Francisco, California, USA, 2004, Rosemont, Illinois, Orthopaedic Research Society, 2004, p. 276.
122 Yau S S, Wang A, Essner A, Manley M and Dumbleton J, 'Sequential irradiation and annealing of highly crosslinked polyethylenes: resist oxidation without sacrificing physical/mechanical properties', in *Transactions of the 51st Annual Meeting of the Orthopaedic Research Society*, Washington, DC, USA, 2005, Rosemont, Illinois, Orthopaedic Research Society, 2005, p. 1670.
123 Essner A, Herrera L, Yau S S, Wang A, Dumbleton J and Manley M, 'Sequentially crollinked and annealed UHMWPE CR knee wear', in *Transactions of the 51st Annual Meeting of the Orthopaedic Research Society*, Washington, DC, USA, 2005, Rosemont, Illinois, Orthopaedic Research Society, 2005, p. 312.
124 Essner A, Herrera L, Yau S S, Wang A, Dumbleton J and Manley M, 'Sequentially crosslinked and annealed UHMWPE knee wear debris', in *Transactions of the 51st Annual Meeting of the Orthopaedic Research Society*, Washington, DC, USA, 2005, Rosemont, Illinois, Orthopaedic Research Society, 2005, p. 71.
125 Collier J P, Currier B H, Kennedy F E, Currier J H, Timmins G S, Jackson S K and Brewer R L, 'Comparison of cross-linked polyethylene materials for orthopaedic applications', *Clin Orthop Relat Res*, 2003 **414** 289–304.
126 Gencur S J, Rimnac C M and Kurtz S M, 'Failure micromechanisms during uniaxial tensile fracture of conventional and highly crosslinked ultra-high molecular weight polyethylenes used in total joint replacements', *Biomaterials*, 2003 **24** 3947–3954.
127 Kurtz S M, Manley M, Wang A, Taylor S and Dumbleton J, 'Comparison of the properties of annealed crosslinked (Crossfire) and conventional polyethylene as hip bearing materials', *Bull Hosp Jt Dis*, 2002 **61** 17–26.
128 Kurtz S M, Hozack W, Turner J, Purtill J, MacDonald D, Sharkey P, Parvizi J, Manley M and Rothman R, 'Mechanical properties of retrieved highly crosslinked crossfire liners after short-term implantation', *J Arthroplasty*, 2005 **20** 840–849.
129 Kurtz S M, Bergstrom J and Rimnac C M, 'Failure property distributions for conventional and highly crosslinked ultrahigh molecular weight polyethylenes', *J Biomed Mater Res Part B: Appl Biomater*, 2005 **73** 214–220.
130 Bergstrom J S, Rimnac C M and Kurtz S M, 'Molecular chain stretch is a multiaxial failure criterion for conventional and highly crosslinked UHMWPE', *J Orthop Res*, 2005 **23** 367–375.
131 Villarraga M L, Kurtz S M, Herr M P and Edidin A A, 'Multiaxial fatigue behavior of conventional and highly crosslinked UHMWPE during cyclic small punch testing', *J Biomed Mater Res Part A*, 2003 **66** 298–309.
132 Muratoglu O K, Mark A, Vittetoe D A, Harris W H and Rubash H E, 'Polyethylene damage in total knees and use of highly crosslinked polyethylene', *J Bone Jt Surg Am*, 2003 **85** S7–S13.

133 Bradford L, Baker D, Ries M D and Pruitt L A, 'Fatigue crack propagation resistance of highly crosslinked polyethylene', *Clin Orthop Relat Res*, 2004 **429** 68–72.
134 Sobieraj M C, Kurtz S M and Rimnac C M, 'Notch strengthening and hardening behavior of conventional and highly crosslinked UHMWPE under applied tensile loading', *Biomaterials*, 2005 **26** 3411–3426.
135 Park K, Mishra S, Lewis G, Losby J, Fan Z and Park J B, 'Quasi-static and dynamic nanoindentation studies on highly crosslinked ultra-high-molecular-weight polyethylene', *Biomaterials*, 2004 **25** 2427–2436.
136 Bragdon C R, Jasty M, Muratoglu O K, O'Connor D O and Harris W H, 'Third-body wear of highly cross-linked polyethylene in a hip simulator', *J Arthroplasty*, 2003 **18** 553–561.
137 Estok D M II, Bragdon C R, Plank G R, Huang A, Muratoglu O K and Harris W H, 'The measurement of creep in ultrahigh molecular weight polyethylene: a comparison of conventional versus highly cross-linked polyethylene', *J Arthroplasty*, 2005 **20** 239–243.
138 Muratoglu O K, Bragdon C R, O'Connor D, Perinchief R S, Estok D M, II, Jasty M and Harris W H, 'Larger diameter femoral heads used in conjunction with a highly cross-linked ultra-high molecular weight polyethylene: a new concept', *J Arthroplasty*, 2001 **16**(Suppl) 24–30.
139 Muratoglu O K, Bragdon C R, Jasty M, O'Connor D O, Von Knoch R S and Harris W H, 'Knee-simulator testing of conventional and cross-linked polyethylene tibial inserts', *J Arthroplasty*, 2004 **19** 887–897.
140 Harris W H and Muratoglu O K, 'A review of current cross-linked polyethylenes used in total joint arthroplasty', *Clin Orthop Relat Res*, 2005 **430** 46–52.
141 Baker D A, Hastings R S and Pruitt L, 'Study of fatigue resistance of chemical and radiation crosslinked medical grade ultrahigh molecular weight polyethylene', *J Biomed Mater Res*, 1999 **46** 573–581.
142 Baker D A, Bellare A and Pruitt L, 'The effects of degree of crosslinking on the fatigue crack initiation and propagation resistance of orthopaedic-grade polyethylene', *J Biomed Mater Res Part A*, 2003 **66** 146–154.
143 Ries M D and Pruitt L, 'Effect of cross-linking on the microstructure and mechanical properties of ultra-high molecular weight polyethylene', *Clin Orthop Relat Res*, 2005 **440** 149–156.
144 Pruitt L A, 'Deformation, yielding, fracture and fatigue behavior of conventional and highly cross-linked ultra high molecular weight polyethylene', *Biomaterials*, 2005 **26** 905–915.
145 Puertolas J A, Medel F J, Cegonino J, Gomez-Barrena E and Rios R, 'Influence of the remelting process on the fatigue behavior of electron beam irradiated UHMWPE', *J Biomed Mater Res Part B: Appl Biomater*, 2006 **76** 346–353.
146 Shen F W and McKellop H, 'Surface-gradient cross-linked polyethylene acetabular cups: oxidation resistance and wear against smooth and rough femoral balls', *Clin Orthop Relat Res*, 2005 **430** 80–88.
147 Oral E, Wannomae K K, Hawkins N, Harris W H and Muratoglu O K, 'Alpha-tocopherol-doped irradiated UHMWPE for high fatigue resistance and low wear', *Biomaterials*, 2004 **25** 5515–5522.
148 Oral E, Wannomae K K, Rowell S L and Muratoglu O K, 'Migration stability of alpha-tocopherol in irradiated UHMWPE', *Biomaterials*, 2006 **27** 3039–3043.

149 Oral E, Greenbaum E S, Malhi A S, Harris W H and Muratoglu O K, 'Characterization of irradiated blends of alpha-tocopherol and UHMWPE', *Biomaterials*, 2005 **26** 6657–6663.
150 Oral E, Christensen S, Malhi A, Wannomae K K and Muratoglu O, 'Wear resistance and mechanical properties of highly crosslinked UHMWPE doped with vitamin E', *J Arthroplasty*, 2006 21 580–591.
151 Shibata N and Tomita N, 'The anti-oxidative properties of alpha-tocopherol in gamma-irradiated UHMWPE with respect to fatigue and oxidation resistance', *Biomaterials*, 2005 **26** 5755–5762.
152 Parth M, Aust N and Lederer K, 'Studies on the effect of electron beam radiation on the molecular structure of UHMWPE under the influence of alpha-tocopherol with respect to its application in medical implants', *J Mater Sci: Mater Med*, 2002 **13** 917–921.
153 Reno F and Cannas M, 'UHMWPE and vitamin E bioactivity: an emerging perspective', *Biomaterials*, 2006 **27** 3039–3043.
154 Reno F, Bracco P, Lombardi F, Boccafoschi F, Costa L and Cannas M, 'The induction of MMP-9 release from granulocytes by vitamin E in UHMWPE', *Biomaterials*, 2004 **25** 995–1001.
155 McKellop H, 'Wear assessment', in *The Adult Hip* (Eds J Callaghan, A Rosenberg and H Rubash), New York, Lippincott–Raven, 1998, pp. 231–246.
156 Gomoll A, Wanich T and Bellare A, '*J*-integral fracture toughness and tearing modulus measurement of radiation crosslinked UHMWPE', *J Orthop Res*, 2002 **20** 1152–1156.
157 Walsh H A, Furman B D, Naab L and Li S, 'Role of oxidation in the clinical fracture of acetabular cups', in *Transactions of the 45th Annual Meeting of the Orthopaedic Research Society*, Anaheim, California, USA, 1999, Rosemont, Illinois, Orthopaedic Research Society, 1999, p. 845.
158 DiMaio W G, Lilly W B, Moore W C and Saum K A, 'Low wear, low oxidation radiation crosslinked UHMWPE', in *Transactions of the 44th Annual Meeting of the Orthopaedic Research Society*, New Orleans, Louisiana, USA, 1998, Rosemont, Illinois, Orthopaedic Research Society, 1998, p. 363.
159 Hopper R H Jr, Young A M, Orishimo K F and McAuley J P, 'Correlation between early and late wear rates in total hip arthroplasty with application to the performance of marathon cross-linked polyethylene liners', *J Arthroplasty*, 2003 **18** 60–67.
160 Heisel C, Silva M, dela Rosa M A and Schmalzried T P, 'Short-term *in vivo* wear of cross-linked polyethylene', *J Bone Jt Surg Am*, 2004 **86** 748–751.
161 Sychterz C J, Engh C A Jr and Engh C A Sr, 'A prospective, randomized clinical study comparing Marathon and Enduron polyethylene acetabular liners: 3 years results', *J Arthroplasty*, 2004 **19** 258–258.
162 Digas G, Karrholm J, Thanner J, Malchau H and Herberts P, 'The Otto Aufranc Award. Highly cross-linked polyethylene in total hip arthroplasty: randomized evaluation of penetration rate in cemented and uncemented sockets using radiostereometric analysis', *Clin Orthop Relat Res*, 2004 **429** 6–16.
163 Bradford L, Kurland R, Sankaran M, Kim H, Pruitt L A and Ries M D, 'Early failure due to osteolysis associated with contemporary highly cross-linked

ultra-high molecular weight polyethylene. A case report', *J Bone Jt Surg Am*, 2004 **86** 1051–1056.

164 Digas G, Karrholm J, Thanner J, Malchau H and Herberts P, 'Highly cross-linked polyethylene in cemented THA: randomized study of 61 hips', *Clin Orthop Relat Res*, **417** 126–138.

165 Dorr L D, Wan Z, Shahrdar C, Sirianni L, Boutary M and Yun A, 'Clinical performance of a Durasul highly cross-linked polyethylene acetabular liner for total hip arthroplasty at five years', *J Bone Jt Surg Am*, 2005 **87** 1816–1821.

166 Martell J M, Verner J J and Incavo S J, 'Clinical performance of a highly cross-linked polyethylene at two years in total hip arthroplasty: a randomized prospective trial', *J Arthroplasty*, 2003 **18** 55–59.

167 D'Antonio J A, Manley M T, Capello W N, Bierbaum B E, Ramakrishnan R, Naughton M and Sutton K, 'Five-year experience with Crossfire® highly cross-linked polyethylene', *Clin Orthop Relat Res*, 2005 **441** 143–150.

168 Della Valle A G, Doty S, Gradl G, Labissiere A and Nestor B J, 'Wear of a highly cross-linked polyethylene liner associated with metallic deposition on a ceramic femoral head', *J Arthroplasty*, 2004 **19** 532–536.

169 Rohrl S, Nivbrant B, Mingguo L and Hewitt B, '*In vivo* wear and migration of highly cross-linked polyethylene cups a radiostereometry analysis study', *J Arthroplasty*, 2005 **20** 409–413.

7
Polymers in biosensors

F DAVIS and S P J HIGSON, Cranfield University, UK

7.1 Introduction

This chapter will be devoted to the incorporation of polymers within biosensors, beginning with a history and descriptions of basic sensor formats, while concentrating on optical and electrochemical sensors. Initially the chapter will discuss the incorporation of polymers as simple coatings for biosensors. These coatings are typically used, firstly, to improve selectivity (by preventing interferents from reaching the active parts of the sensors) and, secondly, to improve the biocompatibility of biosensors. Similar coatings which are used as anchors for biomolecules in various techniques will also be discussed. Following this is a section on polymers that have a more active role. Conducting polymers will be discussed and their structures and use in biosensors will be described. A section follows on redox-active polymers and their use to 'wire' biological moieties to electrodes. Finally, we shall discuss molecularly imprinted polymer (MIPs) and their potential to replace biological molecules as active components within biosensors.

7.2 The development and format of biosensors

A biosensor is a device that measures the presence or concentration of biological molecules, by translating a biochemical interaction at the sensor surface into a quantifiable physical response; this is usually optical or electrochemical in nature. Most sensors consist of three principal components, as described below and detailed in Fig. 7.1.

1 The first of these includes a receptor species, which is usually biological in origin such as an enzyme, antibody or deoxyribonucleic acid (DNA) strand capable of recognising the analyte of interest with a high degree of selectivity; this is usually concurrent with a binding event between a receptor and the analyte. However, receptor species for biological molecules, which are themselves artificial in nature, can also be utilised.

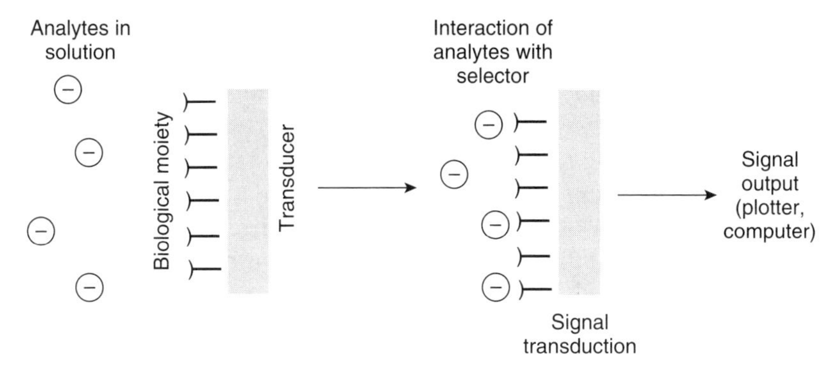

7.1 Schematic diagram of biosensor components.

2 The second component that must be present is a transducer, enabling the translation of the binding event into a measurable physical change; possible events include the generation of electrons, protons, an electrochemically active chemical species such as hydrogen peroxide or simple physical changes such as a change in conductivity, optical absorbance or fluorescence.
3 Thirdly there must be inclusion of a method for measuring the change detected at the transducer and converting this into useful information.

Usually biological molecules are utilised as the active recognition entity within a sensor. These display unsurpassed selectivities. For example, glucose oxidase will interact with glucose and no other sugar, and in this way will act as a highly selective receptor. In the case of glucose oxidase, the electrochemically inactive substrate glucose is oxidised to form gluconolactone together with the concurrent generation of the electroactive species hydrogen peroxide. Enzymes also generally display rapid turnover rates and this is often essential, firstly, to avoid saturation and, secondly, to allow sufficient generation of the active species in order to be detectable.

Antibodies bind solely to their antigens and achieve specificity via a complex series of multiple non-covalent bonds. Since the principle of immunoassays were first published by Yalow and Berson (1959), there has been an exponential growth in both the range of analytes to which the technique has been successfully applied and the number of novel assay designs that have been reported. Development of enzyme-labelled immunoanalytical techniques, e.g. enzyme-linked immunosorbent assay, has provided analytical tests without the safety risks associated with radiolabelling-based techniques.

The rapid measurement of analytes of clinical significance, e.g. towards various disease markers, would permit earlier intervention, which in a medical setting is frequently of utmost importance. There has been much research directed towards the development of direct immunosensors that do not rely on the use of a detectable label. Such a system will lead to simpler assay formats and, ideally, shorter detection times. A reusable and rapid detection system would, moreover, allow for continuous real-time measurement, so helping to maintain optimal homeostatic conditions.

Unfortunately, there are also some disadvantages related to the construction and use of biosensors. Often the biological species can either be extremely expensive or difficult to isolate in sufficient purity. Immobilisation of these species can lead to loss of activity and the presence of various chemical species in the test solution can also cause loss of activity (e.g. enzymes can be easily poisoned by heavy metals). In biological samples such as blood or saliva, there can also be solutes that are electrochemically active and interfere with determinations of the target species. Again, in physiological fluids such as blood, various species may be present which bind to the surface, so causing fouling and loss of sensor response.

A series of extensive reviews on biosensors and their history have been published elsewhere (Hall, 1990; Eggins, 1996; Wang, 2001) and therefore only a brief history will be given here. Easily the most intensively researched area has been towards the development of glucose biosensors (Wang, 2001; Newman *et al.*, 2004). The reason for this is the prevalence of diabetes which has become a worldwide public health problem. The incidence of diabetes is continuing to increase with, at the time of writing, 170 million sufferers diagnosed worldwide (World Health Organisation, www.who.org), with this number being estimated to reach 300 million by 2045 (Newman *et al.*, 2004). Diabetes is related to a number of factors such as obesity and heart disease, all of which make this disease one of the leading causes of death and disability in the world. The world market for biosensors is approximately US $5 billion with approximately 85% of the world commercial market for biosensors currently being for blood glucose monitoring (Newman *et al.*, 2004).

These factors have led to the development of a number of inexpensive disposable electrochemical biosensors for glucose, incorporating glucose oxidase immobilised at various electrodes. They are generally amperometric sensors, with electrodes polarised at a set potential; the oxidation or reduction of a chosen electroactive species at the surface will then lead to generation of a detectable current.

7.3 Polymer membranes in biosensors

Two major problems that can affect the performance of a biosensor are the presence of interferents and also biofouling. Interference from electroactive substances is especially problematic when electrochemical measurements are being made on physiological materials such as blood. For example, glucose sensors can be affected by the presence of species such as ascorbate or acetaminophen (paracetamol), both of which can be oxidised at electrode surfaces. Physiological fluids, especially blood, also have a tendency to deposit materials such as proteins, usually irreversibly, on to solid surfaces. This biofouling process can diminish the response of sensors and in some cases can passivate them completely. This is especially a problem for sensors that we wish to utilise more than once or for sensors that are implanted *in vivo*. A detailed review on enhancing blood compatibility has been recently published elsewhere (Gavalas *et al.*, 2006).

Application of a permselective coating to the sensor can prevent or minimise the access of interfering compounds to the sensor surface, thereby minimising interference from electroactive species. Polymeric materials have led the way, with two of the earliest and most commonly utilised being the fluorinated ionomer Nafion (Turner and Sherwood, 1994) and cellulose acetate (Maines *et al.*, 1997). A beneficial side effect is that these materials can also confer a degree of biocompatibility. The structures of both materials are shown in Fig. 7.2.

Cellulose acetate has been widely utilised as a selective barrier as well as for enhancing biocompatibility within electrochemical sensors (Maines *et al.*, 1997). The cellulose acetate layer permits only small molecules, such as hydrogen peroxide, to reach the electrode, eliminating many

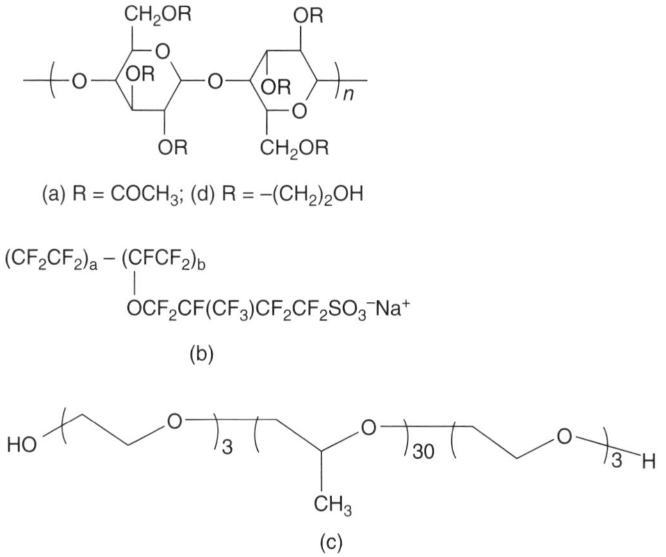

(a) R = $COCH_3$; (d) R = $-(CH_2)_2OH$

$(CF_2CF_2)_a - (CFCF_2)_b$ | $OCF_2CF(CF_3)CF_2CF_2SO_3^-Na^+$

(b)

(c)

7.2 Structures of polymers used within biosensors: (a) cellulose acetate; (b) Nafion; (c) Pluronic-type surfactants; (d) poly(hydroxyethyl methacrylate).

electrochemically active compounds that could interfere with the measurement.

Nafion has also been widely utilised as a coating material, as reviewed here (Wisniewski and Reichart, 2000). The polymer displays the advantages of being chemically inert and easily cast from solution. As shown in Fig. 7.2(b), the polymer is anionic and upon casting forms a structure with hydrophilic channels contained within a hydrophobic matrix. Films formed from this material are reasonably robust, show strong exclusion of anionic interferents and display enhanced biocompatibility (Moussy and Harrison, 1994; Moussy *et al.*, 1994). For example, Nafion-coated electrodes show a much lower rate of signal attenuation when implanted *in vivo* for 2 weeks compared with untreated electrodes (Moussy and Harrison, 1994). Coating a glucose-oxidase-based biosensor with Nafion was found to help to screen out interference from urea and ascorbate (Moussy *et al.*, 1994).

A range of other polymers have also been utilised in the attempted prevention of biofouling as described in the extensive review by Kingschott and Griesser (1999). Some of the most popular materials have been those based on poly(ethylene glycol) (PEG)–poly(ethylene oxide) (PEO) (Kingschott and Grieser, 1999). The reasons why a PEG–PEO surface should resist biofouling so well is a topic for a complete review article in itself; however, it has been widely reported that a very low adsorption of proteins occurs at the surface of these materials (Kingschott and Grieser, 1999). PEG–PEO chains are usually highly solvated in aqueous systems, which means that any incoming protein molecules will experience a surface that is largely composed of water, so mimicking the typical conditions found within biological systems. This is thought to be a major contributor to their biocompatibility.

Simple physical adsorption of Pluronic (Fig. 7.2(c)) surfactants which consist of PEO–poly(propylene oxide) (PPO)–PEO block terpolymers (Green *et al.*, 1998) has been utilised to treat a variety of materials. The PPO section of the chain is more hydrophobic and therefore is absorbed on to the substrate being treated. This leaves the hydrophilic PEO blocks stretching out from the surface into the aqueous phase. The make-up of the surfactant materials affects their biocompatibilities. For example, increasing the length of the PPO section leads to enhanced protein repulsion compared with increasing the length of the PEO section. Possibly only short PEO chains are necessary for effective protein repulsion, and increasing the PPO section leads to better anchoring of the surfactant, thereby preventing either leaching of the coating into the aqueous phase or displacement by protein molecules (Green *et al.*, 1998).

Hydrogels have also been investigated as coatings for use within sensors. A hydrogel is usually based on polymers such as poly(vinyl alcohol) or poly(acrylic acid), which would normally be soluble in water but, either during or after the polymer synthesis, the linear polymer chains become cross-linked into a polymer network. The resultant network has a high affinity for water but does not dissolve, but rather it is capable of adsorbing water with consequent swelling of the polymer matrix. Because of their high water content, hydrogels often show high biocompatibility. Typical materials involve cross-linked PEO or poly(hydroxyethyl methacrylate) (PHEMA) (Fig. 7.2(d)). They are attractive materials not only because of their biocompatibility but also because water-soluble analytes are capable of diffusing quickly through the water-swollen polymer. The swelling behaviour can be easily controlled by the amount of cross-linking; a network with few cross-links will adsorb large amounts of water with a high degree of swelling. Less hydrophilic monomers, incorporation of hydrophobic comonomers or a high degree of cross-linking all act to reduce water adsorption, usually leading to a firmer, more rigid gel.

Hydrogels have been shown to act as stabilising layers when applied to sensors. For example, cross-linked PEO has been used to stabilise an implanted glucose sensor (Csoeregi *et al.*, 1994). A more widely utilised application for hydrogels, however, has been as enzyme-stabilising agents. Enzymes can often denature and lose their efficiency; however, this effect can be mitigated by encapsulating it inside a hydrogel. A swollen hydrogel of high water content mimics an aqueous environment and helps to prevent denaturing. For example, glucose oxidase could be incorporated within a cross-linked PHEMA membrane and enabled formation of a glucose sensor which only showed a 20% loss in activity after continuous operation for 3 months (Doretti *et al.*, 1996). Other polymers have also been utilised (Gibson and Woodward, 1992; Gibson *et al.*, 1992). For example, a variety of enzymes have been stabilised using cationic polymers such as diethyl-amino-modified dextran. Alcohol oxidase retained 100% of its efficiency after 2 months at 37 °C when stabilisers were utilised (Gibson *et al.*, 1992).

Other polymers have also been studied as biocompatible agents. A study of protein deposition on membranes made from poly(vinyl chloride), polyurethane and silicone-rubber-based materials, for utilisation in solid-state ion sensors (Cha *et al.*, 1991), found that polyurethane and silicone-based membranes exhibited less protein adsorption following exposure to blood. More recent research utilises silicone-modified polyurethanes and showed enhanced biocompatibility compared with polyurethane and poly(vinyl chloride) (Berrocal *et al.*, 2001). The modification of poly(vinyl chloride) membranes with anionic surfactants also improves biocompatibility and has been utilised in the development of amperometric enzyme electrodes (Reddy and Vadgama, 1997).

Cell membranes consist mainly of phospholipids and therefore attempts have been made to synthesise polymers that contain phospholipid-type

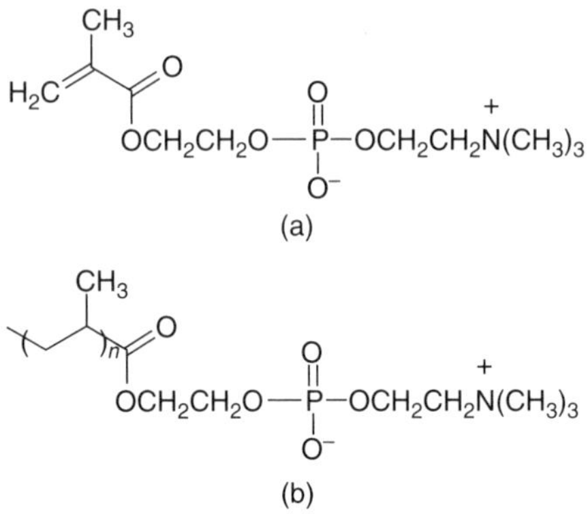

7.3 Structure of methacroyl phosphoryl choline: (a) monomer; (b) polymer.

head groups. Polymers, for example, based on the phospholipid polar group, such as 2-methacryloyloxyethyl phosphorylcholine (Fig. 7.3(a)), copolymerised with other methacrylate monomers, have been pioneered by Ueda *et al.* (1992). By correct selection of the monomers, materials were formulated and found to minimise adsorption of blood proteins greatly on to surfaces. Poly(2-methacroylethyl phosphorylcholine) (Fig. 7.3(b)) could be plasma deposited on to silicone rubber and the adhesion of albumin was found to be minimised by factors of up to 80 (Hsuie *et al.*, 1998). These materials have been successfully applied to the outer membranes of ion-selective electrodes (Berrocal *et al.*, 2002; Yajima *et al.*, 2002) and show enhanced biocompatibility. Glucose biosensors also showed enhanced *in vivo* lifetimes compared with unmodified sensors (Ishihara *et al.*, 1998) with a subcutaneously implanted probe showing lifetimes of up to 14 days. Other 'natural' species can also be grafted on to polymer films; for instance, heparin is found on the inside of vascular walls and can be grafted on to poly(vinyl alcohol)-based coatings (Brinkman *et al.*, 1991).

An alternative approach has been to electropolymerise suitable monomers to form protective coatings. 1,2-Diaminobenzene (Myler *et al.*, 1997), for example, when deposited at the bioelectrode surface, serves both to stabilise the electrode due to its inherent high biocompatibility and also to impart selective exclusion of interferents such as ascorbate. Similar results were also obtained using polypyrrole (Vidal *et al.*, 1999).

Plasma polymers have been the subject of recent interest. Basically, many chemical species if irradiated in a glow discharge or radiofrequency device will form a reactive plasma and deposit as a polymer on almost any surface (Muguruma and Karube, 1999). One advantage of this method is that it will often give pinhole-free, highly cross-linked films which are extremely even over substrates of almost any shape. There has been some work on utilising these materials in biosensors. Ethylenediamine was plasma polymerised on to a quartz crystal microbalance (QCM) chip to give a polymer surface that was very suitable for immobilisation of antibodies (Nakanishi *et al.*, 1995). Plasma polymers are also especially suitable for use in microfluidic type devices because of their deposition even over complex shapes (Hiratsuka *et al.*, 2004). Deposition on to surface plasmon resonance (SPR) chips has also been studied (Mugurama *et al.*, 2000).

This process has also been utilised for the development of immunosensors. For example, butylamine plasma polymer films have been utilised for the electrostatic adsorption of anticeruloplasmin antibody (Wang *et al.*, 2004). This system gave immunosensors capable of detecting 0.15 μg/ml of antigen.

7.4 Polymer coatings for biosensors

Coatings have also been used elsewhere in the biosensing world. The two examples given below are commercial variations on the theme of sensors, although they tend to be used more as research tools rather than as widespread applications.

SPR is a technique widely used for probing immunological interactions. Commercial SPR systems are widely available with Biacore AB being the major systems provider at the time of writing (Karlsson, 2004). SPR is a method that combines optical and electrochemical phenomena at a metal surface and is capable of measuring real-time label-free biomolecular interactions. The nature of the surface of the SPR chip can affect the nature of any interactions. Polymer coatings are often utilised, usually to minimise non-specific interactions. Most commercial chips are coated with carboxymethylated dextran or substituted variants (Karlsson, 2004).

One of the major biotechnology success stories of recent times has been the sequencing of the human genome. The detection of specific DNA sequences has been a major issue in the field of biological sciences for many years. Early methods were intensively laborious, expensive and time consuming and have now been superseded by the appearance of DNA arrays, permitting multiple-sequence detection with high specificity and rapid response times. DNA microarrays are constructed by spotting a variety of known oligonucleotides on to precisely defined locations on a solid substrate, usually a glass microscope slide. Immobilisation of the DNA is often electrostatic, usually by means of a cationic polymer such as polylysine. A wide variety of precoated slides are now commercially available.

7.5 Conducting polymers in biosensors

Conducting polymers are especially suitable for immobilisation of enzymes at electrode surfaces and this process has been reviewed in detail elsewhere

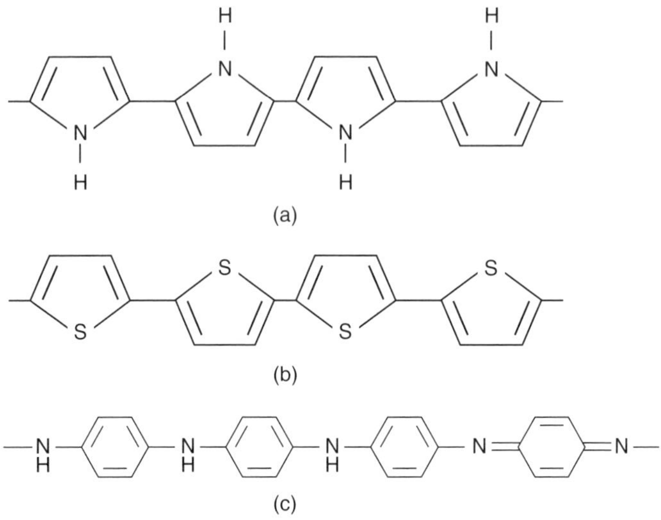

(a)

(b)

(c)

7.4 Structures of conducting polymers: (a) polypyrrole; (b) polythiophene; (c) polyaniline.

(Barisci *et al.*, 1996; Gerard *et al.*, 2002). A variety of monomers can be electropolymerised on an electrode surface and under correct conditions form stable conductive films. Typical conductive polymers include polyaniline, polypyrrole and polythiophenes (Fig. 7.4). Polymers of these types generally contain a highly conjugated backbone and display properties such as electrical conductivity, low-energy optical transitions and a high affinity for electrons. If, during the electrochemical polymerisation process, biological molecules are present in the solution, they can be entrapped within the film during the deposition process (Cosnier, 2003; Geetha *et al.*, 2006). Alternatively, a polymeric film can be deposited electrochemically and then the biological species can be adsorbed on to, or be chemically grafted to, the film (Barisci *et al.*, 1996; Gerard *et al.*, 2002). This leads to a close association between the conductive polymer and the biomolecule, which could potentially facilitate rapid electron transfer between the active species and an electrode surface. Alternatively, should the active species interact in some way with the environment, this could lead to a change in the properties of the conductive film. For example, if an antibody is included in the film and binds its antigen, the resultant conformational changes could affect the film. This then may lead to a measurable change in its electrochemical or optical properties. Therefore, the conductive polymer can be thought in some way to be acting as the transducer element within the biosensor (Fig. 7.1).

One of the simplest methods involves the entrapment of enzymes such as glucose oxidase within polyaniline films (Cooper and Hall, 1992). Aniline was electrochemically polymerised from a solution containing glucose oxidase (3 mg/ml) on to platinum electrodes. Exposure of these electrodes to glucose solution led to the formation of hydrogen peroxide, which could be measured electrochemically. The advantages of this method is that it allows the controlled deposition of biological molecules on to electrodes of just about any size and composition. Further work utilising this system (Skinner and Hall, 1997) utilised an alternating-current (AC) impedance detection technique and showed that not only could the hydrogen peroxide produced by oxidation of glucose be detected but also even in anaerobic conditions the presence of glucose could be detected by the enzyme electrode.

A variety of electrodeposited polymers have been studied as hosts for enzymes (Cosnier, 2003; Geetha *et al.*, 2006). Polyaniline has been used as a host for, amongst others, enzymes such as glucose oxidase (Ramanathan *et al.*, 1995), lactate dehydrogenease (Chaubey *et al.*, 2000) and horseradish peroxidase (Yang and Mu, 1997). Polypyrrole is also a popular material since, like polyaniline, it can be deposited in a variety of oxidation states as well as charged or uncharged, conducting or insulating forms. For example, urease or glutamate dehydrogenase were co-deposited with polypyrrole or physically adsorbed on to preformed films (Gambhir *et al.*, 2002). Polypyrrole films have also been used as hosts for cholesterol oxidase for use as cholesterol biosensors (Kajiya *et al.*, 1991; Kumar *et al.*, 2001; Vidal *et al.*, 2004).

Cholesterol biosensors have also been constructed using polyaniline (Wang and Mu, 1999; Singh *et al.*, 2006). Pyruvate oxidase has been incorporated within a copolymer of a modified pyrrole monomer with thiophene and used to detect pyruvate (Gajovic *et al.*, 1999). A platinum microelectrode was used as the substrate for deposition of polypyrrole containing a three-enzyme mixture (xanthine oxidase, purine nucleoside phosphorylase and adenosine deaminase), with the resultant sensor being capable of detecting adenosine at concentrations down to 100 nM (Llaudet *et al.*, 2003).

Our group has taken this process further, utilising both non-conductive and conductive polymers to fabricate arrays of conductive microelectrodes with entrapped biological molecules such as glucose oxidase (Barton *et al.*, 2004). Basically an insulating film of polydiaminobenzene is electrochemically deposited on an electrode and then sonochemically ablated to create an array of pores. Conductive polyaniline containing enzymes is then deposited within the pores as shown schematically in Fig. 7.5(a), Fig. 7.5(b) and Fig. 7.5(c). Scanning electron microscopy clearly demonstrates formation of pores within the film and mushroom-like protrusions of polyaniline (Fig. 7.5(d) and Fig. 7.5(e)). This technique has been used to develop sensors for pesticides based on acetylcholineesterase immobilised within polyaniline.

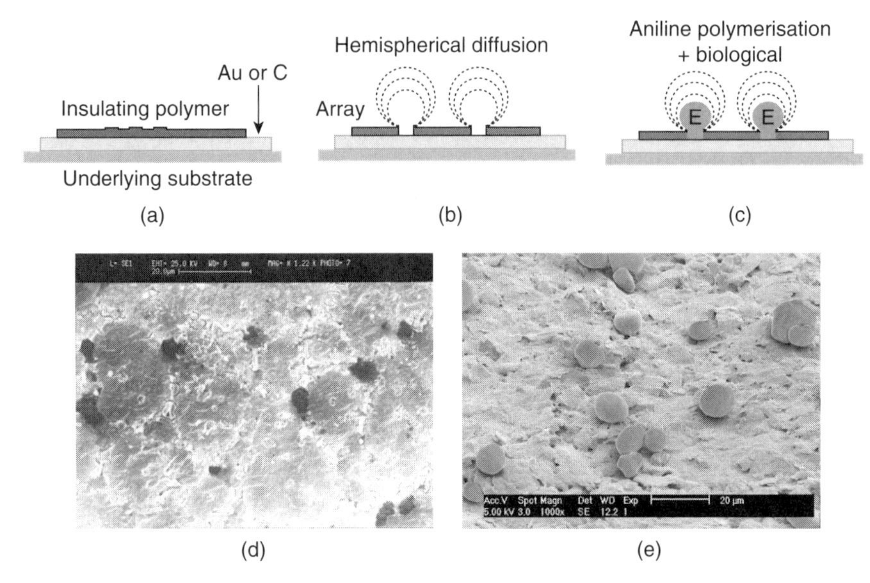

7.5 (a) Deposition of an insulating layer; (b) sonochemical formation of pores; (c) polymerisation of aniline; (d) scanning electron micrograph of pores; (e) scanning electron micrograph of polyaniline 'mushroom' protrusions.

These sensors allowed determination of pesticide concentrations as low as 10^{-17} M (Pritchard *et al.*, 2004; Law and Higson, 2005).

Enzymes are not the only biomolecules that can be immobilised within electrodeposited films. There has been a sustained effort into the development of conducting polymer-based immunosensors as recently reviewed by Cosnier (2005). A wide variety of biomolecules that have been attached to or co-deposited with conducting polymers have been detailed in other reviews (Cosnier, 2003; Geetha *et al.*, 2006), a few of which will be described here.

One of the earliest uses of these techniques was for the entrapment of antihuman serum albumin (anti-HSA) within polypyrrole (John *et al.*, 1991). The resultant films were studied by AC voltammetry and shown to respond to the presence of HSA. Polypyrrole containing cyano groups could be electrodeposited and the resultant films utilised for the electrostatic binding of anti-rabbit immunoglobulin IgG (Ouerghi *et al.*, 2001) with the heavy chains of the antibodies being preferentially bound to the film, thereby orienting the antibody on the surface. The resultant films when studied by AC impedance were found to be capable of detecting rabbit IgG at levels of 10 ng/ml. Polypyrrole could also be used as the host for anti-HSA and when interrogated with pulsed electrometry could detect HSA at levels of 25 pg/ml (Sargent *et al.*, 1990). Antibodies for bovine serum albumin (BSA) and digoxin could also be incorporated into polypyrrole (Grant *et al.*, 2003). Moreover, the use of radiolabelled antibodies allowed accurate quantification of the levels of antibody incorporation within the films and also the optimum method for antibody incorporation to be determined. Similar films containing anti-BSA when combined with AC impedance measurements could detect the antigen with a linear response from 0 to 75 ppm (Grant *et al.*, 2005).

An alternative method involved depositing biotin-functionalised polypyrrole and then utilising the strong biotin–avidin to deposit first a layer of avidin followed by a layer of biotinylated antihuman IgG (Ouerghi *et al.*, 2002). Many other groups have also utilised the biotin–avidin interaction for binding biomolecules to conducting polymers (Cosnier, 2005). Electrostatic interactions have also been utilised since often conductive polymers are charged. Antibodies for species such as digoxin and hepatitis B have been deposited on polypyrrole (Purvis *et al.*, 2003), leading to development of a potentiometric biosensor with detection limits down to picogram per millilitre levels and good stability. Many conducting polymer films can also be generated which contain reactive species such as *n*-hydroxysuccinimide, which can then react with groups such as amines (contained within many enzymes and antibodies), thereby covalently immobilising them on the polymer surface (Cosnier, 2005).

Oligonucleotides have also been widely investigated in conjunction with conducting polymer films (Davis and Higson, 2005). Early approaches used simple adsorption of oligonucleotides on to polypyrrole (Minehan *et al.*, 1994). This was later found to be highly dependent on the oxidation state and therefore the number of positive charges that are available within the polypyrrole film (Minehan *et al.*, 2001). Co-deposition of DNA strands with conducting polymers has also been widely utilised. For example, short single-stranded oligonucleotides could be incorporated within polypyrrole (Wang *et al.*, 1999) to allow the electrochemical detection of their counterstrands. Polyaniline and polydiaminobenzene have also been successfully utilised as hosts for DNA (Davis *et al.*, 2004). When polypyrrole and a single-stranded oligonucleotide were co-deposited on to carbon-nanotube-modified electrodes, the resultant biosensor could detect 10^{-6} mol/l of the counterstrand and was also found to be capable of differentiating between the counterstrands and other oligonucleotides with one, two and three base mismatches (Cai *et al.*, 2003). Other methods such as use of the avidin–biotin pair and chemical grafting have also been utilised to attach oligonucleotides to conducting polymers (Cosnier, 2005).

The majority of the sensors constructed using conductive polymers are electrochemical in nature; however, some alternative methods have been utilised. Various oligonucleotides were synthesised with a pyrrole unit on one end. These were then electropolymerised as copolymers with pyrrole on to individual gold microelectrodes of a 128-electrode array (Livache *et al.*, 1998). Detection of a DNA target could then be determined by fluorescence measurements. Other work involved taking an indium–tin-oxide-coated optical fibre and electrochemically depositing a biotin-substituted polypyrrole layer (Konry *et al.*, 2003). This layer was then used to attach first avidin and then biotinylated cholera toxin. The resultant sensor was capable of detecting anticholera toxin antibodies using a luminol-based assay, with negligible response to other antibodies. Similarly, a pyrrole–benzophenone copolymer was electrodeposited on optical fibres and the HCV-E2 envelope protein antigen immobilised photochemically (Konry *et al.*, 2005) to generate an optical biosensor capable of selectively detecting anti-E2 antibodies.

7.6 Redox-active polymers in biosensors

The earliest electrochemical glucose biosensors relied on detection of either oxygen (Clark and Lyons, 1962) or hydrogen peroxide at an electrode surface. Unfortunately, this leads to the possibilities of interference by electroactive species such as ascorbate. Also, the active site of the enzyme may be insulated from the electrode by the surrounding protein shell. These problems can be circumvented by utilising an artificial electron charge transfer moiety known as a mediator. Use of mediators lead to the development of so-called 'second-generation biosensors' with a typical example being shown in Fig. 7.6 where a ferrocene compound is utilised to 'shuttle' electrons between the enzyme and the electrode (Cass *et al.*, 1984). As an alternative to the use of mediators, it has been proposed that a suitable polymer could 'wire' the enzyme to the electrode. Conducting polymers have been utilised for this purpose, although another possible method that has been studied utilises a polymer that does not conduct electrons along the polymer backbone but rather shuttles electrons between electroactive groups bound along the polymer chain.

One of the earliest proposed methods was that of Heller in 1990 who suggested the use of a composite material containing polypyridine and

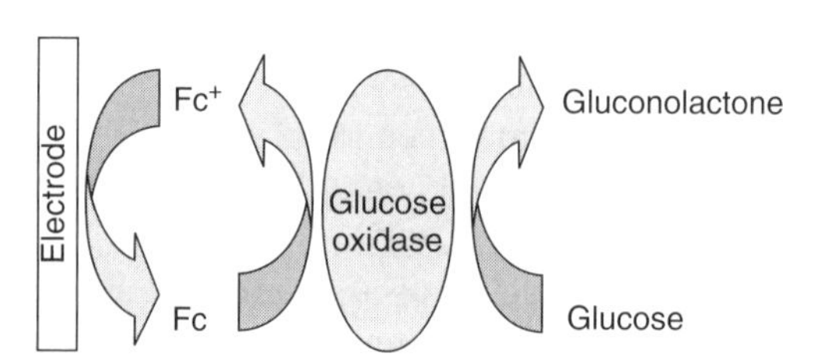

7.6 The oxidation of glucose at an electrode, mediated by a ferrocene derivative (Fc).

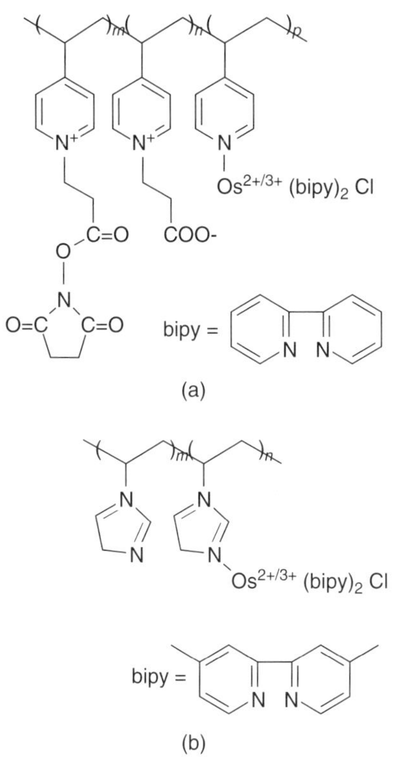

7.7 Structures of redox active polymers based on osmium bipyridyl complexes substituted on to (a) poly(vinyl pyridine) and (b) poly(vinyl imidazole).

osmium 2,2-bipyridine (Fig. 7.7(a)). The resultant substituted polymer was deposited at an electrode surface as an electrostatic complex with glucose oxidase and shown to respond to glucose in the physiological range. Polymers of a similar type containing reactive groups such as succinimide were used to immobilise enzymes covalently (Heller, 1990). This gave rise to the construction of films of up to 1 μm thickness, which gave a strong electrochemical response to glucose. Similar polymers were used to immobilise horseradish peroxidase on glassy carbon for the measurement of hydrogen peroxide at much lower potentials than normally required (Yang *et al.*, 1995). Pyruvate sensors have also been constructed using these systems (Gajovic *et al.*, 1999).

An alternative system was developed based on osmium-modified polyvinyl imidazole (Fig. 7.7(b)) which, when mixed with a polyethylene glycol-based cross-linker, could be used to immobilise glucose or lactase oxidase on to electrodes. Again, this led to the formation of sensors for their respective substrates (Ohara *et al.*, 1994). The performance of these sensors could be improved by adding a second polymer, Nafion, and allowed constructions of sensors with linear ranges of 6–30 mM (glucose) and 4–7 mM (lactate). In both cases, only a negligible response to common interferents was observed (Ohara *et al.*, 1994). Similar polymers were used to immobilise glutamate oxidase and horseradish peroxidase and, in conjunction with a high-performance liquid chromatography technique, were used to determine levels of the neurotoxin *N*-oxalyl-diamino propionic acid (Belay *et al.*, 1997). Using oligosaccaride dehydrogenase as the enzyme, electrodes capable of detecting a range of sugars and saccarides were developed (Tessema *et al.*, 1997).

This technique is highly versatile, where the behaviour of the polymers can be fine tuned by variation in their substituents. For example, using a layered enzyme electrode where both glucose oxidase and bilirubin oxidase are 'wired' by polyvinyl pyridine–osmium polymers to a glassy carbon electrode, concentrations of glucose as low as 2 fM were detected in the presence of atmospheric oxygen (Mano and Heller, 2005). In a similar way, single-stranded DNA was complexed with a redox polymer and bound at an electrode surface. Hybridisation of this strand with a probe DNA, which then had horseradish peroxidase attached, allowed detection of DNA down to levels of just 3000 copies (Zhang *et al.*, 2003).

Hydrogels containing redox-active groups could be generated by the photochemically initiated polymerisation of poly(ethylene glycol dimethacrylate) and vinyl ferrocene. These materials were utilised to immobilise glucose oxidase on gold electrodes (Sirkar and Pishko, 1998) with the resulting glucose sensors showing good linearity between 2 and 20 mM. It was also possible to produce patterned sensors using these materials and photolithographic techniques. Vinyl ferrocene could also be plasma polymerised on to a needle-type electrode to give a redox layer on to which further plasma processes could be used to deposit acetonitrile to give a hydrophilic surface, suitable for the immobilisation of glucose oxidase and construction of a glucose sensor (Hiratsuka *et al.*, 2005).

7.7 Molecularly imprinted polymers in biosensors

The use of biological molecules within sensors can lead to problems. The molecules can be difficult to purify, can be expensive and often display limited stability. One possibility to try to address this problem is to make artificial systems that mimic the behaviour of biologicals such as enzymes or antibodies. MIPs represent a possibly solution (Whitcombe and Vulfson, 2001; Hillberg *et al.*, 2005; Alexander *et al.*, 2006). Basically, a template molecule, which can be biological in nature, is mixed in solution with a variety of polymerisable monomers, some of which will interact with it. The monomers are then polymerised and cross-linked to create a network with

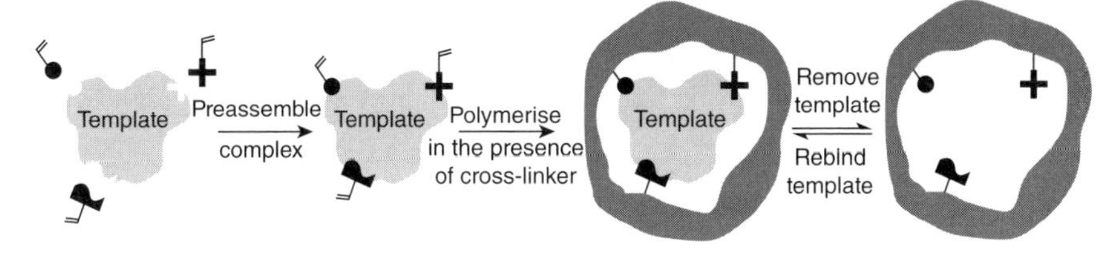

7.8 Schematic representation of the imprinting process. A template is complexed, either covalently or non-covalently with functional monomers. The complex is polymerised with an excess of cross-linker to form a rigid porous shell around the template. Removal of the template creates a recognition site or cavity capable of reversibly rebinding the template. (Reproduced with permission from Whitcombe and Vulfson (2001) and Wiley–VCH.)

the template complexed within it. If the template is then washed out, a 'pocket' remains and this could then potentially selectively entrap more template molecule. This is summarised in Fig. 7.8.

Although sensors which contain MIPs are not biosensors in the classical sense, i.e. there is no biological molecule contained within the polymer, they can be synthesised containing recognition sites for biological molecules by using a biological template, although not as selectively as their biological counterparts. MIPs have shown some promise as sensors for biological molecules. For example, an inorganic polymer film containing glucose was deposited on a QCM by a sol–gel process. If the template is removed, this allowed the resultant film to act as a sensor, giving a change in mass when exposed to aqueous glucose (Lee and Kunitake, 2001). Vanillylmandelic acid, which can be a marker for some tumours, was incorporated as a template into a cross-linked methacrylic acid polymer film, cast on an electrode (Blanco-Lopez *et al.*, 2003) and washed. Voltametric measurements were then made on the system when immersed into solutions of vanillylmandelic acid. The resultant sensor was capable of detecting the analyte at concentrations between 1×10^{-4} and 1.7×10^{-3} M. Later work refined this to permit a linear response between 5×10^{-8} and 1×10^{-5} M (Dineiro *et al.*, 2005). An amperometric detector for fructosylamine utilising a poly(vinyl imidazole)-based MIP has also been described (Sode *et al.*, 2003).

Electrochemically generated polymers have also been used and, if deposited in the presence of a template which is later removed, have allowed the resultant film to detect a target analyte. For example, poly(*o*-phenylene diamine) could be electrochemically deposited from a glucose solutions on to a QCM chip. When washed, the resultant chip showed a sensitivity for glucose (Malitesta *et al.*, 1999). Also sensors for atropine (with a linear range between 8×10^{-6} and 4×10^{-3} M (Peng *et al.*, 2000)) and sorbitol (which is thought to cause complications for diabetes patients (Feng *et al.*, 2004)) have been developed, both being based on poly(*o*-phenylene diamine). The sorbitol sensor had a range 0–16 mM and was selective with respect to other sugars.

An interesting development of this technology is that MIPs have been used to sense cells as well as molecules. Coating a QCM with a cross-linked polymer into which yeast cells had been impressed gave a selective sensor for yeast over other bacterial strains (Dickert and Hayden, 2002). Sensors for enzymes and viruses could also be obtained by this method (Hayden *et al.*, 2003) and could be applied successfully to the detection of viruses in tobacco plant sap (Dickert *et al.*, 2004).

7.8 Summary and future trends

We have, within this chapter, surveyed some of the applications of polymers in biosensors. It is obvious that this is a field which will command much interest over the years to come. The versatility of polymers available, conductive or insulating, hydrophobic or hydrophilic, rigid or flexible and impervious to water or swellable gives rise to a wide range of potential applications. This is aided by their processability, the wide range of synthetic and deposition methods and the ability to fine-tune their properties by changes in the chemical and physical structures of the polymers.

The most relevant fields for polymer research in the future in the field of biosensors, we feel, are those focused towards designing 'smart' polymers. We have seen attempts to replace the biological components of biosensors with MIPs, which has the potential for eliminating the problems of stability and supply of biological molecules. The use of conducting polymers will also be of great interest, whether of the conjugated type, e.g. polypyrrole, or the redox hydrogel polymers developed by Heller and others, to 'wire' biomolecules directly to the electrode.

Finally, the vast majority of these biosensors will be required to deal with physiological samples such as blood or potentially to be implanted as functional components within *in vivo* devices. It is obvious that such sensors, unless they are designed for single use only, must show biocompatibility and stability over extended periods of time.

7.9 Sources of further information and advice

Cooper J and Cass A E G (2004), *Biosensors (The Practical Approach Series)*, Oxford, Oxford University Press.

Eggins B R (2002), *Chemical Sensors and Biosensors (Analytical Techniques in the Sciences)*, Chichester, West Sussex, Wiley.

Yan M and Ranstrom O (2004), *Molecularly Imprinted Materials: Science and Technology*, London, Taylor & Francis.

7.10 References

Alexander C, Andersson H S, Andersson L I, Ansell R J, Kirsch N, Nicholls I A, O'Mahony J and Whitcombe M J (2006), 'Molecular imprinting science and technology: a survey of the literature for the years up to and including 2003', *J Mol Recognit*, **19** 106–180.

Barisci J N, Conn C and Wallace G G (1996), 'Conducting polymer sensors', *Trends Polym Sci*, **4** 301–311.

Barton A C, Collyer S D, Davis F, Gornall D D, Law K A, Lawrence E C D, Mills D W, Myler S, Pritchard J A, Thompson M and Higson S P J (2004), 'Sonochemically fabricated microelectrode arrays for biosensors offering widespread applicability Part I', *Biosens Bioelection*, **20** 328–337.

Belay A, Ruzgas T, Csöregi E, Moges G, Tessema M, Solomon T and Gorton L (1997), 'LC-biosensor system for the determination of the neurotoxin-*N*-oxalyl-L-diaminopropionic acid', *Anal Chem*, **69** 3471–3475.

Berrocal M J, Badr I H A, Gao D and Bachas L G (2001), 'Reducing the thrombogenicity of ion-selective electrode membranes through the use of a silicone-modified segmented polyurethane', *Anal Chem*, **73** 5328–5333.

Berrocal M J, Johnson R D, Badr I H A, Liu M, Gao D and Bachas L G (2002), 'Improving the blood compatibility of ion-selective electrodes by employing poly(MPC-co-BMA), a copolymer containing phosphorylcholine, as a membrane coating', *Anal Chem*, **74** 3644–3648.

Blanco-Lopez M C, Lobo-Castanon M J, Miranda-Ordieres A J and Tunon-Blanco P (2003), 'Voltammetric sensor for vanillylmandelic acid based on molecularly imprinted polymer-modified electrodes', *Biosens Bioelection*, **18** 353–362.

Brinkman E, van der Does L and Bantjes A (1991), 'Poly(vinyl alcohol)–heparin hydrogels as sensor catheter membranes', *Biomaterials*, **12** 63–70.

Cai H, Xu Y, He P G and Fang Y Z (2003), 'Indicator free DNA hybridization detection by impedance measurement based on the DNA-doped conducting polymer film formed on the carbon nanotube modified electrode', *Electroanalysis*, **15** 1864–1870.

Cass A E G, Davis G, Francis G D, Hill A O, Aston W J, Higgins I J, Plotkin E V, Scott L D L and Turner A P F (1984), 'Ferrocene-mediated enzyme electrode for amperometric determination of glucose', *Anal Chem*, **56** 667–671.

Cha G S, Liu D, Meyerhoff M E, Cantor H C, Midgley A R, Goldberg H D and Brown R B (1991), 'Electrochemical performance, biocompatibility and adhesion of new polymer matrixes for solid-state ion sensors', *Anal Chem*, **63** 1666–1672.

Chaubey A, Pande K K, Singh V S and Malholtra B D (2000), 'Co-immobilisation of lactate oxidase and lactate dehydrogenase on conducting polyaniline films', *Anal Chim Acta*, **407** 97–103.

Clark L and Lyons C (1962), 'Electrode systems for continuous monitoring in cardiovascular surgery', *Ann NY Acad Sci*, **102** 29–45.

Cooper J C and Hall E A H (1992), 'Electrochemical response of an enzyme-loaded polyaniline film', *Biosens Bioelection*, **7** 473–485.

Cosnier S (2003), 'Biomolecule immobilization on electrode surfaces by entrapment or attachment to electrochemically polymerized films. A review', *Biosens Bioelection*, **14** 443–456.

Cosnier S (2005), 'Affinity biosensors based on electropolymerized films', *Electroanalysis*, **17** 1701–1715.

Csoeregi E, Quinn C P, Schmidtke D W, Lindquist S E, Pishko M V, Ye L, Katakis I, Hubbell J A and Heller A (1994), 'Design, characterization, and one-point *in vivo* calibration of a subcutaneously implanted glucose electrode', *Anal Chem*, **66** 3131–3138.

Davis F and Higson S P J (2005), 'Structured thin films as components in biosensors', *Biosens Bioelection*, **21** 1–20.

Davis F, Nabok A V and Higson S P J (2004), 'Species differentiation by DNA-modified carbon electrodes using an AC impedimetric approach', *Biosens Bioelection*, **20** 1531–1538.

Dickert F L and Hayden O (2002), 'Bioimprinting of polymers and sol–gel phases. Selective detection of yeasts with imprinted polymers', *Anal Chem*, **74** 1302–1306.

Dickert F L, Hayden O, Bindeus R, Mann K J, Blaas D and Waigmann E (2004), 'Bioimprinted QCM sensors for virus detection – screening of plant sap', *Anal Bioanal Chem*, **378** 1929–1934.

Dineiro Y, Menendez M I, Blanco-Lopez M C, Lobo-Castanon M J, Miranda-Ordieres A J and Tunon-Blanco P (2005), 'Computational approach to the rational design of molecularly imprinted polymers for voltammetric sensing of homovanillic acid', *Anal Chem*, **77** 6471–6476.

Doretti L, Ferrara D, Gattolin P and Lora S (1996), 'Covalently immobilized enzymes on biocompatible polymers for amperometric sensor applications', *Biosens Bioelection*, **11** 365–373.

Eggins B R (1996), *Biosensors*, Chichester, West Sussex, Wiley.

Feng L, Liu Y, Tan Y and Hu J (2004), 'Biosensor for the determination of sorbitol based on molecularly imprinted electro synthesized polymers', *Biosens Bioelection*, **19** 1513–1519.

Gajovic N, Habermuller K, Warsinke A, Schuhmann W and Scheller F W (1999), 'A pyruvate oxidase electrode based on an electrochemically deposited redox polymer', *Electroanalysis*, **11** 1377–1383.

Gambhir A, Gerard M, Mulchandani A K and Malhotra B D (2002), 'Coimmobilization of urease and glutamate dehydrogenase in electrochemically prepared polypyrrole–polyvinyl sulfonate films', *Appl Biochem Biotechnol*, **96** 249–257.

Gavalas Y G, Berrocal M J and Bachas L G (2006), 'Enhancing the blood compatibility of ion-selective electrodes', *Anal Bioanal Chem*, **384** 65–72.

Geetha S, Rao C R K, Vijayan M and Trivedi D C (2006), 'Biosensing and drug delivery by polypyrrole', *Anal Chim Acta*, **568** 119–125.

Gerard M, Chaubey A and Malhotra B D (2002), 'Application of conducting polymers to biosensors', *Biosens Bioelection*, **17** 345–359.

Gibson T D, Higgins I J and Woodward J R (1992), 'Stabilization of analytical enzymes using a novel polymer–carbohydrate system and the production of a stabilized, single reagent for alcohol analysis', *Analyst*, **117** 1293–1297.

Gibson T D and Woodward J R (1992), 'Protein stabilization in biosensors systems', in *Biosensors and Chemical Sensors* (Eds P G Edelman and J Wang), Washington, DC, American Chemical Society, pp. 40–55.

Grant S, Davis F, Law K A, Barton A C, Collyer S D, Higson S P J and Gibson T D (2005), 'Label-free and reversible immunosensor based upon an AC impedance interrogation protocol', *Anal Chim Acta*, **537** 163–168.

Grant S, Davis F, Pritchard J A, Law K A, Higson S P J and Gibson T D (2003), 'Labeless and reversible immunosensor assay based upon an electrochemical current-transient protocol', *Anal Chim Acta*, **495** 21–32.

Green R J, Davies M C, Roberts C J and Tendler S J B (1998), 'A surface plasmon resonance study of albumin adsorption to PEO–PPO triblock copolymers', *J Biomed Mater Res*, **42** 165–171.

Hall E A C (1990), *Biosensors*, Maidenhead, Open University Press.

Hayden O, Bindeus R, Haderspock C, Mann K J, Wirl B and Dickert F L (2003), 'Mass-sensitive detection of cells, viruses and enzymes with artificial receptors', *Sens Actuators B*, **91** 316–319.

Heller A (1990), 'Electrical wiring of redox enzymes', *Acc Chem Res*, **23** 128–134.

Hillberg A L, Brain K R and Allender C J (2005), 'Molecular imprinted polymer sensors: implications for therapeutics', *Adv Drug Deliv Rev*, **57** 1875–1889.

Hiratsuka A, Kojima K, Muguruma H, Lee K H, Suzuki H and Karube I (2005), 'Electron transfer mediator micro-biosensor fabrication by organic plasma process', *Biosens Bioelection*, **21** 957–964.

Hiratsuka A, Muguruma H, Lee K H and Karube I (2004), 'Organic plasma process for simple and substrate-independent surface modification of polymeric bioMEMS devices', *Biosens Bioelection*, **19** 1667–1672.

Hsuie G H, Lee S D, Chang P C and Kao C Y (1998), 'Surface characterization and biological properties study of silicone rubber material grafted with phospholipid as biomaterial via plasma induced graft copolymerization', *J Biomed Mater Res*, **42** 134–147.

Ishihara K, Nakabayashi N, Sakakida M, Nishida K and Shichiri M (1998), 'Biocompatible microdialysis hollow-fiber probes for long-term *in vivo* glucose monitoring', *ACS Symp Ser*, **690** 24–33.

John R, Spencer M, Wallace G G and Smyth M R (1991), 'Development of a polypyrrole-based human serum albumin sensor', *Anal Chim Acta*, **249** 381–385.

Kajiya Y, Tsuda R and Yoneyama H (1991), 'Conferment of cholesterol sensitivity on polypyrrole films by immobilization of cholesterol oxidase and ferrocene carboxylate ions', *J Electroanal Chem*, **301** 155–164.

Karlsson R (2004), 'SPR for molecular interaction analysis: a review of emerging application areas', *J Mol Recognit*, **17** 151–161.

Kingschott P and Grieser H J (1999), 'Surfaces that resist bioadhesion', *Curr Opin Solid State Mater Sci*, **4** 403–412.

Konry T, Novoa A, Cosnier S and Marks R S (2003), 'Development of an "electroptode" immunosensor: indium tin oxide-coated optical fiber tips conjugated with an electropolymerized thin film with conjugated cholera toxin B subunit', *Anal Chem*, **75** 2633–2639.

Konry T, Novoa A, Shemer-Avni Y, Hanuka N, Cosnier S, Lepellec A and Marks R S (2005), 'Optical fiber immunosensor based on a poly(pyrrole-benzophenone) film for the detection of antibodies to viral antigen', *Anal Chem*, **77** 1771–1779.

Kumar A, Rajesh, Chaubey A, Grover S K and Malhotra B D (2001), 'Immobilization of cholesterol oxidase and potassium ferricyanide on dodecylbenzene sulfonate ion-doped polypyrrole film', *J Appl Polym Sci*, **82** 3486–3491.

Law K A and Higson S P J (2005), 'Sonochemically fabricated acetylcholinesterase micro-electrode arrays within a flow injection analyser for the determination of organophosphate pesticides', *Biosens Bioelection*, **20** 1914–1924.

Lee S W and Kunitake T (2001), 'Adsorption of TiO_2 nanoparticles imprinted with D-glucose on a gold surface', *Mol Cryst Liq Cryst*, **371** 11–114.

Livache T, Bazin H, Caillat P and Roget A (2001), 'Electroconducting polymers for the construction of DNA or peptide arrays on silicon chips', *Biosens Bioelection*, **13** 629–634.

Llaudet E, Botting N P, Crayston J A and Dale N (2003), 'A three-enzyme microelectrode sensor for detecting purine release from central nervous system', *Biosens Bioelection*, **18** 43–52.

Maines A, Ashworth D and Vadgama P (1997), 'Diffusion restricting outer membranes for greatly extended linearity measurements with glucose oxidase enzyme electrodes', *Anal Chim Acta*, **323** 223–231.

Malitesta C, Losito I and Zambonin P G (1999), 'Molecularly imprinted electrosynthesized polymers: new materials for biomimetic sensors', *Anal Chem*, **71** 1366–1370.

Mano N and Heller A (2005), 'Detection of glucose at 2 fM concentration', *Anal Chem*, **77** 729–732.

Minehan D S, Marx K A and Tripathy S K (1994), 'Kinetics of DNA-binding to electrically conducting polypyrrole films', *Macromolecules*, **27** 777–783.

Minehan D S, Marx K A and Tripathy S K (2001), 'DNA binding to electropolymerized polypyrrole: the dependence on film characteristics', *J Macromol Sci Pure, Appl Chem*, **38** 1245–1258.

Moussy F and Harrison J D (1994), 'Prevention of the rapid degradation of subcutaneously implanted Ag/AgCl reference electrodes using polymer coatings', *Anal Chem*, **66** 674–679.

Moussy F, Jakeway S, Harrison J D and Rajotte R V (1994), '*In vitro* and *in vivo* performance and lifetime of perfluorinated ionomer-coated glucose sensors after high-temperature curing', *Anal Chem*, **66** 3882–3888.

Mugurama H and Karube I (1999), 'Plasma-polymerised films for biosensors', *Trends Anal Chem*, **18** 63–68.

Muguruma H, Nagata R, Nakamura R, Sato K, Uchiyama S and Karube I (2000), 'Sensor chip using a plasma-polymerized film for surface plasmon resonance biosensors: reliable analysis of binding kinetics', *Anal Lett*, **16** 347–348.

Myler S, Eaton S and Higson S P J (1997), 'Poly(*o*-phenylenediamine) ultra-thin polymer-film composite membranes for enzyme electrodes', *Anal Chim Acta*, **357** 55–61.

Nakanishi K, Muguruma H and Karube I (1995), 'Novel method of immobilizing antibodies on a quartz crystal microbalance using plasma-polymerized films for immunosensors', *Anal Chem*, **68** 1695–1700.

Newman J D, Tigwell L J, Turner A P F and Warner P J (2004), *Biosensors: A Clearer View, Biosensors 2004 – The 8th World Congress on Biosensors*, New York, Elsevier.

Ohara T J, Rajagopalan R and Heller A (1994), 'Wired enzyme electrodes for amperometric determination of glucose or lactate in the presence of interfering substances', *Anal Chem*, **66** 245–2457.

Ouerghi O, Senillou A, Jaffrezic-Renault N, Martelet C, Ben Ouada H and Cosnier S (2001), 'Gold electrode functionalized by electropolymerization of a cyano *N*-substituted pyrrole: application to an impedimetric immunosensor', *J Electroanal Chem*, **501** 62–69.

Ouerghi O, Touhami A, Jaffrezic-Renault N, Martelet C, Ben Ouada H and Cosnier S (2002), 'Impedimetric immunosensor using avidin–biotin for antibody immobilization', *Bioelectrochemistry*, **56** 131–133.

Peng H, Liang C D, Zhou A H, Zhang Y Y, Xie Q J and Yao S Z (2000), 'Development of a new atropine sulfate bulk acoustic wave sensor based on a molecularly imprinted electrosynthesized copolymer of aniline with *o*-phenylenediamine', *Anal Chim Acta*, **423** 221–228.

Pritchard J, Law K, Vakurov A, Millner P and Higson S P J (2004), 'Sonochemically fabricated enzyme microelectrode arrays for the environmental monitoring of pesticides', *Biosens Bioelection*, **20** 765–774.

Purvis D, Leonardova O, Farmakovsky D and Cherkasov V (2003), 'An ultrasensitive and stable potentiometric immunosensor', *Biosens Bioelection*, **18** 1385–1390.

Ramanathan K, Ram M K, Malholtra B D and Murthy A S N (1995), 'Application of polyaniline Langmuir–Blodgett films as a glucose biosensor', *Mater Sci Eng C*, **3** 159–163.

Reddy S M and Vadgama P M (1997), 'A study of the permeability properties of surfactant modified poly(vinyl chloride) membranes', *Anal Chim Acta*, **350** 67–76.

Sargent A, Loi T, Gal S and Sadik O A (1999), 'The electrochemistry of antibody-modified conducting polymer electrodes', *J Electroanal Chem*, **470** 144–156.

Singh S, Solanki P R, Pandey M K and Malhotra B D (2006), 'Covalent immobilization of cholesterol esterase and cholesterol oxidase on polyaniline films for application to cholesterol biosensor', *Anal Chim Acta*, **568** 126–132.

Sirkar K and Pishko M V (1998), 'Amperometric biosensors based on oxidoreductases immobilized in photopolymerized poly(ethylene glycol) redox polymer hydrogels', *Anal Chem*, **70** 2888–2894.

Skinner N G and Hall E A H (1997), 'Investigation of the origin of the glucose response in a glucose oxidase:polyaniline system', *J Electroanal Chem*, **420** 179–188.

Sode K, Ohta S, Yanai Y and Yamazaki T (2003), 'Construction of a molecular imprinting catalyst using target analogue template and its application for an amperometric fructosylamine sensor', *Biosens Bioelection*, **18** 1485–1490.

Tessema M, Csöregi E, Ruzgas T, Kenausis G, Solomon T and Gorton L (1997), 'Oligosaccharide dehydrogenase-modified graphite electrodes for the amperometric determination of sugars in a flow injection system', *Anal Chem*, **69** 4039–4044.

Turner R B F and Sherwood C S (1994), 'Biocompatibility of perfluorosulfonic acid polymer membranes for biosensor applications', *ACS Symp Ser*, **556** 211–221.

Ueda T, Oshida H, Kurita K, Ishihara K and Nakabayashi N (1992), 'Preparation of 2-methacryloyloxyethyl phosphorylcholine copolymers with alkyl methacrylates and their blood compatibility', *Polym J*, **24** 1259–1269.

Vidal J C, Espuelas J, Garcia-Ruiz E and Castillo J R (2004), 'Amperometric cholesterol biosensors based on the electropolymerization of pyrrole and the electrocatalytic effect of prussian-blue layers helped with self-assembled monolayers', *Talanta*, **64** 655–664.

Vidal J C, Mendez S and Castillo J R (1999), 'Electropolymerization of pyrrole and phenylenediamine over an organic conducting salt based amperometric sensor of increased selectivity for glucose determination', *Anal Chim Acta*, **385** 203–211.

Wang H, Li D, Wu Z Y, Shen G L and Yu R Q (2004), 'A reusable piezo-immunosensor with amplified sensitivity for ceruloplasmin based on plasma-polymerized film', *Talanta*, **62** 201–208.

Wang H Y and Mu S L (1999), 'Bioelectrochemical characteristics of cholesterol oxidase immobilized in a polyaniline film', *Sens Actuators B*, **56** 22–30.

Wang J (2001), 'Glucose biosensors: 40 years of advances and challenges', *Electroanalysis*, **13** 983–988.

Wang J, Jiang M, Fortes A and Mukherjee B (1999), 'New label-free DNA recognition based on doping nucleic-acid probes within conducting polymer films', *Anal Chim Acta*, **402** 7–12.

Whitcombe M J and Vulfson E N (2001), 'Imprinted polymers', *Adv Mater*, **13** 467–478.

Wisniewski N and Reichert M (2000), 'Methods for reducing biosensor membrane biofouling', *Colloids Surf B: Biointerfaces*, **18** 197–219.

Yajima S, Sonoyama Y, Suzuki K and Kimura K (2002), 'Ion-sensor property and blood compatibility of neutral-carrier-type poly(vinyl chloride) membranes coated by phosphorylcholine polymers', *Anal Chim Acta*, **463** 31–37.

Yalow R S and Berson S A (1959), 'Assay of plasma insulin in human subjects by immunological methods', *Nature*, **184** 1648–1649.

Yang L, Janle E, Huang T, Gitzen J, Kissinger P T, Vreeke R and Heller A (1995), 'Applications of Wired peroxidase electrodes for peroxide determination in liquid chromatography coupled to oxidase immobilized enzyme reactors', *Anal Chem*, **67** 1326–1331.

Yang Y and Mu S (1997), 'Biolectrochemical responses of polyaniline horseradish peroxidase electrodes', *J Electroanal Chem*, **432** 71–78.

Zhang Y C, Kim H H and Heller A (2003), 'Enzyme-amplified amperometric detection of 3000 copies of DNA in a 10 μL droplet at 0.5 fM concentration', *Anal Chem*, **75** 3267–3269.

8
Tissue engineering using natural polymers

V M CORRELO, M E GOMES, K TUZLAKOGLU, J M OLIVEIRA, P B MALAFAYA, J F MANO, N M NEVES and R L REIS, University of Minho, Portugal

8.1 Introduction

Although several important advances have been made through the years in the bone and cartilage substitution and regeneration field, most serious injuries are still unrecoverable. Tissue engineering has been emerging as one of the most promising techniques in orthopaedic surgery and biomedical engineering, offering promising alternatives to current therapies. This new research area was defined by Langer and Vacanti[1] in 1993 as 'an interdisciplinary field of research that applies the principles of engineering and the life sciences towards the development of biological substitutes that restore, maintain, or improve tissue function'.

The most common strategy for tissue engineering of hard tissues combines the use of autogenous cells (which can be fully differentiated cells, such as osteoblasts and chondrocytes, or undifferentiated cells, such as mesenchymal stem cells) obtained from the patient's hard or soft tissues that are seeded on to a scaffold that will slowly degrade and resorb as the tissue structures grow *in vitro* and/or *in vivo*. In this context, the development of appropriate three-dimensional (3D) porous structures (scaffolds) that will provide the necessary support for cells to proliferate and maintain their differentiated phenotype and to permit the convenient delivery of cells into the patients is one of the important keys for the success of hard tissue engineering.

There are some requirements that an ideal scaffold to be used in tissue engineering of hard tissues should accomplish as follows: the material (and its degradation products) must be biocompatible and biodegradable with an adjustable degradation rate to mach the rate of tissue regeneration; it should have appropriate mechanical properties that should match as closely as possible those of the neotissue; there must be appropriate surface chemistry to promote cell attachment, proliferation and differentiation; moreover, the scaffold should possess appropriate pore size and interconnected pore network to enhance cell or tissue growth, facilitate vascularisation, improving oxygen and nutrients supply and waste removal.[2]

The development of appropriate materials for this kind of application is a hard and very demanding task. In the past decade there has been an extensive research on the application of biodegradable polymers, of both synthetic and natural origin, in this field. The synthetic polymers most often employed on the development of 3D porous scaffolds for tissue engineering applications are aliphatic polyesters derived from the polymerization of lactones, such as poly(lactic acid),[3] poly(glycolic acid),[4] polycaprolactone[5] and their copolymers. A major drawback of these polymers is that, during the degradation process, the mass loss is accompanied by a release gradient of acidic by-products that results in *in vivo* inflammatory reactions.[6,7]

8.2 Chitosan and starch-based polymers in tissue engineering

In the past few years, several polymers of natural origin have been proposed as alternative materials for application within the tissue engineering field. Among the natural polymers, chitosan has been one of the most widely studied biodegradable polymers. Chitosan is a cationic natural biopolymer produced by alkaline *N*-deacetylation of chitin, the second most abundant natural polymer after cellulose. It is an interesting biomaterial because of its good biocompatibility, biodegradability and bioactivity.[8,9] Owing to its positively charged surface and biocompatibility, chitosan is considered to be effective for supporting cell functions, proliferation and differentiation without additives, even *in vitro*.[10,11] One of the most promising features of chitosan is its excellent ability to be processed into porous structures for use in cell transplantation and tissue regeneration.[12]

Starch-based polymers constitute another potential alternative material that may find different uses in biomedical applications. These natural-origin materials were originally proposed by Reis and his co-workers[13–15] at 3B's Research Group at the University of Minho as alternatives for hard tissue applications. Starch-based polymers are degradable and biocompatible polymers, with distinct structural forms and properties that can be tailored by the synthetic component of the starch-based blend, their processing methods and the incorporation of additives and reinforcement materials.[16–18] For this reason, together with their low cost and abundance of raw materials, starch-based polymers have been suggested for a wide range of biomedical applications.

Nevertheless, the properties of a scaffold are dependent not only on the selected material but also on the chosen processing technology. It is well known that the use of different processing technologies allows the production of 3D porous structures with different characteristics, namely porosity and porous interconnectivity, mechanical properties, surface properties and biocompatibility. Several processing methodologies have been developed by the 3B's Research Group: Biomaterial, Biodegradables and Biomimetics at the University of Minho to produce natural-origin polymeric scaffolds based on starch and chitosan polymers, with different properties and porous architectures. This chapter will therefore describe some of those technologies. The achieved structures and their physical, morphological and biological behaviour will also be discussed.

8.3 Production of 3D porous scaffolds by extrusion and injection moulding with a blowing agent

Melt moulding has normally been used in combination with porogen techniques or to produce a preshape of the final material, e.g. to produce fibres that will be used in fibre-bonding methods that will be described later in this chapter. However, it is also possible to produce 3D scaffolds using melt moulding as a single method based on traditional melting technologies, such as injection moulding and extrusion with blowing agents. In these processes, the polymers are mixed with blowing agents, which are previously selected according to their decomposition temperatures, toxicity, etc., and then processed in an extruder or in an injection moulding machine. The blowing agents react by heating releasing gases, usually CO_2, that are dissolved in the polymer melt, leading to the formation of pores within the material. These methods allow for the productions of highly reproducible scaffolds with very complex 3D structures, since it is possible to obtain scaffolds with the precise shape of the mould designed for specific applications.[13,14,19,20] This type of technology also offers the possibility of using a wide range of currently available equipment that can be used to produce, for example, bimaterial scaffolds, i.e. scaffolds that may combine two different polymers and/or two different structures. Starch-based scaffolds have been developed on the basis of these methods.[13,14,19]

Several different blowing agents and processing conditions have been studied to obtain porous structures with adequate porosities. However, as the porous structure of the samples obtained by extrusion or injection moulding of the polymers combined with blowing agents results from the gases released by decomposition of the blowing agent during processing, it is difficult to have full control over the pore size and the interconnectivity between the pores of the materials obtained by these methods. Nevertheless, the optimisation of processing parameters and of the type and amount of blowing agent, allowed scaffolds to be obtained with a subsequent higher porosity, with interconnectivity between pores and with pore sizes that can vary from roughly between 50 and 1000 μm.[21] Moreover, the scaffolds obtained by these melt-based methods present a microporosity throughout the whole structure, which can play an important role in the flow of nutrients during cell culture and/or the implantation of the scaffolds. A thin layer of compact material surrounds the porous structure of the material obtained with both processes, but this outershell can be removed easily as a final step in the processing of the scaffolds.

The starch-based scaffolds obtained by these methodologies present very promising mechanical properties when compared with other scaffolds, obtained from other biodegradable polymers, and proposed for applications in tissue engineering. In fact, several studies performed using osteoblast-like cells and marrow stromal cells using these starch-based scaffolds obtained by these methodologies have shown very promising results regarding their application in bone tissue engineering.[22–25]

8.4 Producing 3D porous scaffolds using fibre bonding

Fibre meshes consist of individual fibres either woven or knitted into 3D patterns of variable pore sizes.[26–30] The most important advantageous features of scaffolds obtained by fibre-bonding processes, i.e. fibre meshes, are a large surface area for cell attachment and a rapid diffusion of nutrients which enhances cell survival and growth.[26–30] This, of course, results from a high interconnectivity between pores. A drawback of these scaffolds might be the difficulty in controlling accurately the porosity.[26–28,30]

Several studies have demonstrated that scaffolds obtained by fibre-bonding processes have adequate structure for use in tissue engineering strategies that utilise bioreactor cultures, probably because they provide highly interconnected porosity that allows the creation of hydrodynamic micro-environments with minimal diffusion constraints that closely resemble natural interstitial fluid conditions *in vivo*, allowing large and well-organised cell communities to be achieved.[22,31–35] On the contrary, most of the porous structures obtained with other methodologies exhibit lower interconnectivity which is very likely to generate complex fluid flow pathways thought the scaffolds and which does not allow for the distribution of cells throughout the whole construct.

Fibre-bonding methods include a great variety of processing methods that involve the knitting or physical bonding (by means of casting or compression procedures) of fibres prefabricated by wet or dry spinning from polymeric solutions or by melt spinning.

Starch-based fibre mesh scaffolds have been obtained by a fibre-bonding process consisting in cutting and sintering melt-spun fibres with a diameter of about 180 μm and used in several tissue-engineering studies.[22,31] In one of these studies, the influence of the porosity of the scaffolds on the proliferation and osteogenic differentiation of marrow stromal cells cultured under static and flow perfusion conditions was assessed. For this study, fibre mesh scaffolds based on a 30–70 wt% blend of starch with poly(ε-caprolactone) with different porosities, namely 50% and 75% of the fibre mesh scaffolds, were obtained using different amounts (by weight) of fibres.

This study demonstrated that the use of fibre mesh scaffolds with higher porosity promotes improvement in cell proliferation under both static and flow perfusion culture conditions. Another study has addressed the effect of scaffold architecture in the cell proliferation and distribution by seeding and culturing rat bone marrow stromal cells seeded on to starch–polycaprolactone (SPCL) fibre meshes and starch–ethylene vinyl alcohol (SEVA-C) scaffolds obtained by extrusion using blowing agents.[22] Histological analysis and confocal images of the cultured scaffolds showed a much better distribution of cells within the SPCL scaffolds than within the SEVA-C scaffolds, which had limited pore interconnectivity, indicating that scaffold architecture and especially pore interconnectivity affect the homogeneity of the tissue formed by *in vitro* tissue-engineering approaches. Based on the same polymer, we have developed nano- and micro-fiber combined scaffolds from the same blend in our group.[36] The basic point of this concept was to use nanofibers for mimicking the physical structure of natural ECM. The micro support for cells was provided by SPCL microfiber meshes produced by melt spinning. The presence of nanofibers in the structure showed great influence by means of cell morphology, viability and differentiation. Human osteoblast-like cell line (SaOs-2) and rat bone marrow stromal cultured on combined scaffolds presented different cell organization than that on SPCL fiber meshes without nanofibers. The cells tended to stretch themselves along the nanofibers and to bridge between microfibers. This stretched morphology led to a difference in differentiation rate which could be related with the different gene expression. Furthermore, the presence of nanofibers seemed to be an advantage for increasing the cell seeding efficiency, resulting in an increase in cell viability. Consequently, the developed structures are believed have a great potential in the 3D organisation and guidance of cells that is provided for the engineering of 3D bone tissues.

In other studies, fibre mesh scaffolds based on a chitosan–poly(butylene succinate) blend were obtained using the extrusion of microfibres and a further processing step of fibre bonding using pressure and temperature. These fibre mesh scaffolds supported bovine articular chondrocytes proliferation, differentiation and hyaline-like cartilage matrix formation, being therefore considered adequate to serve as a support for articular cartilage repair.[37] Another study demonstrated that new chitosan–poly(butylene succinate) fibre mesh scaffolds produced by this method support the adhesion, proliferation and osteogenic differentiation of mesenchymal stem cells, being therefore suitable for bone tissue-engineering applications.[38]

Wet spinning is the oldest method of fibre spinning and is mostly used to produce natural fibres, such as chitin and chitosan fibres, which cannot be formed by either melt- or dry-spinning methods. This technique was used to prepared chitosan fibres and 3D fibre meshes having an average pore size in the range 100–500 μm.[39] Cell-culturing studies using osteoblast-like cells showed that, after culture for 7 days, cells presented adequate morphology and good proliferation, demonstrating that the developed scaffolds might be used for bone tissue-engineering applications.

8.5 Producing 3D porous scaffolds by melt based compression moulding with particulate leaching

Methods based on the leaching of soluble particulates are widely employed in the fabrication of 3D porous structures (scaffolds).[40–52] By these methods the porosity can be controlled by varying the amount of leachable particles and the pore size; the pore morphology can be adjusted, independently of the porosity, by using particles of different sizes and different morphologies.[40,41]

To improve the structure and to increase the pore interconnectivity of the porous scaffold, particulate leaching has been used in combination with other techniques, namely solvent casting,[41,42] gas forming,[43,44] freeze-drying,[45] injection moulding,[46] extrusion[47] and compression moulding.[40,48,49] However, some of these methods require the use of organic solvents (e.g. the solvent-casting and particulate-leaching methods), which might be harmful. In fact, organic solvents used in these methodologies can remain in the scaffold and may damage cells transplanted on to the scaffolds or tissues near the transplantation site.[50,51]

Many efforts have been made to manufacture porous scaffold without organic solvents for tissue-engineering applications.[43,44,50–52] One such technology is known as melt-based compression moulding with particulate leaching. The first step in this methodology consists in mixing a polymer (usually in the powder form) with calibrated leachable particles and loading it into a mould. This mould is then heated above the glass transition temperature (in the case of amorphous polymers) or above the melting temperature (in the case of semicrystalline polymers). During the heating process the mould should be pressed to maximise packaging. The heating process causes the fusion of the polymer particles and promotes the formation a continuous matrix. In the end, the moulded polymer–porogen composite is immersed in a solvent for selective dissolution of the porogen.

This methodology was applied in the production of natural-origin starch-based scaffolds.[14] The obtained scaffolds have been demonstrated to possess an open network of pores, with sizes from 10 to 500 μm and a porosity of about 50%. More recently, this approach was used to produce novel chitosan–polyester-based scaffolds that can be processed by melt-based routes and are aimed at bone and cartilage tissue-engineering applications.[53] Materials used consisted of blends of chitosan with poly(butylene succinate), poly(butylene terepthalate adipate) and poly(ε-caprolactone). All the scaffolds were produced by melt-based compression moulding followed by salt leaching. For the production of scaffolds for chondrogenic applications, the chitosan–polyester blends were dry mixed with salt (80 wt%) with a granulometric size between 65 and 125 μm (Fig. 8.1(a)). In the case of the scaffolds for osteogenic applications the three developed blends were mixed with salt (60 wt%) with a larger granulometric size between 250 and 500 μm (Fig. 8.1(b)). The compression-moulded samples were immersed in distilled water for periods of up to 7 days in order to dissolve the salt and to form, in this sense, the porous network. The scaffolds disclosed levels of porosity similar to the ratios of porogen used, with quite reasonable degrees of interconnectivity.

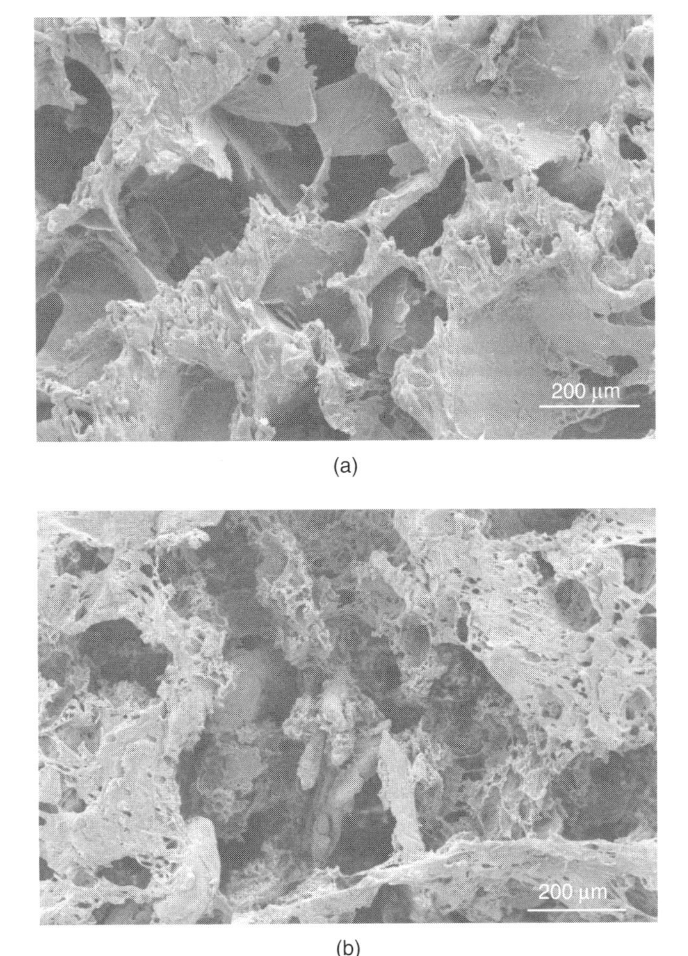

8.1 Scanning electron micrographs of the scaffold's surface: (a) chondrogenic applications; (b) osteogenic applications.

Later studies confirmed that the chitosan–polyester-based scaffolds developed support adhesion, viability and proliferation, and osteogenic or chondrogenic differentiation of a mouse mesenchymal stem cell line (BMC-9) and therefore may be used for cell-based approaches in the bone or cartilage tissue-engineering field.[54–56]

8.6 3D porous scaffolds produced by freeze-drying

Several methods have been reported for producing highly porous and interconnected polymeric scaffolds to find applications in tissue engineering of bone and cartilage.[57,58] Among these, freeze-drying has been attracting a great deal of attention owing to the versatility of the technique.[59] In fact, freeze-drying allows highly porous structures to be obtained by means of freezing a polymer solution, at temperatures varying between –20 and –196 °C, followed by the removal of solvent through lyophilisation.[45,60–62] Thus, during freeze-drying, the space occupied by the frozen solvent will become empty after evaporation and, by this means, pores will originate.[63] In practice, the polymer solutions should be previously transferred into a mould and frozen before freeze-drying at temperatures which are typically in the range from –20 to –80 °C.[60] The relevant aspect of this processing route consists in guaranteeing that the final freezing temperature is adequate to maintain all the molecules of solvent in the solid state.[64] Otherwise, the final structure will shrink during the drying process, resulting in the formation of a dense external skin-like layer.[64] In certain applications this is an undesired goal since this skin layer will prevent the ingrowth of cells during seeding, for example. Therefore, after freezing, special drying conditions are required at the freeze-dryer equipment. Usually, this equipment among other functions should control the temperatures of the sample, the surface, the plate and the ice condenser.[64] Additionally, the place where the sample will be kept for drying, the so-called 'vacuum chamber', should be at a low pressure (less than 100 mTorr) for several days to allow complete sublimation of solvent.[65] The low temperatures needed and the required drying regimes involved in the freeze-drying process explain the high energy costs, which is the major disadvantage of the technique. Thus, the main drawbacks of the freeze-drying technique are the time and energy consumed.[66] Despite this, when compared with other methodologies such as freeze extraction (an economical process), the main advantage of the freeze-drying technique lies in the capacity to retain the final porous structure, i.e. to prevent the disintegration of the scaffolds.[63] However, the great advantage of freeze-drying consists on the possibility of tailoring the typical foam-like structures by varying several experimental parameters. For example, by varying the polymer concentration,[59,67–69] type of solvent,[70] freezing temperature[45,60,65,70,71] and types of mould[62,72] and by incorporating porogens,[45,60,67] it is possible to obtain scaffolds with different densities, shapes, porosities and pore size distributions.[65,68,71] A parameter that can also be controlled is the cooling rate, which influences considerably the final structure of the scaffolds. Since the freezing rate induces the formation of ice crystals of different sizes, after freeze-drying the space occupied by these ice crystals will become empty and consequently affect the geometry and size of the pores in the dry material.[60,65,73]

Another advantage of the freeze-drying technique consists of the possibility of incorporating the features of thermosensitive molecules or cells such as growth factors directly into the porous scaffolds without any detriment to their behaviour.[74] Consequently, these types of delivery system, which can support cell attachment and cell functions and simultaneously deliver, in a controlled manner, therapeutic molecules to promote tissue regeneration are of great interest. On the other hand, when developing scaffolds by the freeze-drying technique, we face some limitations. Since there is a compromise between the porosity of the scaffolds and its final mechanical properties, it seems quite obvious that the highly porous scaffolds obtained by means of freeze–drying will possess very low mechanical properties. Therefore, the applications of this type of scaffold are not adequate for applications in the tissue engineering of hard tissues, such as bone. However, this problem can be circumvented to a certain extent by means of increasing the polymer concentration or developing composite materials, i.e. reinforcement with ceramics.[75–77] Maquet *et al.*[77] have reported that the mechanical properties of poly(D,L-lactic acid) and poly(lactic acid-co-glycolic acid) (PLGA) became improved by mixing with bioactive glass (45S5 Bioglasss). In a different study, Malafaya and Reis[78] also reported that, by means of the freeze-drying processing route, it was possible to develop natural-origin composite chitosan–hydroxyapatite scaffolds. It was demonstrated that the chitosan–hydroxyapatite porous structures developed were bioactive and possess an adequate porosity and good adhesion at the polymer–ceramic interface, among other features. Therefore, this work has shown that these structures have a great potential to find applications as bone engineering scaffolding and can be further loaded with biologically active agents. Other studies have shown that several foam-like structures obtained by means of freeze-drying may also act as excellent supports for cell attachment and maintenance of their functions with the possibility of subsequent transplantation to repair or regenerate bone and cartilage defects.[65,79–81] While bone and cartilage have been studied for a long time, other clinical problems have been more recent subject of investigation, namely osteochondral defects. A promising osteochondral approach has been recently reported by Oliveira *et al.*[72] This work has shown that it is possible to develop 3D macroporous hydroxyapatite–chitosan bilayer

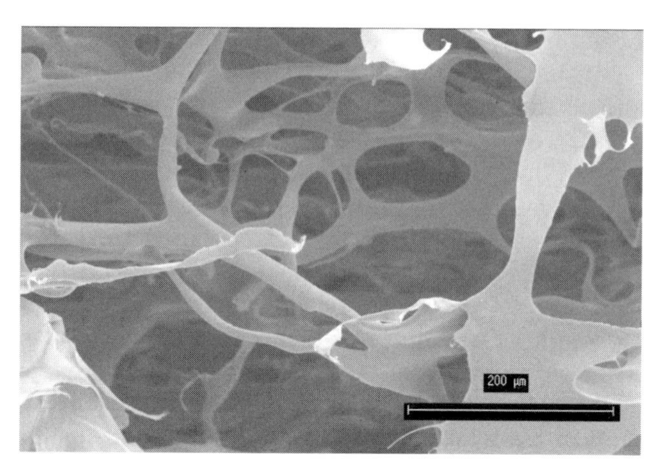

8.2 Scanning electron micrograph of the microstructure of a chitosan porous structure obtained by freeze-drying technique.

scaffolds which are mechanically stable, by means of combining a sintering and a freeze-drying technique. Figure 8.2 shows a typical scanning electron micrograph of the chitosan porous layer obtained by freeze-drying a 3 wt% chitosan solution. It shows that the chitosan layer possesses an anisotropic porosity, high interconnectivity and pores with size in the range 50–350 μm.

Furthermore, the hydroxyapatite–chitosan bilayer scaffolds developed exhibit very promising properties, suggesting that these materials provide adequate support for the seeding and culturing of marrow cells (data not shown). These cells can differentiate into osteoblasts and chondrocytes in the hydroxyapatite and chitosan porous layers, respectively, towards the formation of bone- and cartilage-like tissue.

To summarise, the freeze-drying processing route has been shown to be an effective and bioclean technique to find applications in many fields. Much attention has been given to the development of a variety of foam-like scaffolds, i.e. to the production of a wide variety of porous structures that can act as supports for cell attachment, cells ingrowths and functions, which ultimately are expected to repair or regenerate damaged or diseased tissues. The versatility of the technique not only allows the materials' properties, namely the scaffold's shape, density, pore size, pore morphology and pore distribution, to be tailored but also possibly combines with other techniques to develop more suitable supports. On the other hand, scientists face many application scenarios where the release of therapeutic molecules is required at a controlled rate, for example. Fortunately, the freeze-drying technique also allows therapeutic molecules (either thermosensitive or not) to be incorporated directly into the bulk of many biodegradable polymeric matrices. Therefore, freeze-drying has been shown to be a reliable technique for developing porous structures, which can act simultaneously as supports and drug delivery matrices for tissue-engineering applications.

8.7 Particle aggregation techniques to produce 3D porous scaffolds

Scaffolds need to be developed for sustaining *in vitro* tissue reconstruction as well as for *in vivo* cell-mediated tissue regeneration. It is almost impossible to repair tissue defects if the cells are not supplied with some kind of an ECM substitute. Bearing this in mind, several different methodologies have been used and described herein to produce a variety of 3D synthetic or naturally based scaffolds suitable for tissue-engineering applications.

Nevertheless, further research on the scaffold design is still needed because the chemical nature and structure of the 3D constructs significantly affect the success of tissue engineering approaches both *in vitro* and *in vivo*. Moreover, an optimal scaffold has not been identified yet. Towards this goal, an innovative methodology is being developed in some groups, based on the agglomeration of prefabricated polymeric or composite microspheres. The technique is generally based on the random packing of microspheres with further aggregation by physical, chemical or thermal means to create a 3D porous structure. The porosity obtained in this type of scaffold can be controlled by the microsphere diameter that will create the interstices when the particles aggregate. If an increased pore size is desired, it is also possible to use microspheres with increased sizes as has been achieved by our group.[82,83] This technique is being used to construct scaffolds directly,[82,84,85] or it could be used indirectly by producing a negative structure that will serve as a reverse template to obtain the scaffolds.

The research group of Laurencin[84–87] has been applying this technique for the development of matrices based on PLGA microspheres for bone repair. These researchers have tried different approaches by developing matrices based on sintered microspheres,[84,85] or matrices based on gel microspheres.[86] Composite microspheres containing hydroxyapatite were also used for the fabrication of polymer–ceramic 3D matrices for bone applications.[87] In the case of matrices based on sintered microspheres, the microspheres were first obtained by a solvent evaporation technique. The 3D structures were then further processed by heating the prefabricated PLGA microspheres above the glass transition temperature. The polymer chains were activated to interlink with neighbouring polymer chains and thus to form contacts between neighbouring microspheres.[86] In the gel microspheres matrix methodology, the PLGA gel microspheres were obtained by emulsion with poly(vinyl alcohol). The subsequent agglomeration is based on multiple-step production that includes air-drying, freeze-drying, rehydration with salt leaching and freeze-drying again. In general, microsphere-based matrices show very interesting properties for possible application in bone repair.

In the 3B's Research Group, chitosan-based scaffolds have been produced by aggregating previously developed chitosan microspheres.[82] One drawback of the particle aggregation method is that the porosity generated by using microspheres is low but, as was mentioned before, the interstices between the aggregated particles are directly related to the particle diameter. The main advantage is the high degree of interconnectivity obtained using this method. In fact, Fig. 8.3 shows the high degree of interconnectiv-

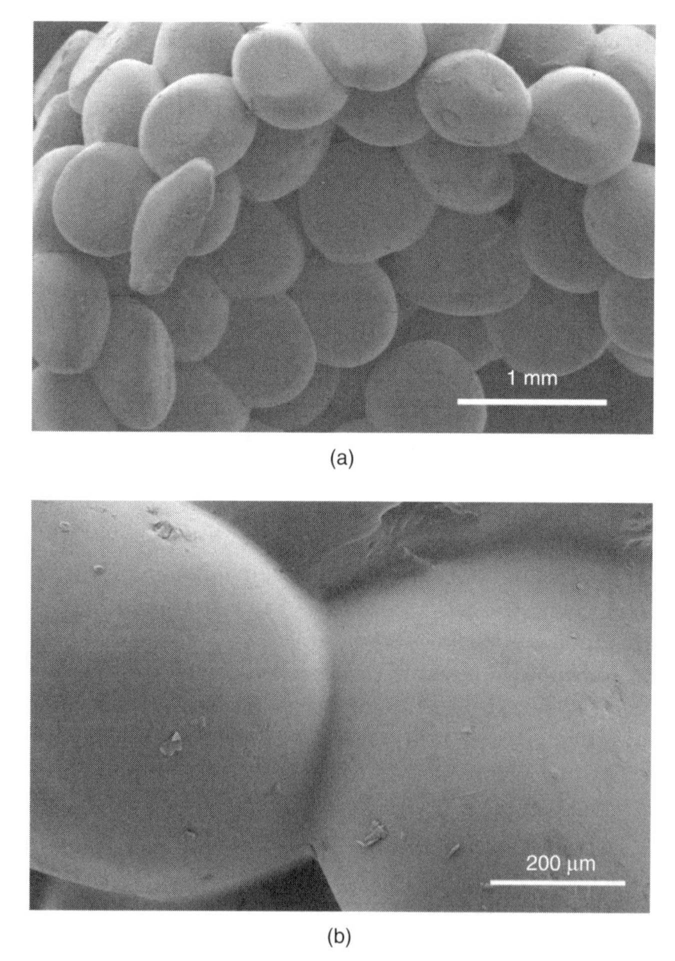

8.3 (a) Typical morphology of chitosan-based agglomerated scaffolds highlighting (b) the interface between adjacent microspheres.

ity and 3D structure of the chitosan scaffolds developed. The bonding of the chitosan particles is achieved owing to the bioadhesive character of the chitosan polymer that resulted in the union of adjacent particles at their contact points to form the chitosan porous matrices (Fig. 8.3(b)). This chitosan particle bonding leads to a very stable interface between the particles, which assures the mechanical integrity of the developed scaffolds. These scaffolds exhibit very promising mechanical properties (a compressive modulus of around 300 MPa depending on the matrix processing). These values can be further increased to 400 MPa with the incorporation of a bioactive reinforcement phase (in this study,[83] hydroxyapatite was used). One main advantage of this method is the possibility of controlling the water uptake ability by cross-linking the chitosan polymer; this decreases the hydration degree significantly and will obviously influence the drug release, allowing for a wide range of release profiles depending on the required application. The developed scaffolds seem to be very adequate for cell ingrowth. The developed scaffolds demonstrate no cytotoxicity as evaluated by 3-(4,5-dimethylthiazol-2-yl)-5-(3-carboxymethoxyphenyl)-2-(4-sulphophenyl)-2H-tetrazolium (MTS) assay. Preliminary cell seeding and differentiation tests with mesenchymal stem cells isolated from adipose tissue were also carried out, indicating cells with osteogenic and chondrogenic morphology in the 3D particle-agglomerated scaffolds.[82]

To create constructs having more favourable integration properties that might be used for osteochondral tissue-engineering applications, we have also investigated the development of osteochondral bilayered porous materials by using the particle aggregation method. Bilayered scaffolds were successfully developed by means of aggregating polymeric and composite chitosan-based particles (Fig. 8.4).

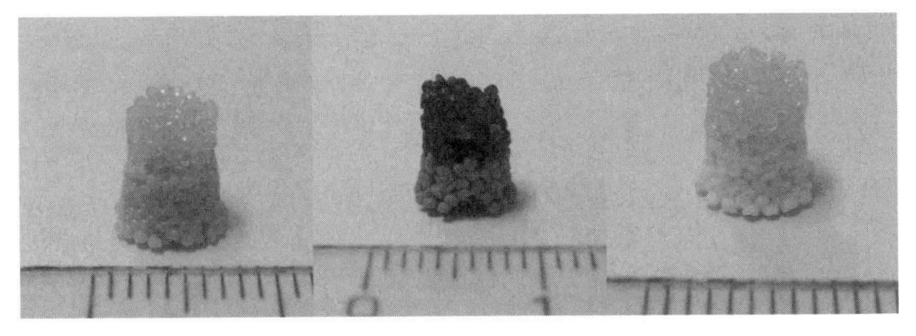

8.4 Different compositions of bilayered chitosan-based agglomerated scaffolds consisting of a polymeric component aimed at the cartilage part and a composite component for the bone part.

8.8 Microwave processing of 3D polymeric scaffolds

Another innovative methodology for producing porous biodegradable and natural-origin (starch-based) 3D architectures based on microwave processing was also developed by our research group.[15] The porous scaffolds produced by a microwave-based technique present an interesting combination of morphological and mechanical properties (matching the compressive behaviour of human cancellous bone) and may find uses in tissue-engineering applications and drug delivery applications which have an important role in tissue engineering.

Figure 8.5 shows the typical structure of the starch-based degradable scaffolds produced. It was possible to produce materials with interconnecting pores, and an interesting combination of macroporosity (between 200 and 900 μm) and microporosity (20–100 μm). The typical density of the biodegradable porous structures was in the 0.40–0.50 g/cm^3 range. The measured mechanical properties are in some way remarkable. The best results were a compression modulus of 530 MPa and a maximum compressive strength of 60 MPa. These values, obtained for blowing-agent (containing corn starch, sodium pyrophosphate and sodium bicarbonate) amounts of 10%, in the presence of hydrogen peroxide, are very similar to those of the cancellous bone. Better results are obtained in the presence of hydrogen peroxide because of partial oxidation of the starch molecule.

Finally it is very important to stress that the materials are degradable, and their loss of weight is about 40% after immersion for 30 days in an isotonic saline solution. The developed morphologies seem to be adequate for use as tissue-engineering scaffolds, or as drug delivery carriers. In the latter case the water-uptake capability of materials is a very important issue

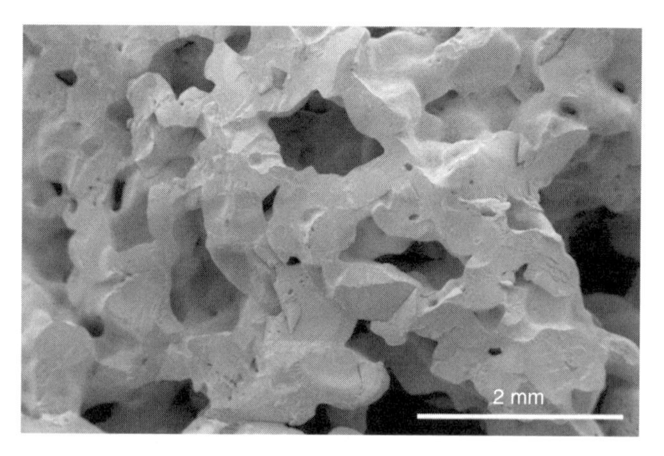

8.5 Starch-based scaffolds produced by a microwave technique.

since it is controllable by the porosity, as discussed further later in this chapter. Work was also carried out in our group for the development of composite porous structures, using hydroxyapatite as filler, by means of a similar microwave technique. The improvement in the mechanical properties and *in vitro* bioactive behaviour of these porous structures were the main goals of the approach. As described herein, a new simple processing route to produce starch-based scaffolds was developed by the 3B's Research Group, based on a microwave baking methodology. This innovative processing route was also used to obtain loaded drug delivery porous carriers, incorporating a non-steroid anti-inflammatory agent. This bioactive agent was selected as a model drug, and it is expected that the developed methodology might be used for other drugs and growth factors that play a crucial role in tissue engineering. More information can be found in the paper by Malafaya *et al.*[15]

The prepared systems were characterised by ^{1}H and ^{13}C nuclear magnetic resonance spectroscopy, which permitted the interactions between the starch-based materials and the processing components, namely the blowing agents, to be studied. The behaviour of the porous structures, while immersed in aqueous media, was studied in terms of swelling and degradation, which are intimately related to their porosity.

Finally, the systems exhibit a controlled release of the drug with clear different stages. The *in vitro* drug release studies that were performed showed two stages: first a clear burst effect controlled by the porosity, followed by a slow controlled release of the drug during several days. The first stage corresponds to a period of 10 h with a release of 40–55% (depending on porosity) of the loaded meclofenamic sodium salt (MS) and the second stage, which is much slower, is dynamically controlled by the degradation of the polymeric matrix, leading to a release of 55–70% of the loaded MS during a release period of 10 days.

8.9 Conclusion

In this chapter a range of processing methodologies and technologies that have been used to to develop tissue-engineering scaffolds from natural-origin polymers have been described. Tissue-engineering scaffolds consisting of naturally derived macromolecules have the potential advantages of biocompatibility, cell-controlled degradability and intrinsic cellular interaction. However, they may exhibit batch variations and, in many cases, possess a narrow and limited range of mechanical properties. Nevertheless, the processing technologies presented herein can tailor, to a great extent, the final properties of natural-origin scaffolds. Furthermore, in the same way that no material alone will satisfy all design parameters in all applications within the tissue-engineering field, it is also true that a wide range of materials can be tailored for discrete applications, through the use of the most appropriate processing methodologies and processing parameters selected.

Despite all the difficulties of working with natural based materials, it was shown that by using different process routes it is possible to obtain a range of microstructures and mechanical properties that can accomplish many of the requirements of 3D scaffolds for different tissue engineering applications.

8.10 References

1 Langer R and Vacanti J P, 'Tissue engineering', *Science*, 1993 **260** 920–926.

2 Hutmacher D W, 'Scaffold design and fabrication technologies for engineering tissues – state of the art and future perspectives', *J Biomater Sci, Polym Edn*, 2001 **12**(1) 107–124.

3 Howard D, Partridge K, Yang X B, Clarke N M P, Okubo Y, Bessho K, Howdle S M, Shakesheff K M and Oreffo R O C, 'Immunoselection and adenoviral genetic modulation of human osteoprogenitors: *in vivo* bone formation on PLA scaffold', *Biochem Biophys Res Commun*, 2002 **299**(2) 208–215.

4 Freed L E, Vunjaknovakovic G, Marquis J C and Langer R, 'Kinetics of chondrocyte growth in cell–polymer implants', *Biotechnol Bioeng*, 1994 **43**(7) 597–604.

5 Williams J M, Adewunmi A, Schek R M, Flanagan C L, Krebsbach P H, Feinberg S E, Hollister S J and Das S, 'Bone tissue engineering using polycaprolactone scaffolds fabricated via selective laser sintering', *Biomaterials*, 2005 **26** 4817–4827.

6 Bergsma J E, De Bruijn W C, Rozema F R, Bos R R M and Boering G, 'Late degradation tissue response to poly(L-lactide) bone plates and screws', *Biomaterials*, 1995 **16**(1) 25–31.

7 Bergsma E J, Rozema F R, Bos R R M and De Bruijn W C, 'Foreign body reactions to resorbable poly(L-lactide) bone plates and screws used for the fixation of unstable zygomatic fractures', *J Oral Maxillofac Surg*, 1993 **51**(6) 666–670.

8 Chandy T and Sharma C P, 'Chitosan – as a biomaterial', *Biomater Artif Cells Artif Organs*, 1990 **18**(1) 1–24.

9 Goosen M F A, *Applications of Chitin and Chitosan*, Lancaster, Pennsylvania, Technomic Publishing, 1997.

10 Hamano T, Teramoto A, Lizuka E and Abe K, 'Effects of polyelectrolyte complex (PEC) on human periodontal ligament fibroblast (HPLF) function. I. Three-dimensional structure of HPLF cultured on PEC', *J Biomed Mater Res*, 1998 **41** 257–269.

11 Inui H, Tsujikubo M and Hirano S, 'Low molecular weight chitosan stimulation of mitogenic response to platelet-derived growth factor in vascular smooth muscle cells', *Biosci Biotechnol Biochem*, 1995 **59**(11) 2111–2114.

12 Suh J K F and Matthew H W T, 'Application of chitosan-based polysaccharide biomaterials in cartilage tissue engineering: a review', *Biomaterials*, 2000 **21**(24) 2589–2598.

13 Gomes M E, Ribeiro A S, Malafaya P B, Reis R L and Cunha A M, 'A new approach based on injection moulding to produce biodegradable starch-based

polymeric scaffolds: morphology, mechanical and degradation behaviour', *Biomaterials*, 2001 **22**(9) 883–889.
14 Gomes M E, Godinho J S, Tchalamov D, Cunha A M and Reis R L, 'Alternative tissue engineering scaffolds based on starch: processing methodologies, morphology, degradation and mechanical properties', *Mater Sci Eng C*, 2002 **20**(1–2) 19–26.
15 Malafaya P B, Elvira C, Gallardo A, San Roman J and Reis R L, 'Porous starch-based drug delivery systems processed by a microwave route', *J Biomater Sci, Polym Edn*, 2001 **12**(11) 1227–1241.
16 Gomes M E, Reis R L, Cunha A M, Blitterswijk C A and de Bruijn J D, 'Cytocompatibility and response of osteoblastic-like cells to starch-based polymers: effect of several additives and processing conditions', *Biomaterials*, 2001 **22** 1911–1917.
17 Marques A P, Reis R L and Hunt J A, 'The biocompatibility of novel starch-based polymers and composites: in vitro studies', *Biomaterials*, 2002 **23** 1471–1478.
18 Mendes S C, Reis R L, Bovell Y P, Cunha A M, van Blitterswijk C A and de Bruijn J D, 'Biocompatibility testing of novel starch-based materials with potential application in orthopaedic surgery: a preliminary study', *Biomaterials*, 2001 **22** 2057–2064.
19 Gomes M E, Godinho J, Tchalamov D, Cunha A M and Reis R L, 'Design and processing of starch based scaffolds for hard tissue engineering', *J Appl Med Polym*, 2002 **6** 75–80.
20 Thomson R C, Yaszemski M J, Powers J M and Mikos A G, 'Fabrication of biodegradable polymer scaffolds to engineer trabecular bone', *J Biomater Sci, Polym Edn*, 1995 **7**(1) 23–38.
21 Gomes M, Salgado A and Reis R, 'Bone tissue engineering using starch based scaffolds obtained by different methods', in *Polymer Based Systems on Tissue Engineering, Replacement and Regeneration* (Eds R Reis and D Cohn), Amsterdam, Kluwer, 2002, pp. 221–249.
22 Gomes M E, Sikavitsas V I, Behravesh E, Reis R L and Mikos A G, 'Effect of flow perfusion on the osteogenic differentiation of bone marrow stromal cells cultured on starch-based three-dimensional scaffolds', *J Biomed Mater Res Part A*, 2003 **67**(1) 87–95.
23 Salgado A J, Coutinho O P and Reis R L, 'Novel starch-based scaffolds for bone tissue engineering: cytotoxicity, cell culture, and protein expression', *Tissue Eng*, 2004 **10**(3–4) 465–474.
24 Salgado A J, Figueiredo J E, Coutinho O P and Reis R L, 'Biological response to pre-mineralized starch based scaffolds for bone tissue engineering', *J Mater Sci: Mater Med*, 2005 **16**(3) 267–275.
25 Salgado A J, Gomes M E, Coutinho O P, Reis R L and Hutmacher D W, 'Preliminary study on the adhesion and proliferation of human osteoblasts on starch-based scaffolds', *Mater Sci Eng C*, 2002 **20**(1–2) 27–33.
26 Lu L and Mikos A G, 'The importance of new processing techniques in tissue engineering', *MRS Bull*, 1996 **21**(11) 28–32.
27 Thompson R, Yaszemski M and Mikos A G, 'Polymer scaffold processing', in *Principles of Tissue Engineering* (Eds R Lanza, R Langer and W Chick), 1st edition, New York, Academic Press, 1997, p. 263.

28 Thompson R, Wake M C, Yaszemski M and Mikos A G, 'Biodegradable polymer scaffolds to regenerate organs', *Adv Polym Sci*, 1995 **122** 218–274.
29 Langer R, 'Selected advances in drug delivery and tissue engineering', *J Control Release*, 1999 **62**(1–2) 7–11.
30 Maquet V and Jerome R, 'Design of macroporous biodegradable polymer scaffolds for cell transplantation', *Mater Sci Forum*, 1997 **250** 15–42.
31 Gomes M E, Holtorfc H L, Reis R L and Mikos A G, 'Influence of the porosity of starch-based fiber mesh scaffolds on the proliferation and osteogenic differentiation of bone marrow stromal cells cultured in a flow perfusion bioreactor', *Tissue Eng*, 2006 **12** 801–809.
32 Gomes M E, Bossano C M, Johnston C M, Reis R L and Mikos A G, '*In vitro* localization of bone growth factors in constructs of biodegradable scaffolds seeded with marrow stromal cells and cultured in a flow perfusion bioreactor', *Tissue Eng*, 2006 **12** 177–188.
33 Sikavitsas V I, Bancroft G N, Holtorf H L, Jansen J A and Mikos A G, 'Mineralized matrix deposition by marrow stromal osteoblasts in 3D perfusion culture increases with increasing fluid shear forces', *Proc Natl Acad Sci USA*, 2003 **100** 14 683–14 688.
34 Bancroft G N, Sikavitsas V I, van den Dolder J, Sheffield T L, Ambrose C G, Jansen J A and Mikos A G, 'Fluid flow increases mineralized matrix deposition in 3D perfusion culture of marrow stromal osteoblasts in a dose-dependent manner', *Proc Natl Acad Sci USA*, 2002 **99** 12 600–12 605.
35 van den Dolder J, Bancroft G N, Sikavitsas V I, Spauwen P H M, Jansen J A and Mikos A G, 'Flow perfusion culture of marrow stromal osteoblasts in titanium fiber mesh', *J Biomed Mater Res Part A*, 2003 **64** 235–241.
36 Tuzlakoglu K, Bolgen N, Salgado A J, Gomes M E, Piskin E and Reis R L, 'Nano- and micro-fiber combined scaffolds: a new architecture for bone tissue engineering', *J Mater Sci: Mater Med*, 2005 **16** 1099–1104.
37 Oliveira J T, Correlo V M, Crawford A, Mundy J M, Bhattacharya M, Neves N M, Hatton P V and Reis R L, 'Chitosan–polyester scaffolds seeded with bovine articular chondrocytes for cartilage tissue engineering applications', *Artif Organs*, 2005 **29**(9) 774.
38 Pinto A R, Correlo V M, Bhattacharya M, Charbord P, Reis R L and Neves N M, 'Behaviour of human bone marrow mesenchymal stem cells seeded on fiber bonding chitosan polyester based for bone tissue engineering scaffolds', in *Proceedings of the 8th Tissue Engineering Society International (TESI) Annual Meeting*, Shanghai, PR China, 2005, p. 206.
39 Tuzlakoglu K, Alves C M, Mano J F and Reis R L, 'Production and characterization of chitosan fibers and 3-D fiber mesh scaffolds for tissue engineering applications', *Macromol Biosci*, 2004 **4**(8) 811–819.
40 Zhang J, Wu L, Jing D and Ding J, 'A comparative study of porous scaffolds with cubic and spherical macropores', *Polymer*, 2005 **46**(13) 4979–4985.
41 McGlohorn J B, Holder W D Jr, Grimes L W, Thomas C B and Burg K J L, 'Evaluation of smooth muscle cell response using two types of porous polylactide scaffolds with differing pore topography', *Tissue Eng*, 2004 **10**(3–4) 505–514.
42 Lee W K, Ichi T, Ooya T, Yamamoto T, Katoh M and Yui N, 'Novel poly(ethylene glycol) scaffolds crosslinked by hydrolyzable polyrotaxane for cartilage tissue engineering', *J Biomed Mater Res Part A*, 2003 **67**(4) 1087–1092.

43 Kim S S, Sun Park M, Jeon O, Yong Choi C and Kim B S, 'Poly(lactide-co-glycolide)/hydroxyapatite composite scaffolds for bone tissue engineering', *Biomaterials*, 2006 **27**(8) 1399–1409.
44 Riddle K W and Mooney D J, 'Role of poly(lactide-co-glycolide) particle size on gas-foamed scaffolds', *J Biomater Sci, Polym Edn*, 2004 **15**(12) 1561–1570.
45 Hou Q, Grijpma D W and Feijen J, 'Preparation of interconnected highly porous polymeric structures by a replication and freeze-drying process', *J Biomed Mater Res Part B*, 2003 **67**(2) 732–740.
46 Wu L, Jing D and Ding J, 'A "room-temperature" injection moulding/particulate leaching approach for fabrication of biodegradable three-dimensional porous scaffolds', *Biomaterials*, 2006 **27**(2) 185–191.
47 Jeong S I, Kim S H, Kim Y H, Jung Y, Kwon J H, Kim B S and Lee Y M, 'Manufacture of elastic biodegradable PLCL scaffolds for mechano-active vascular tissue engineering', *J Biomater Sci, Polym Edn*, 2004 **15**(5) 645–660.
48 Wu L, Zhang H, Zhang J and Ding J, 'Fabrication of three-dimensional porous scaffolds of complicated shape for tissue engineering. I. Compression molding based on flexible-rigid combined mold', *Tissue Eng*, 2005 **11**(7–8) 1105–1114.
49 Malda J, Woodfield T B F, Van Der Vloodt F, Wilson C, Martens D E, Tramper J, Van Blitterswijk C A and Riesle J, 'The effect of PEGT/PBT scaffold architecture on the composition of tissue engineered cartilage', *Biomaterials*, 2005 **26**(1) 63–72.
50 Lee S H, Kim B S, Kim S H, Kang S W and Kim Y H, 'Thermally produced biodegradable scaffolds for cartilage tissue engineering', *Macromol Biosci*, 2004 **4**(8–9) 802–810.
51 Jung Y, Kim S S, Young H K, Kim S H, Kim B S, Kim S, Cha Y C and Soo H K, 'A poly(lactic acid)/calcium metaphosphate composite for bone tissue engineering', *Biomaterials*, 2005 **26**(32) 6314–6322.
52 Sun J, Wu J, Li H and Chang J, 'Macroporous poly(3-hydroxybutyrate-co-3-hydroxyvalerate) matrices for cartilage tissue engineering', *Eur Polym J*, 2005 **41**(10) 2443–2449.
53 Correlo V M, Boesel L F, Pinto A R, Bhattacharya M, Reis R L and Neves N M, 'Novel 3-D chitosan/polyester scaffolds for bone and cartilage tissue engineering', in *Proceedings of the 19th European Conference on Biomaterials (ESB 2005)*, Sorrento, Italy, 2005, Naples, Effe Erre Congressi, 2005, p. 323.
54 Oliveira J T, Salgado A J, Correlo V M, Pinto A R, Battacharya M, Charbord P, Neves N M and Reis R L, 'Preliminary assessment of the potential of chitosan/polyester based scaffolds for bone and cartilage tissue engineering', in *Proceedings of the 30th Annual Meeting and Exposition: New Applications and Technologies (SFB 2005)*, Memphis, Tennessee, USA, 2005, Mt Laurel, New Jessey, Society for Biomaterials, 2005, p. 154.
55 Oliveira J T, Salgado A J, Correlo V M, Pinto A R, Battacharya M, Charbord P, Neves N M and Reis R L, 'Preliminary assessment of the behaviour of chitosan/poly(butylene succinate) scaffolds seeded with mouse mesenchymal stem cells for cartilage tissue engineering', in *Proceedings of the 19th European Conference on Biomaterials (ESB 2005)*, Sorrento, Italy, 2005, Naples, Effe Erre Congressi, 2005, p. T54.
56 Pinto A R, Salgado A J, Oliveira J T, Correlo V M, Bhattacharya M, Charbord P, Reis R L and Neves N M, 'Evaluation of the adhesion, proliferation and

differentiation of a mouse mesenchymal stem cell line on novel chitosan/polyester based scaffolds', in *Proceedings of the 19th European Conference on Biomaterials (ESB 2005)*, Sorrento, Italy, 2005, Naples, Effe Erre Congressi, 2005, p. 172.

57 Hutmacher D W, 'Scaffolds in tissue engineering bone and cartilage', *Biomaterials*, 2000 **21** 2529–2543.

58 Kawanishi M, Ushida T, Kaneko T, Niwa H, Fukubayashi T, Nakamura K, Oda H, Tanaka S and Tateishi T, 'New type of biodegradable porous scaffolds for tissue-engineered articular cartilage', *Mater Sci Eng C*, 2004 **24**(3) 431–435.

59 Chen G, Ushida T and Tateishi T, 'Development of biodegradable porous scaffolds for tissue engineering', *Mater Sci Eng C*, 2001 **17**(1–2) 63–69.

60 Kang H W, Tabata Y and Ikada Y, 'Fabrication of porous gelatin scaffolds for tissue engineering', *Biomaterials*, 1999 **20**(14) 1339–1344.

61 Park S N, Park J C, Kim H O, Song M J and Suh H, 'Characterization of porous collagen/hyaluronic acid scaffold modified by 1-ethyl-3-(3-dimethylaminopropy l)carbodiimide cross-linking', *Biomaterials*, 2002 **23**(4) 1205–1212.

62 Ren L, Tsuru K, Hayakawa S and Osaka A, 'Novel approach to fabricate porous gelatin–siloxane hybrids for bone tissue engineering', *Biomaterials*, 2002 **23**(24) 4765–4773.

63 Ho M H, Kuo P Y, Hsieh H J, Hsien T Y, Hou L T, Lai J Y and Wang D M, 'Preparation of porous scaffolds by using freeze-extraction and freeze-gelation methods', *Biomaterials*, 2004 **25**(1) 129–138.

64 Mladenov D A, Tsvetkov Ts D and Vulchanov N L, 'Freeze drying of biomaterials for the medical practice', *Cryobiology*, 1993 **30**(3) 335–348.

65 O'Brien F J, Harley B A, Yannas I V and Gibson L J, 'The effect of pore size on cell adhesion in collagen–GAG scaffolds', *Biomaterials*, 2005 **26**(4) 433–441.

66 Ho M-H, Kuo P-Y, Hsien H-J, Hsien T-Y, Hou L-T, Lai J-Y and Wang D-M, 'Preparation of porous scaffolds by using freeze-extraction and freeze-gelation methods', *Biomaterials*, 2004 **25**(1) 129–138.

67 Weng J and Wang M, 'Producing chitin scaffolds with controlled pore size and interconnectivity for tissue engineering', *J Mater Sci Lett*, 2001 **20** 1401–1403.

68 Silva S S, Oliveira J M, Mano J F and Reis R L, 'Preparation and characterization of novel chitosan/soy protein porous for tissue engineering applications', *Adv Mater Forum*, 2006 **514–516** 1000–1004.

69 Blacher S, Maquet V, Pirard R, Pirard J P and Jérôme R, 'Image analysis impedance spectroscopy and mercury porosimetry characterization of freeze-drying porous materials', *Colloids Surf A*, 2001 **187–188** 375–383.

70 Madihally S V and Matthew H W T, 'Porous chitosan scaffolds for tissue engineering', *Biomaterials*, 1999 **20**(12) 1133–1142.

71 Mao J S, Zhao L G, Yin Y J and Yao K D, 'Structure and properties of bilayer chitosan–gelatin scaffolds', *Biomaterials*, 2003 **24**(6) 1067–1074.

72 Oliveira J M, Silva S S, Mano J F and Reis R L, 'Innovative technique for the preparation of porous bilayer hydroxyapatite/chitosan scaffolds for osteochondral applications', in *Bioceramics 18, Key Engineering Materials*, Vols 309–311 (Eds T Nakamura, K Yamashita and M Neo), Kyoto, Japan, 2006, Zurich, Trans Tech, 2006, pp. 927–930.

73 O'Brien F J, Harley B A, Yannas I V and Gibson L, 'Influence of freezing rate on pore structure in freeze-dried collagen–GAG scaffolds', *Biomaterials*, 2004 **25**(6) 1077–1086.

74 Whang K, Goldstick T K and Healy K E, 'A biodegradable polymer scaffold for delivery of osteotropic factors', *Biomaterials*, 2000 **21**(24) 2545–2551.

75 Coviello T, Alhaique F, Parisi C, Matricardi P, Bocchinfuso G and Grassi M, 'A new polysaccharidic gel matrix for drug delivery: preparation and mechanical properties', *J Control Release*, 2005 **102**(3) 643–656.

76 Mao J S, Zhao L G, Yin Y J and Yao K D, 'Structure and properties of bilayer chitosan–gelatin scaffolds', *Biomaterials*, 2003 **24**(6) 1067–1074.

77 Maquet V, Boccaccini A R, Pravata L, Notingher I and Jérôme R, 'Porous poly([alpha]-hydroxyacid)/Bioglass(R) composite scaffolds for bone tissue engineering. I: preparation and *in vitro* characterization', *Biomaterials*, 2004 **25**(18) 4185–4194.

78 Malafaya P B and Reis R L, 'Porous bioactive composites from marine origin based in chitosan and hydroxyapatite particles', in *Bioceramics 15, Key Engineering Materials*, Vols 240–242 (Eds D S B Ben-Nissan and W Walsh) Sydney, Australia, 2003, Zurich, Trans Tech, 2003, pp. 39–42.

79 Shapiro L and Cohen L, 'Novel alginate sponges for cell culture and transplantation', *Biomaterials*, 1997 **18**(8) 583–590.

80 Lee S B, Kim Y H, Chong M S and Lee Y M, 'Preparation and characteristics of hybrid scaffolds composed of [beta]-chitin and collagen', *Biomaterials*, 2004 **25**(12) 2309–2317.

81 Gravel M, Gross T, Vago R and Tabrizian M, 'Responses of mesenchymal stem cell to chitosan–coralline composites microstructured using coralline as gas forming agent', *Biomaterials*, 2006 **27**(9) 1899–1906.

82 Malafaya P B, Pedro A, Peterbauer A, Gabriel C, Redl H and Reis R L, 'Chitosan particles agglomerated scaffolds for cartilage and osteochondral tissue engineering approaches with adipose tissue derived stem cells', *J Mater Sci: Mater Med*, 2005 **16**(12) 1077–1085.

83 Malafaya P B and Reis R L, 'Development and characterization of pH responsive chitosan and chitosan/HA scaffolds processed by a microsphere-based aggregation route', in *Transactions of the 7th World Biomaterials Congress*, Sydney, Australia, 2004, Mt Laurel, New Jersey, Society for Biomaterials, 2004, p. 1285.

84 Borden M, El-Amin S F, Attawia M and Laurencin C T, 'Structural and human cellular assessment of a novel microsphere-based tissue engineered scaffold for bone repair', *Biomaterials*, 2003 **24**(4) 597–609.

85 Borden M, Attawia M and Laurencin C T, 'The sintered microsphere matrix for bone tissue engineering: *in vitro* osteoconductivity studies', *J Biomed Mater Res*, 2002 **61**(3) 421–429.

86 Borden M, Attawia M, Khan Y and Laurencin C T, 'Tissue engineered microsphere-based matrices for bone repair: design and evaluation', *Biomaterials*, 2002 **23**(2) 551–559.

87 Devin J E, Attawia M A and Laurencin C T, 'Three-dimensional degradable porous polymer–ceramic matrices for use in bone repair', *J Biomater Sci, Polym Edn*, 1996 **7**(8) 661–669.

Index